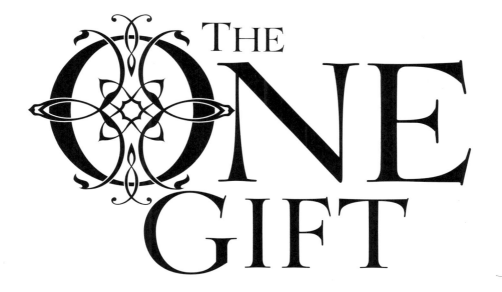

Published in Orem, Utah, by YL Wisdom.

Second Edition December 2010

Copyright @ 2010 YL Wisdom
www.ylwisdom.com

ISBN 0-9845959-0-2

Printed in the United States of America

The information contained in this book is for education
and entertainment purposes only. It is not provided to
diagnose, prescribe, or treat any condition of the body.
The stories in this book should not be used as a
substitute for medical counseling. Neither the author
nor the publisher accepts responsibility for such use.

Illustrations by Hugh Butterfield

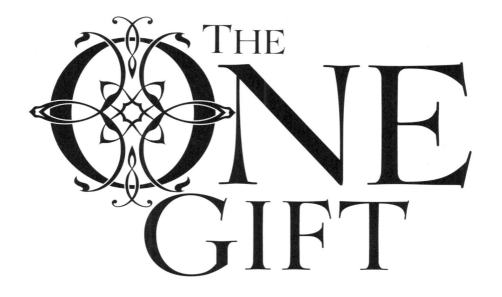

THE ONE GIFT

by

D. Gary Young, N.D.

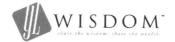

WISDOM

share the wisdom; share the wealth

Love and Appreciation

An age-old adage says that behind every good
man is a greater woman. A truer statement
could not be made in my life!

My wife, Mary, is the "wind beneath my wings."
She is the stabilizing force in our home and the anchor
for Jacob and Josef, teaching, encouraging, and helping
them to understand why I was away from home for
so many days and weeks, traveling, studying, and
researching to discover the vastness of this world and
what God has given to us to help His children.

This book would not have been possible without
her constant encouragement, her countless hours of
typing all that I had written, and then her directing
the editing of the whole project.

This book became a masterpiece because
of her touch and her gift of language.
Thank you, my sweetheart!

Contents:

Dedication

This book and related documentary are dedicated to all of the beautiful people who are seeking understanding, who may not be sure about their purpose and life's path, and who may be questioning their relationship with their Divine Creator. My hope is that in the pages of this novel, the individuals and families who struggle with growth, life, and learning about God might touch your heart and lead you to deeper and more fulfilling relationships.

Many of the challenges and successes in this novel have been taken from real-life experiences, which helped give me greater insight into the development of the characters portrayed in this book.

The proceeds from the sale of this book and related documentary film will go to the D. Gary Young Foundation, which builds schools in rural areas of Third World countries, where little or no education is available.

Acknowledgments

I wish to thank all of the people in my life who gave encouragement and support and my many friends and employees who helped in various areas of this project over the years.

Alene Frandsen: Executive Editor, who carried a double load while fulfilling her teaching responsibilities at Brigham Young University and who made meeting our deadlines possible. Thank you, Alene.

Karen Boren: Executive Researcher and Editor, who spent many sleepless nights verifying ancient names, locations, and dates in order to keep the historical information as accurate as possible. Thank you, Karen.

Dr. Leida Argüello, Medical Director; Tamara Packer, Director of Therapies; and Vallorie Judd, Director of Patient Services: For taking over the management and responsibilities of the NovaVita Research Center in Guayaquil, Ecuador, where we develop new therapies and conduct clinical research on the usage and efficacy of essential oils. Their dedication and loyalty in my absence enabled me to travel and do the research that was needed to write this book.

Marc Schreuder, John Whetten, and Don Muirhead: Who traveled many times with me to Arabia to film and photograph during the research and development phase of this book and the documentary film.

My friend and CEO of Young Living Essential Oils, Doug Nelson, Ph.D.: Who has given me constant encouragement and unending support.

The 118 personal friends, the Young Living employees and distributors: Who participated in the filming project in Egypt and Jordon for the documentary that was created as a companion to this book. Many photos of them taken during the filming have been used to create the illustrations that you will enjoy as you read from chapter to chapter.

Preface

In my quest to find the truth about the legendary frankincense, I found myself traveling to study and conduct research in faraway places such as the Hebrew University in Jerusalem, where I did biblical research into the ancient historical writings of frankincense and the association with Christ. I was also able to study biochemistry and essential oil sciences at the Cairo University, which led me to spend several weekends in Upper Egypt. It was here where I started discovering some of the oldest recorded uses of oils and aromatics and the transplanting of frankincense trees from the Land of Punt, which I believe to be within the boundaries of present-day Yemen and Oman.

This motivated me to start studying the Qur'an and cross-referencing it with the Bible. From there I began searching in the archaeological departments of the libraries that I visited and spent many wonderful hours studying ancient manuscripts and rare books in the museums of Egypt, Israel, France, Turkey, England, and even the Smithsonian Institute in Washington, D.C.

Then my most recent studies in the universities in Muscat and Salalah, Oman, and Sana'a, Yemen, brought fascinating, new discoveries. I was greatly rewarded in my research when I spent time in the historical societies and antiquities departments as well as interviewing historians and archaeologists in Salalah, Oman, and Ataq, Yemen. I found the information available from the Dead Sea Scrolls to be very revealing as well.

Through all of this research, though, I discovered that many of the stories written about frankincense and other ancient oils contradicted each other. There seemed to be many inaccuracies and false assumptions about these precious gifts. One false statement is that *Boswellia frereana*, one of the many species of frankincense, grows in Oman.

The truth was easy to find and document through such agencies as the Ministry of Agriculture in Salalah, Oman, the Chamber of Commerce and Trade Ministry in Muscat, Oman, as well as the Aden Trade Commission in Aden, Yemen.

Dr. Abdirizak Osman, Minister of Post and Telecommunications in Somalia, was very willing to talk with me and answered my questions and enlightened me with other interesting facts about the frankincense industry.

When I was in Ethiopia conducting research, I learned much about the frankincense market from Mr. Teklehaimanot Nigatu, the general manager of Natural Gum Processing and Marketing Enterprise in Addis Ababa.

The dating for the domestication of the camel was also a subject of much controversy, varying from the year 600 B.C. to 1,100 B.C., depending on the author. The Bible clearly tells us that the camel was domesticated for packing and riding before 2,000 B.C. The Book of Genesis, written about 1,896 B.C., indicates that the Ishmaelites were using camels for packing at that time. This could then validate that camels were well domesticated before 1,896 B.C. and could have been used for caravan travel from Gilead to Cairo, when the brothers of Joseph cast him into a pit from which Midianite merchants took and sold him to a passing caravan traveling to Egypt (Genesis 37:28).

Ancient writings and drawings found recently in China show camels pulling a cart about 3,500 B.C. Therefore, we cannot assume that just because a drawing on a cave or rock wall depicting the hunt of the camel for meat, dating 1,100 B.C. to 600 B.C., would indicate that the camel was not domesticated until after people quit hunting it for meat. It would be the same as if we were to say that since horses and cattle are used for meat today, they have not yet been domesticated.

I felt very drawn to find the truth about these precious commodities that for 3,000 years or more commanded a price higher than gold. This era marked the beginning of international trade and commerce. The frankincense trade easily could have brought about the beginning of writing, the development of the first alphabet, and the rudimentary beginning of reading and arithmetic followed by laws, taxation, courts and judges, architecture, and irrigation. Land and sea trade routes were also discovered and mapped. Ships were built to carry the merchandise, and roads were built all along the caravan routes.

Cities grew with their policies, governments, and surveying of territorial boundaries. Villages grew out of military posts and forts that were first built to guard and resupply the caravans. Many small villages and seaports like Petra, Aqaba, Najran, Marib, Salalah, Aden, Wubar, and Ur grew into large cities, and some still thrive today, 3,000 to 4,000 years later.

The caravaners had to cross mountainous terrain and arid wadis that were very harsh and rugged. The Wadi Andhur was a mountaintop fortress, apothecary, and way station going northwest over the Al-Hasik Mountains.

The Wadi Hanoon was the first caravan stop going north over the Jebal Al-Awast Mountains. Most caravan routes converged at the second stop in Wubar, which took ten days to two weeks and at that time was considered the edge of the world.

The mountains north of Habban, Yemen, another main supply station, were heavily covered with flourishing frankincense trees. Today, sadly only 10 percent of those mighty trees remain. Because of so much harvesting, the reproduction of the trees decreased greatly, weakening them so much that they eventually died out.

Shabwah was the first taxation port going north where Queen Balkis, the Queen of Sheba, collected her 25 percent tax to pay for her opulent lifestyle. Very few caravaners dared evade the taxation port because the penalty was death.

The frankincense trade was the main economic foundation for Southern Arabia during ancient times, as the resin became a commodity that commanded a very high price in world trade. Overland caravan routes, the Silk Road, ocean ports, and many shipping routes opened up because of the demand for this precious resin. Whole cities were built to accommodate the frankincense business.

This began the separation of territories that later became provinces and/or regions out of which grew rivalry and dissention. Wars were eventually fought over land ownership. How little we realize that so much of our society came from the quest for the mighty frankincense.

The frankincense tree was regarded as a sacred gift from God by the people of the Land of Zofar, the Land of Frankincense. In the King James edition of the Bible, more than 50 references are made to frankincense, incense, myrrh (which was also called bdellium), and *levonah*, which is the Hebrew equivalent of the Arabic word for frankincense, *luban*.

These resins, and the oils that were extracted from them, were the very essence of healing and purifying and were valued greater than any other commodity at that time. They were considered God's holy oils to be used in sacred healing and spiritual rituals.

Frankincense was so mysterious and intriguing that it was talked about by prophets, kings, and wise men. God even gave recipes and formulas for healing through worship (Exodus 30:20-30).

A legend is told in Yemen that when Adam and Eve were banished from the Garden of Eden, God gave them three gifts: frankincense, myrrh, and balsam. Could this have contributed to Adam's long life of 930 years and Shem's of 600 years, unlike Moses, who did not have the gifts and lived only 120 years?

Alexander the Great was planning to conquer the Land of Frankincense in 325 B.C. but died before he was able to start his siege. Cleopatra and her entourage sailed down the Nile with the white smoke of frankincense — the smoke of the gods — billowing from incense burners on each ship, sending its exotic fragrance into the air.

Kings like Tutankhamun, Tuthmosis III, and the great Pharaohs like Ramses and many others measured their wealth in the abundance of aromatic resins. Queen Hatshepsut and her royal navy brought frankincense and myrrh to Upper Egypt some 1,500 years B.C.

The frankincense tree is one of the oldest trees written about in the world, with a myriad of stories and legends; and because of those writings, incense began an historical journey through the minds of people worldwide. Moreover, its rich, pungent aroma has evolved into a billion dollar fragrance industry.

The gum resin is gathered from stout, hardy trees that grow in northern Kenya, Somalia, India, Sudan, Ethiopia, the island of Socotra, and, of course, in Yemen and Oman. There are 27 main species of frankincense with another 16 less-known subspecies. Today, it is used for religious ceremonies, exotic perfumes, aromatherapy, and the treatment of a variety of diseases.

Do all species of frankincense have healing properties? No! For example: *Boswellia neglecta* and *Boswellia paferifia* were never used in ancient times for healing, nor was *Boswellia frereana*, which was used only for perfume. In our modern world, it is easy to recognize and validate the species that contain healing constituents through gas chromatography and masspectrometry analysis. Today, the only frankincense species that are recognized for their healing properties are *B.sacra*, *B. carteri*, and *B. serrata*. In ancient times only *B. sacra and B. carteri* were used for healing.

Through distillation, we learn that there is a water-soluble chemical component called boswellic acid that has been found to kill cancer as well as reverse arthritis. However, through further studies, we see that *B. frereana* contains little to no boswellic acid, while *B. carteri and B. sacra* contain 25 to 30 percent.

Research shows that other family compounds like sesquiterpenes work directly on the anterior pituitary, stimulating human growth hormone (hGH) production, which slows the aging process and has been said by some scientists to reverse it. With this scientific research, it is evident that the healing properties of frankincense are determined by its chemical components.

Why has this tree from the arid, hot desert created such a mysterious fascination for over 5,000 years? Why have wars been fought over this precious resin, camel caravans raided, and trade ships sunk by pirates who lusted after this cargo that was considered more valuable than gold? Frankincense was much more than just a substance with an exotic fragrance surrounded by an alluring mystery and a luxury available only to royalty.

Millions of Christians look to Jesus Christ as the Messiah, who brought forth the fulfillment of scriptural prophecies made by ancient prophets who taught the belief of "One God." Millions of non-Christians still believe that Jesus was a great prophet and teacher and respect what He taught. Even the symbolism of the three gifts brought to Him at birth by the Magi is recognized throughout the world.

When King Herod heard of the great journey of the Magi, he may have wanted to know why these gifts were taken instead of precious stones and silk. Traditionally, the Magi, known as Balthazar, Melchior, and Caspar, whose names and story were translated into Latin from an early Fifth Century Greek tale, were the bearers of gifts that have been talked about, sung about, and written about as part of the Christmas story that has been read by millions of people worldwide.

The spiritual component of frankincense is perhaps one of its more profound aspects. Anciently, it was believed to drive away evil spirits and to bring God or the gods (as some believed) closer. Frankincense became a powerful symbol of spirituality as it was used in many religious ceremonies and rituals.

For some 5,000 years, the white purifying smoke of frankincense was used in prayers and healing and was first recorded in the Sumerian temples in 3,500 B.C., located in southern Mesopotamia (modern Iraq). This area is considered by many archaeologists to be the "cradle of civilization." History records that Emperor Nero bought thousands of tons of resin. It is said that he burned so much at one time that the people could not see through the streets of Rome because the smoke of the burning frankincense was so thick.

Frankincense was even more legendary for its healing power, which ranged from treating psychological conditions such as stress, depression, and insomnia to physical conditions like asthma, arthritic pain, menstrual irregularity, and many other problems, including cancer. Diodorus of Sicily wrote in the First Century B.C. that frankincense was good for "broken heads . . . and to bind bloody wounds." Indeed, it has held the world captive for thousands of years with its enticing aroma and mysterious past.

Introduction

kept asking myself what it was that compelled me to keep returning to the land of Arabia again and again, searching for more answers. Is it possible that the ancient people knew something that we don't know? Could frankincense cure every conceivable illness? A lot of laboratory and university research is being conducted with frankincense right now, and science is beginning to document its reversal of cancer, depression, insomnia, arthritis, and autoimmune diseases, as well as building the immune system and repairing DNA breakdown. Is this a possible answer to why the ancient prophets of so long ago lived to such an old age?

The country of Yemen has been looked upon as a warring, hostile nation. Little is known about its vast wealth in ancient history that seems to have been lost to the modern world. I felt driven to find the secrets that these ancient people must have known. Why was this knowledge lost? The thought of new discoveries from out of the past was exhilarating. I knew that a great gift awaited me.

My return to the land of God's precious resins filled me with anxiousness and excitement. As the plane landed in the capital city of Sana'a, Yemen, a strange feeling came over me as I pondered my return to Southern Arabia for the 11th time during the past 15 years in pursuit of my quest to discover the truth about God's ancient oils–frankincense, myrrh, and balsam.

I quickly changed planes and flew to the island of Socotra, where seven unique species of frankincense and four unique species of myrrh were growing that I wanted to investigate. My research companion and I covered the entire island and even hired a boat to take us on a 1½-hour boat ride to the west side of the island. There were no roads, so we had to hike five hours into the mountains to photograph the trees of the socotrana and elongata species of frankincense, as well as two of the myrrh species and any others we might discover that were unknown to the scientific world.

Three days later we flew back to Mukalla and drove to Shibam in the Hadhramaut. When I arrived, I asked about myrrh and was told that we had to go back to Mukalla and take another road to Bayhan and then to the Mawsaqah Mountains to find the myrrh trees. Finding myrrh had been very elusive in the past because every time we thought we were close, we'd find there was none. After two weeks of hiking in the mountains of Oman, Yemen, and the island of Socotra, we were beginning to understand why myrrh was such a highly prized commodity.

When we arrived in Seiyun, we were immediately hustled off the street to the airport office to buy tickets to Aden in the morning. The military police said the road through Bayhan and the Mablaqah Pass going to Shabwah was closed, and travel was very dangerous. Then they whisked us off to the hotel and told us not to go outside.

Our rooms were relatively clean and each had two single beds with futon-like mattresses just 3 inches thick made by local people. As I lay down, I could feel every board under the mattress, not to mention spotting the 3-inch-long guest that was sharing the bed next to mine. It soon became apparent that my bed wasn't going to offer me a very comfortable night's sleep, similar to the beds from the hotels of the previous nights since I had left home.

I decided to wrestle my uninvited guest for his mattress as well. To my joy, I won. He retreated to a safe place under the TV cabinet, only to reappear in the dark of the night scurrying across my chest, up my arm, and off my shoulder just fast enough that I couldn't hit him but slowly enough to make sure that I felt him and came fully awake. In an instant I grabbed my shoe, but my unwanted friend retreated back under the cabinet as my shoe smacked the floor a split second too late to bag my trophy. Now the battle was on as he retraced his steps. As the clock ticked past 3 a.m., it became evident that he was going to make sure I didn't enjoy his mattress.

At 7 a.m. I bid my "roommate" good-bye and went out the door to be greeted by six military police, who escorted us to the airport. We flew to Aden, the main seaport on the eastern coast of Yemen, to meet with the president of The Chamber of Commerce and Industrial Trade. As we landed one hour later, I couldn't help but marvel how short the flying time was from Seiyun to Aden, while it took the great caravans four to five weeks to travel the same distance.

As I stepped off the plane, I felt a bit of a tingling sensation as I pondered the possibility that perhaps we were standing on the ground that once was the home of Adam and Eve, not having realized that the name Aden had evolved from Eden.

Legends passed down for thousands of years claimed that this land was once the Garden of Eden and could be cross-referenced in Genesis where it says "the whole land of Havilah, [the present day Hadhramaut], where there is gold; and the gold of that land is good: there is bdellium [myrrh] . . ." (Genesis 2:11-12). The local people, who are mostly Muslim, know the story of Adam and Eve from their sacred book, the Qur'an and are very proud of the fact that, as they believe, the city of Aden was the location of the Garden of Eden.

We drove through the city heading toward the Alarakhia Warehouse from where the largest amount of resin is exported in the world. They market over a million tons of various resins each year. We could easily imagine that at one time the beauty of the ancient architecture of the old buildings must have been magnificent. But now the landscape was just a terrain of rugged, rocky mountains, which would be difficult for most goats to cross.

I could hardly imagine that this was the land of the Garden of Eden, although archaeologists and geologists have reported that the area was once a tropical garden stretching from the Euphrates River to the Dead Sea to Aden. The Bible describes this region very well as the Garden of Eden.

I was grateful I had been able to explore this country with its vast secrets of ancient times. Yemen has been recognized as the oldest inhabited country in the world today and, sadly, one of the poorest and least peaceful with much hostility and warring. I knew my research would require that I return in my quest to unravel the mysteries hidden in the forbidden and ancient territories of Yemen.

Having been in Yemen once before, I knew what I needed for my return trip. After filling out mountains of paperwork that would allow me to take in my video equipment, I was finally able to obtain a journalist visa, after waiting for six months.

After I cleared customs, I was met at the airport by Yasser, my interpreter and government escort. Even though I was able to get my camera through customs that time, he informed me that I couldn't travel to the interior because the government had closed the roads due to terrorist and rebel activities.

I wanted so much to go into the heart of the country because I knew that there was much to see and learn about the caravan routes and their way of traveling. But foreigners were not allowed into the "forbidden zone." However, I was determined and kept talking and waiting. I had a thick, black beard, was dressed in native attire, and looked just like one of them. I emphasized that I was not a tourist but a researcher who wanted to write about their country. Perhaps that is what made the difference.

It seemed like a triumphant moment when I was granted my special permit to go into the forbidden zone of the Hadhramaut interior and hike the mountains north of Habban where now small groves of frankincense trees were growing on the steep, rugged, limestone mountains that challenge the most nimble-footed goats, rising from an elevation of 500 meters to 2,000 meters in brain-baking heat of 48 degrees Celsius (118 degrees Fahrenheit).

We hiked for four hours up the mountain to the frankincense groves, where I was able to harvest the resin from the trees growing on the steep wadi banks. Strangely, I seemed to know exactly how to cut the bark. It all felt so familiar. Yasser, my translator, wanted to know how I knew to make the right cuts. I didn't answer him as I pondered his question.

The family of the young man who accompanied us up the mountain had been harvesting frankincense for 10 to 12 generations. He was also amazed and asked, "Yasser, how is it that the American doctor knows how to harvest frankincense the ancient way?"

I looked straight at him and shrugged my shoulders as I answered, "It just seems to be the logical way to do it."

By the time we left the top, it had become very dark. Even the seven military soldiers assigned to guard me wondered how I knew the way off the mountain in the pitch black of the night. I just smiled, remembering my many midnight rides as a young boy on my horse, Cannonball, through the mountains of Challis, Idaho. I looked into their quizzical faces and had a peculiar thought come to me as I said, "I grew up in the mountains and feel right at home here!" But as I said it, my own answer felt strange.

The next day I had a most unusual feeling standing at the south gate that led into the ancient city of Shabwah. A rock sat at the entrance with

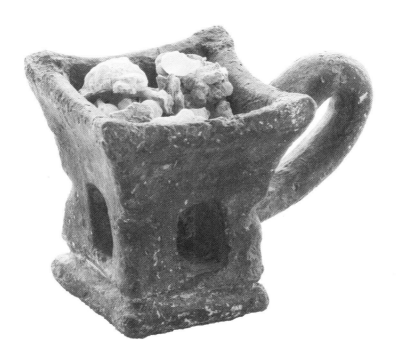

what appeared to be Shahri writing that welcomed the caravans into the city. It was like the whole scene transformed before my eyes, and I could see the camels being led to the Treasury House across from the king's palace. Here they off-loaded their merchandise to be weighed and taxed. The taxes were usually paid for with frankincense resin. I blinked my eyes and again the old ruins were there in view, but the same feeling of having been there before was still so strong.

After two visits to the old ruins of Shabwah, filming, digging, and looking for evidence of the frankincense trade, I dug down about a meter, wanting to evaluate how deep the Treasury House footings were, and made a most unexpected discovery. There I unearthed a stone incense burner that the minister of antiquities allowed me to keep and bring home. He estimated it to be between 3,000 and 4,000 years old.

The antiquities minister from Ataq, who accompanied me on my second visit to Shabwah, said that local archaeologists and historians believe that the ruins under old Shabwah could be the lost ruins of Sodom and Gomorrah.

Later that day Bedouin shepherds from the desert took me 20 minutes from Shabwah to the ancient salt mines of 5,000 years ago. They said this was the mountain where Lot's wife was turned into a pillar of salt, and the mountain on which she stood was in eyesight of the old city of Shabwah. My curiosity intensified, bringing many more questions to my mind.

I felt so blessed to have walked and driven much of the original caravan trail. It was a fabulous opportunity to travel in the world's oldest country, the country of Yemen, where many people believe the world's history began. Shabwah was one of the most fascinating places that I was able to explore, where so much caravan history took place. It was very real and seemed to come alive for me.

The next week I climbed the Al-Mashat Mountains with some Bedouins who lived in rock houses above the old city. It was there that I first found the tree of the sweet myrrh, *Commiphora molmol*, that is mentioned in the Bible (Psalm 45:8). It had a magnificent, sweet fragrance that was almost perfume-like, not the heavy, musky fragrance of the most familiar myrrh. After smelling its sweet fragrance, I could easily understand why it was favored of God. This myrrh was preferred for the healing of women's problems from childbearing, to menstrual pain, to depression, as well as for a very powerful aphrodisiac.

During this day the Saudi Arabia military was bombing villages just to the north, making the road to Sana'a forbidden to travel at night by any foreigner. I told Yasser that I had to be at the Sana'a University in the morning, and because it was a six-hour drive, we had to travel through the night. In a fearful tone he clamored, "You can't! It is forbidden!" He said he would not go, so I told him that was all right with me, but I was going.

When he saw that I could not be persuaded, he stayed in the car and we continued our drive. We drove through 15 military check stations, and at each station they looked in the car, flashed their lights in my eyes, and waved us on through. Not once did they ask for my I.D. We arrived in Sana'a without a problem, and I was able to make it to my meetings on time. I could have spent many more days there, but my time had come to an end, and I had to leave.

As I loaded the 50 kilos (110 lbs.) of frankincense that I had collected onto the plane, I was enveloped in the euphoria of the amazing time I had spent in the interior—the "forbidden zone." The traveling had been challenging, but the research and discoveries were exciting, and the knowledge from the past that I was taking back with me was priceless.

Now it was time to fly back to Oman to continue my research there and to secure my relationship with my new partners with whom I was to start building my distillery, my own distillery in Salalah—the realization of a vision I had had the first time I went to Oman nearly 15 years ago. What a thrilling moment of anticipation. As the plane became airborne, I thought that for my next grand adventure, I would go into the Empty Quarter and camp, to sleep under the stars. I wondered what new discoveries would be awaiting me. I could never have envisioned what I was about to experience.

I had to fly first to Muscat, the capital of Oman, and then catch a flight to Salalah. As soon as I landed, I rented a jeep and drove to Wubar, the lost city of the desert, which was the last civilization before reaching Fort Yabrin in present-day Saudi Arabia. Today it is identified only by its ruins and is nothing more than a crossroad at an oasis, a place to rest and water.

On my quest for the frankincense, I wanted to follow the original trail into the Empty Quarter and experience sleeping in this most treacherous land of desert vipers, deadly scorpions, and frightening camel spiders. I wanted to experience what these ancient caravaners might have felt as they made camp at night.

I felt an indescribable excitement as the Empty Quarter loomed in the distance. Reaching my destination about 200 kilometers inland from Salalah, I started to climb one of the highest sand dunes, about 250 meters high. I felt miniature in size as I reached the top and looked at the immensity of the barren desert around me. Once again I surveyed the surrounding terrain and marveled as the shimmering heat waves danced so close that I felt I could reach out and touch them. The sweat ran down my back and soaked my shirt as the temperature climbed above 45 degrees Celsius (113 F.).

The scarab beetles scurried across the desert as if the hot sand scorched their feet. Beyond that, there was a stillness that sent shivers up my spine as the feeling of loneliness settled into my nerve centers, spiking the adrenaline, creating almost a giddy feeling. Again, I had that most unusual feeling that I had been here before. It was so familiar—a sense of returning—like I was at home.

The realization was almost overwhelming that some 3,500 years ago, caravaners with merchandise from ships, now heavily loaded on camels, crossed here as they headed into the desert northeast to Fort Yabrin, entering the most brutal and feared desert wilderness in the world, the Rub al Khali—the Empty Quarter—that spread out over approximately 600,000 square kilometers to the north, northeast, and northwest, a desert wilderness that was never crossed until about 1,000 B.C. This was a land that without question was the most unforgiving wasteland ever to be conquered by man.

Seventy kilometers to the south from where I was standing lay the ruins of the lost city of Wubar, which, because of an earthquake, had sunk into an underground cavern, leveling the largest and richest city in the Arabian Peninsula, which they had claimed to be the richest in the world. This wild and decadent city was said to be the Sodom and Gomorrah of the desert. It was a pivotal connection for the caravaners—a place where they could rest and take on fresh supplies for the arduous, six-week journey to Fort Yabrin.

The 1,000 meter climb up out of Fort Sumhuram at the Khor Rori Port over the Zophar Mountains with 600-pound pack loads must have been exhausting for man and beast. The 14-day journey from the fort to Wubar was an emotional adjustment for the men as they left their families and friends behind, knowing it would be four to five months at best before they returned. Wubar was the place to adjust and balance the packs and for the new camels to work out any stubborn or high-spirited attitude before entering the Empty Quarter.

At this point, before the discovery of the northern route to Fort Yabrin, the caravans turned west and skirted the northern slopes of the mountains, where both men and animals suffered from the heat along the winding trail westward to Shabwah and then to Marib, the home of the Queen of Sheba. From there they made the journey northward, intercepting the coastline trail at Makka (Mecca) and then traveling along the coastline of the Red Sea to Petra and on to Damascus or Jerusalem. The second route left Najran, skirting the Empty Quarter northeast to Fort Yabrin and continuing on to Gerrha some 750 miles away.

The new route to Fort Yabrin that went north across the Rub al Khali, shortened the trip by almost six weeks and bypassed the taxation ports of Shabwah, Timna, and Najran. This was significant in cost savings to the caravaners and merchants. The compacted ground caused by thousands of camels and men trudging across the desert over these ancient caravan routes was the means by which satellite thermography was able to discover the location of the "Lost City of Ubar" in 1992, which was aired as a Nova Documentary on PBS.

As I stood on the dunes reminiscing over some of the stories I had read about the frankincense trade routes, a queasy feeling started to come over me. The dunes started to spin as I looked through the shifting sand, and I could see a huge camel caravan approaching through the shimmering heat waves not more than a quarter mile away. It seemed so real and yet unbelievable at the same time that I thought I was going to lose my lunch. I took a deep breath, closed my eyes, and rubbed them with both hands. I felt much better as I let my breath out slowly, trying to calm myself. When I opened my eyes, thankfully, everything was normal—no caravan.

I walked pensively down off the dune, trying to make sense of what had just happened, but at the moment I didn't have an answer. There were two smaller dunes in the near distance where I could drive to set up my camp for the night, which I thought would be good protection from the wind. Darkness was rapidly falling on the vast desert as I prepared my sleeping bag and settled in for what I thought would be a peaceful night's sleep in the Rub al Khali. As the night blanketed the desert, the day temperature of 45 degrees Celsius (113 F.) plummeted quickly to a cool 20 degrees Celsius (68 F.).

To my surprise, the wind started to blow with such force that I wondered if my tent would hold as the sand pelted against the sides. But then I thought, "Of course, it will, because, after all, it was designed for harsh conditions and purchased from a well-known sporting goods store at home." The wind continued to blow even stronger, which I thought was typical of a Rub al Khali desert sandstorm that could bury an entire caravan of 1,000 camels overnight. But I was so exhausted from traveling that I couldn't keep my eyes open any longer, and feeling warm and comfortable in my sleeping bag, I drifted into dreams about camels and the Empty Quarter.

I jolted awake with a gripping fear that made me want to run. I told myself, "This is too much. Tomorrow I'm driving to the airport and taking the first plane home." But the howling wind with the rhythmic pelting of the sand against the tent walls again lulled me back into an exhausted state of sleep.

Sometime later I was startled awake again by some strange sound. As I lay listening, I realized that the wind had stopped. At first the sound was unknown to me, but as it grew louder, it became faintly familiar. Then I recognized it! It was the sound of camels. I looked outside my tent and breathed a sigh of relief as several camels had been roped together, like in a corral, near my campsite.

I started to lie back down, thinking I might be able to go back to sleep. Then the realization struck me like a sledgehammer, causing me to break out into a cold sweat. I bolted up out of my wool and cotton-woven blanket and stared in shock at this Bedouin tent that looked like it was made from something like spun flax, horsehair, and coconut fiber. What happened to my modern-day sleeping bag and my tent from that well-known sporting goods store?

I looked down at my feet strapped in leather sandals and looked around for my hiking boots—and where were my long pants with my tucked-in, long-sleeved shirt? I could hardly believe that I was wearing something that looked more like a skirt or a dress. What was happening? A feeling of panic came over me as my head reeled with confusion. I felt faint and more nauseous as I dropped to my knees; and falling over onto the blanket, I closed my eyes and tried to escape into a deep sleep, where I thought I was safe, hoping that when I awakened, everything would be back to normal.

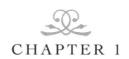

CHAPTER 1

The Caravan

I heard the sound of Jona's voice calling from the distance, "Captain Shutran." He waved to signal me that he was ready. I waved back to let him know I would be coming. Jona was my second-in-command, and I needed to meet with him for his morning report. I had ridden up to the crest of a lonely sand dune as the morning sun had begun to color the vast desert that lay before us.

I ran my hands over my commander's cross belt, thinking about the first time I had buckled it on and what it represented. Many years had passed since that time, but the memory of my father watching with great pride was still vivid. How I missed him, but I often felt him with me. As the Commander, the responsibility was great because so much depended upon my decisions. My father had prepared me well, and I often reflected upon the things that I had learned from him.

I looked out across the expansiveness of 300 camels sprawled in the sand as my men were beginning to put on the pack saddles. Many times my eyes had gazed upon the immensity of the caravan in the early morning as preparations were being made for the day's journey, but every time was like the first, with a feeling of awe and wonder of such an undertaking.

The morning was peaceful as I prepared myself mentally for the day. Jona always waited for me and knew I would come when I was ready. When I started down the dune, he rode towards me and called out, "Captain, everything is in order and we will be ready to move when you give the command."

"Good, Jona. Come to the fire so we can eat while we talk."

The breakfast fires were flickering brightly as daylight was overtaking the night, and the temperature was still refreshingly cool by half of the daytime temperature. It was a most beautiful time of the day. My appetite awakened as I smelled the camel fat frying over the fire while breakfast was being prepared with beans and rice. The luban was boiling in a pot of water on the fire for fresh tea, which most of us drank every morning because it seemed to sharpen the mind and was greatly invigorating with the dawning of a new day.

The men were grabbing their breeches that had been draped over a pyramid-like frame made with four sticks tied together and standing about 1 meter high over the incense burner so that the smoke from the luban could saturate their clothing throughout the night. Everyone liked the aroma because it covered the unpleasant smell of both men and animals after sweating all day in the hot sun as well as sending sand fleas and other hungry critters running in the opposite direction.

The camels, when fully packed with their colorful halters and breast collars, beautifully embroidered packs, and blankets and pads of many colors, were a stunning sight, especially when lined out across the reddish, tan-colored sand. The first morning when the caravan began to move out was always a time of great anticipation for everyone.

For me, the feeling was exhilarating because it challenged my leadership to know what was ahead. It was a new morning and the beginning of a new journey that held the promise of exciting adventures that would be retold around the campfires and in the family circles at home. The men and camels were now ready for the 60- to 70-day arduous trek ahead, leaving Wubar to cross the vast, unforgiving, harsh wasteland that lay before us, a challenge beyond the experience of most of the caravaners.

I had crossed the desert many times, but each time I wondered if this would be the journey when the water in the oasis would be dried up or if we would encounter desert pirates attacking out of the dunes with their marauding band of thieves wanting to take our precious cargo, regardless of the cost of life. With these dangers I knew that some of these men, perhaps even me, might not live to make the return trip home. Even those who journeyed only to Fort Yabrin on the north side of the Empty Quarter, expecting to return with a southbound caravan to Fort Sumhuram, wondered about their fate.

The immense challenges of the unknown always lingered in the minds of the caravaners. The fear of encountering a blinding sandstorm that could drive man and beast absolutely mad was always a possibility, and if the Bedouin scouts were to lose the trail, we might have to travel three or four days before reaching the next water hole.

One mistake and the whole caravan could possibly perish. We carried enough water for only three days for all of the men and horses. The camels could go for about four days in the heat carrying 200- to 300-kilo pack loads and traveling 35 to 45 kilometers a day, but for the men and the other animals, a single day without water could be disastrous.

It was almost impossible to rest in the heat with no shade and the sun beating down at 45 degrees. We could travel for days and not find a rock to give shade or a blade of grass for the animals to eat. Sometimes the gutrah head wrap increased the temperature so much that it felt as though the sun were drilling a large hole through our heads, but it was the only protection we had, and without it our heads would simply burn up as though they were being cooked on a campfire. Wetting the gutrah helped reduce the temperature a couple of degrees, but it wasn't a good idea to use our precious water that way. The desire to drink was almost overpowering, but when it became a question of good sense and survival, it could be a death issue if the balance was broken.

I couldn't help but think about the caravaners who went screaming mad because of the intense heat and the illusion of a beautiful, green oasis just beyond them. If that became fixed in their minds, they could start to run, and any attempt to stop them could put one's own life in jeopardy. The thought of seeing water could become infectious and put the entire caravan at risk. There was nothing like heat and dehydration to alter the mind so quickly. I had seen many men go crazy and even kill a best friend for one drop of water.

I felt both the anticipation and anxiety of the men, especially those making the journey for the first time. The excitement was contagious while the returning caravaners told stories around the campfires, romanticizing the encounters with raiders and the battles fought. But that didn't lessen the reality for the scouts and sentries, who were at risk with their responsibility to watch for bandits.

They told of the exciting and fancy things to see in the cities they passed through; and, of course, the stories of the beautiful, loose, wild women in the other countries were always alluring, even when they weren't true. After a few weeks away from home, their imagination made the women even more beautiful.

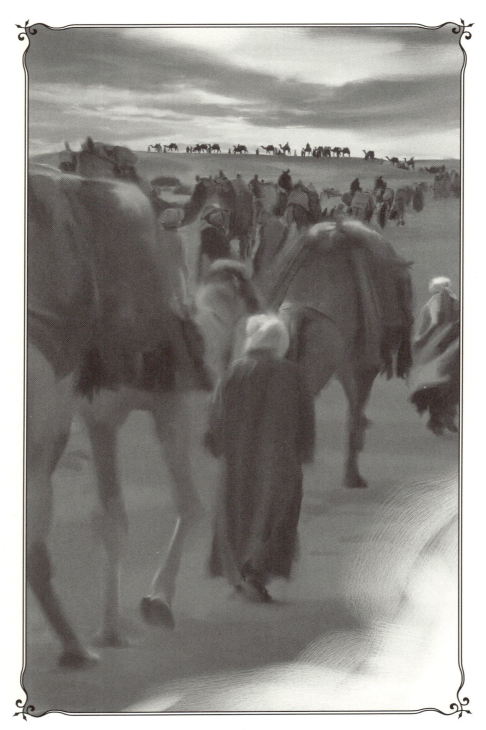

The caravaners were the younger men's heroes, traveling the world and bringing back the tales of other cultures and tribal customs. As usual, the men competed among themselves to see who could embellish the stories in the most sensationalized fashion, becoming the center of attention, as the young men sat around listening with adoration and expectation of the time that they would make the great 2,500 kilometer trek.

They carried on about the lush money they saw being spent in the taverns at night or paid at the taxation ports when the caravans came from another country. The mere fact that the caravaners made three times more money than a fisherman or than the families gathering the incense resin was very enticing to the young and ambitious, who might want to put together a bride price for their first marriage.

Of course, there was no mention about why the caravaners made three to four times more money than those from the village working in the fields or tending the animals. All the danger, the harshness, the tremendous difficulties, and even the possibility of death were of no concern in anticipation of the adventure, the money, and the excitement of the unknown.

But for the experienced caravaners, the dangers were very real. The thoughts of life-threatening disasters always passed through their minds. Arriving at a water hole that had dried up or was buried under 100 meters of sand meant that the water had to be rationed to 1 liter per day for each man and 3 liters for each horse. We would be forced to travel at night, when the temperatures dropped 15 to 20 degrees, so that the camels could go another three to four days, with hope that water would be found at the next stop.

There was always the concern that one of the men might get sick on the journey and die or that we might have to kill him to stop the intense pain of a spreading infection that would only delay his death and prolong his suffering. Sometimes the pain was so terrible that he would beg for someone to take his life. He might have been a most trusted and loyal friend or even the son of one of the villagers where you live. To kill a comrade was the most terrible thing a caravan commander had to do, creating a memory that would stay in his mind forever while he tried to justify it so that he could go on with life.

But the most fearful danger of the night is an encounter with the dreaded camel spider, which can grow to a length of as much as 15 centimeters and can run up to 16 kilometers per hour. This desert predator hunts at night and feeds on blood and flesh. It first injects a serum that numbs the nerves so that it can quietly feast until it satisfies its appetite, which could result in the loss of part of a foot, forearm, or face, which has happened to many men.

It was a moment of horror to be awakened early in the morning by the screaming of a man who discovered that part of his nose and cheek were missing, causing him to take his own life with his curved dagger, the jambiyya, as everyone stood by watching, stunned at the sight and not fully awake to respond in time to stop him.

On one of the caravans that I led, one of my men lost his ear and part of his cheek during the midnight meal. He was almost delirious with the terrible pain and blood running everywhere. It was a shock for all of us to see such a horrible sight. But we moved fast and quickly packed his face and the side of his head with crushed myrrh resin, which stopped the bleeding and the pain. We left him with the villagers so that they could take care of him and wondered what his face would look like when we returned.

On our way back from Gerrha, about six and a half months later, we were amazed to see that he was completely healed and that much of his cheek had grown back. He rejoined us and made another eight journeys with the caravan, even though he lived the rest of his life with only one ear.

Reflecting back, I asked myself, "Why? Why do I continue to put my life at risk when I have a family that I love more than life itself—a beautiful wife, two growing young boys who need their father, and a little princess-like daughter?" I looked at my men, knowing it was the same for them as well; they just wanted to provide a better life for their families—better than the life they had growing up. The young men making the journey for the first time had great hopes of one day owning their own caravan with four or perhaps even as many as two dozen camels.

Three or four small caravans always seemed to join me along the way. Some owners had only 1 or 2 camels, and some had 20 to 30 camels. My caravans were large and I was known to have a lot of experience, so they traveled with me for their safety and protection. It was interesting meeting up with men of different cultures and learning new things, as long as they followed my command and didn't try to do things their way.

The men were eager and wanted something better for their lives and had their own dreams. I was glad I could help with my knowledge and experience. They brought back memories of my beginning days when my father let me take my first caravan to Qana, which charted my path to this time in my life.

I looked at the slaves, busily helping with the packing and preparation, with their hopes for a better life than the one they had left. The slaves had no idea how immensely important they were to the caravan, not only to help with the burden of packing every morning and unpacking at the day's end but also fighting and defending the caravan. Without the free labor of the slaves, the cost of the caravan would have been three or four times greater, which naturally would have increased the cost of goods for the buyer.

Yes, I wanted to give my boys a better life than my own and hoped they would never have to lead a caravan and be away from their families on such long journeys as I went on. I was always happy when I received a dispatch just to go to Wubar, which I could do in four to five weeks.

How long would I continue to lead the caravan? Yes, it was in my blood and I loved the vastness of the desert with all its mysteries. I had always been fascinated by the unknown, and who knows, perhaps that unknown would bring me to a new way, where I could be with my family, and we could work together. I pondered my own question with hope.

But now it was time. The sun was rising and filling the sky with the brilliant colors of the morning. With a wave of my hand, I gave Jona the command to start moving. The dust began swirling about the camels' feet until it looked like sandy water rippling over the desert. It was a glorious sight.

As I watched the caravan move in a wave-like motion, I thought about the dreams I had had from the time I was a young boy. As early as I could remember, I wanted to be a caravaner and travel into the desert of the unknown, making new discoveries and seeing the other side of the world. It seemed so long ago when I sat with my mother in our Bedouin cave and listened as she encouraged me to follow my dreams. I wondered what she would say to me now, knowing that I was the commander of this great caravan.

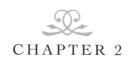

CHAPTER 2

From Bedouin
to Commander

For some reason I kept thinking about the last time my mother spoke to me. After birthing my second brother, she kept bleeding. I remember my father making a tea from the cistus he had gathered and giving it to her. I will never forget the soothing, uplifting aroma that filled our tent. The bleeding stopped quickly but she had lost so much blood and was so weak that she could not regain her strength and passed on to God three days later.

One night before she passed, she called me to her bedside. She knew I was curious about so many things and that my dreams were big for such a young boy who had seen little of the world. I loved her very much and there was a special feeling between us. She must have known that she would soon pass to the world beyond because her words had a tone of urgency in them.

"Shutran," she said, taking hold of my hand, "you are my firstborn and with that comes much responsibility. You have the ability to do great things, like your ancestor Great-grandfather Abdul, who tamed the camel. Believe in yourself and follow your dreams. Create a good life for the family that you will have one day. Your father has taught you well. Take care of your younger sister and brothers while your father is away in the mountains. Remember how much I love you and that I will always be with you wherever you are."

I looked into her gentle eyes and pulled her hand to my heart. With tears running down my cheeks, I said, "Mother, I love you, and I will always carry your words in my heart."

I wanted to be a caravaner and take the incense to the world, even though I had heard the horrifying stories about what happened to those who went into the Empty Quarter and never came out. Many people thought they were eaten by a "sand devil" that buried itself in the drifting sand and waited for unsuspecting travelers to cross its path. Others said they had been caught in a raging sandstorm that in the blink of an eye would tear the flesh off and strip a camel so clean that the wind would whistle through his ribs before he knew he was dead.

Those stories sometimes gave my younger brothers, Asif and Elazar, nightmares, but I only wondered about the strangeness of it all. As I grew older, those stories became more and more intriguing until I was driven with a desire to cross the mysterious unknown. I wasn't afraid. I just wanted to know what was there—to see it—to cross it. I just knew I could find a way to conquer the fierceness of the great Rub al Khali, the Empty Quarter.

My mother's words never quit echoing in my head, "Follow your dreams."

Grandfather Shutran, after whom I was named, used to say, "If you dream about it long enough, it will become real." Little did I know that my dream would start to become a reality that fateful day when Father and I were unloading at Siahd's marketplace in Timna, where we came to sell the resins that we had harvested and brought down from the mountains.

Siahd came up to Father and said, "Shudulla, the demand for incense is growing every day, and I have an order for myrrh to go to Egypt. I need eight to ten camels to carry the load to Qana, where the myrrh will be loaded on the ship. Since you and your son have ten camels, could you take this shipment to Qana for me?"

"Siahd, I would like to help you if you are not in a hurry and could wait. I have two more months in the Al-Mawsaqah Mountains to finish with this season's harvest."

Siahd looked disappointed and asked Father, "Would you consider expanding your caravan?"

"That is more difficult. Since my wife died, I can't be gone that long as I still have children at home."

As they talked, I could see the vision of my opportunity. I almost yelled in my excitement, "Father, I could do it!"

Father turned with a surprised look on his face and without a thought emphatically said, "No, Son! You are too young and we do not have the money to buy more camels and pack equipment."

"But, Father, I've been working with you for five years, and I can pack a camel as well as anyone."

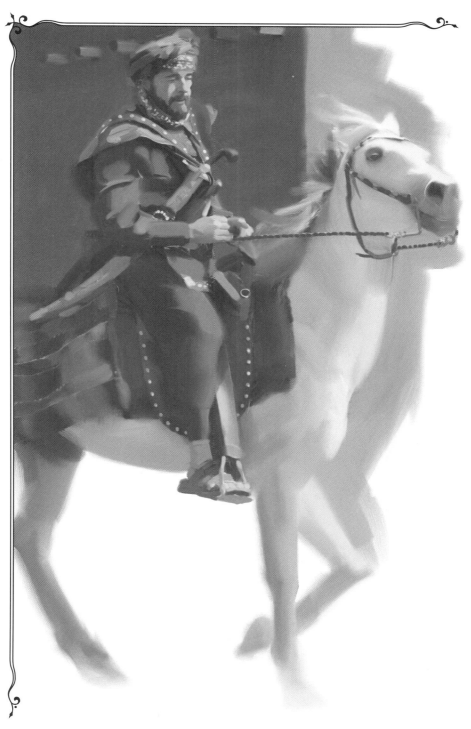

"Yes, Son, you can, but where are you going to get the camels?"

Father thought his question would stop me, but I quickly answered, "Father, it is my dream. I'll find a way; I know I can!"

"Son, you don't know the trail to Qana."

"That's true, but I know how to travel in the desert, and I can ask someone who does know the trail. Father, I know I can do it. Let me try. This has been my dream all my life, and I know Mother would be happy for me."

Siahd finished weighing our sacks of myrrh and then walked over to us as we unloaded the last camel. "Shudulla, I have a question."

"Yes?"

"What would you do if today you broke your leg and could not return to the mountains?"

"I would send Shutran. He is as good as any man!"

"Do you feel he could barter with the mountain people to secure more resin?"

"Yes, of course. I've taught him well."

At that moment I felt like I grew 2 meters tall. That was the first time I had ever heard my father tell someone else that he was proud of me and saw me as a man.

"Shudulla, I have watched Shutran since he was 12 years old coming with you to market. I remember when his mother was sick, and you had to be with her. He brought your caravan in twice by himself, and he was only 14. Shudulla, I believe he could take a caravan to Qana."

"Yes, I believe that also, but how do we get the money we need? What happens if he gets attacked by brigands near the coast or the port?"

"Father, you have taught me well with the sword, better than any Bedouin."

Siahd spoke again, "Shudulla, your firstborn son is talking like a man. You have taught him the two most important things any father could teach a son. First is how to work hard, and second is to be honest in all things. I know if Shutran takes my myrrh to Qana, it will get there just the same as if you took it, so this is my offer.

"Shutran, I will buy the camels and pack equipment and pay for everything except your wages. You work for free for one year, and at the end of the year, I will give you credit for one-half interest in the caravan if you continue to work. At the end of the second year, you will have made enough money to buy the other half of the caravan if you want it, but you must agree to continue to work for me for seven years. No exception."

Father spoke up, "Siahd, that is a good offer, but what does he live on if he has no wage?"

"Father, I have some money. I have sold the myrrh that you let me harvest for myself after our loads had been delivered. When I sold it to Siahd, he always paid me the same price. I have saved enough money to buy two camels, and with what the other merchants pay me for delivering their goods, I can live on that. Father, I know I can make this work."

"If I allow you to do this, who is going to take your place in helping me?"

"Father, I have two brothers, who are now older than I was when I started working with you."

"Yes, you're right! Son, I can see your heart is set."

"Father, I will give you 10 percent of my earnings to help take care of our family until my brothers start to work!"

"Shutran, you are a good son, but that is not necessary. You will have a hard enough time as it is."

Siahd hired two men to go with me for the first six months. Almuk, an older man, who loved date wine and was not sober very often, had traveled on the caravan trails for years and had a lot of experience. I was young and he knew he could teach me a lot. He had been a good caravaner, but after his wife died, he lost his reason to live and turned to wine. But once he started working with me, he never drank again. He had a new purpose: teaching a young man how to become a great caravaner. He became invaluable to me as a trusted companion and taught me many things as I pursued my dream.

I knew that the money I had saved to buy my first two camels would go fast. I didn't take any of it with me on my first trip but killed a deer and made jerky and gathered wild fruit to eat. When we arrived just outside of Qana, I left the caravan in camp with Almuk and walked into the village. I spent three days watching other caravaners to see how they loaded and unloaded their camels. I learned the names of the port people and listened to stories in the taverns at night.

I found the man I was to sell the myrrh to who was shipping it to Egypt. He told me that the price of myrrh was going up and that he needed frankincense as well, but there was none to buy. He said it was all going to Shabwah. I asked him what he would pay for frankincense and myrrh. When he told me, I acted as though I was not interested. His offer was only 2 denarii more per kilo than what Siahd expected to receive.

The next day I found him in the tavern bragging that he would pay the highest price for frankincense and myrrh, so I asked him again, "What would you pay for myrrh today?"

"This time I will pay you 4½ denarii per kilo."

I told him, "I can bring you 1,840 kilos of the finest myrrh in all of the Hadhramaut, but I want 5 denarii per kilo, and I can deliver it in two days." He agreed too easily.

I was excited, but yet an uneasiness made the hair stand up on the back of my neck. I was curious about the feeling I had, but the excitement of getting 5 denarii quickly pushed it to the back of my mind. "You have a deal," I said. "Pay me half now and I will deliver in two days."

"No," he said, "I won't pay until I see the myrrh."

"I can bring it in so you can see it, and then if you don't pay me, what do I do?" Father always said that a man who cannot look you in the eye while making a deal and not trust you is a man who himself cannot be trusted.

So I said to him, "This is my deal. I will bring my caravan within one day's ride of the city. You bring your money, we make the deal, and you ride back with my caravan. If we don't make a deal, I won't bring my caravan to the city."

He finally agreed and two days later I arrived with my caravan as planned. After he inspected the myrrh, he agreed that it was the very best he had seen and asked if I could bring more. "Yes," I said, "in two months."

"What about frankincense?"

"Yes, I can also bring it as well."

After he paid me the money, he asked, "Will you lead your camels to my warehouse to unload?"

"Yes," I answered, but felt reluctant.

There was a change in the tone of his voice that gave me chills again. I walked around my camels as if to put the coins in my pack. Almuk was about to leave to take most of the camels back with him to the mountains where we had camped two nights before. When the merchant wasn't looking, I handed Almuk the pack with the money to take with him where I knew it would be safe. We had agreed that he would return to meet me in two days so that we could buy new merchandise and begin our return journey.

It was dark by the time we finished unloading the last few camels. The merchant told me that my servant and I could sleep in the stable and then leave in the morning. I wasn't able to sleep because I had a feeling something might happen. I laid down in such a way that anyone could see that I didn't have a pouch with me. I had slipped my sword into the straw, where it was hidden but close to my fingers if I needed it.

I heard the door creak and what sounded like three or maybe four men came in, but I didn't make a move. I could hear them walk up close to us but assumed they had determined we were deep enough in sleep that they could search the packs. I listened as they rifled through everything, but to their surprise, they found nothing.

My heart was beating fast and I wondered what they would do next. I found myself silently asking God to just send them away. It was quiet for a moment, and then I heard the creaking door again and the faint sound of their feet as they left. I carefully opened my eyes and, looking around, gratefully thanked Father, the Almighty, for protecting us. I had a hard time going back to sleep, so I just patiently waited for morning to come, thinking about all the things I had to do.

The next day I walked along the dock talking to people and looking at all of the merchandise coming in from other countries. I decided to barter for some silk from India, a few brass ornaments, and some curry and cumin. With the extra 3 denarii per kilo increase over Siahd's expected price of 2 denarii per kilo, I could buy this new merchandise to take back to him to sell in his market. When Almuk returned, I paid for the new goods, loaded the camels, and headed for home.

I was certain that this would be the first time that Siahd would have spices and beautiful silk to sell, which would certainly bring more people to his market. This would give him another 60 percent increase, and as we agreed, for any amount that I made over the set prices, I would receive 75 percent credit toward the purchase of the caravan.

On the return home, I stopped in Habban to inquire about frankincense and secure 500 kilos at 1½ denarii per kilo to pick up on my return trip next month. I was anxious to tell my father about my trip, my first one, which had been so successful. I had earned enough money to buy my first two camels to add to Siahd's caravan, and I had my first shipment of frankincense to be delivered.

Siahd was excited to be the first in Timna to have silk cloth, brass, curry, and cumin. This started him thinking about opening new markets in other cities. For five years my father let me continue to harvest myrrh every day that I could when we didn't have loads to be delivered.

On my next trip for Siahd a few weeks later, I walked into the tavern to look for the Egyptian merchant to let him know that I was back with another 1,840 kilos of myrrh and 500 kilos of frankincense. I was anxious to collect my money and return home. However, I was about to experience the cold reality of being in business.

The merchant wasn't in the tavern, and nobody had seen him or knew his whereabouts. When I walked down to the docks, other merchants ignored me and wouldn't talk to me because I had had the myrrh that they wanted to buy but had sold it to another merchant, who had paid a higher price. I went up to the warehouse where we had unloaded, and no one was there. I walked over to the stable where I slept the night the thieves came to rob me and my servant.

The owner of the stable informed me that this merchant had been paying caravaners for their resins and then at night had been getting them drunk and robbing them, or he had his men wait outside the village and rob them as they left. Two caravaners accused him of being in on the robbery, and in the fight that followed, the merchant was killed.

I asked what I should do with my myrrh and frankincense. The stable owner said that there was another merchant buying for Egypt, but not at the same price. When I found him, he offered me 1½ denarii less than what Siahd had paid Father for the myrrh.

I knew this would end my caravan business if I didn't find an answer. I walked back to the tavern, started asking questions, and learned that ships were coming into Aden and that the merchants were buying incense that was going to the Emperor in India, but that meant the journey would be two weeks longer down the coast.

The Egyptian merchant came in asking arrogantly, "Well, are you going to sell me your incense?"

"No, Sir," I replied. "I'll take it back to Timna first," and I walked out.

Following me outside, he yelled, "Don't be stupid, boy! You might not even make it to Aden." I never even acknowledged that I heard him and kept walking.

"All right, all right!" he yelled. I'll buy your myrrh for 2 denarii!" But I just kept walking.

Two weeks later we arrived in Aden, and I sent Almuk down to the docks to inquire about a ship going to India. They were happy to be able to buy a shipment. They had been waiting for one that never arrived. We agreed on 4½ denarii. As soon as we were unloaded, Almuk found a shipper who needed a caravan to take merchandise to Wadi Dawan and Shabwah, which meant we would need 15 camels. Turning to Almuk, I said, "We need to buy 5 more camels so that we have 15 we can pack. But where can we buy 5 camels?" The money from the sale of the frankincense and myrrh wasn't enough.

Almuk and I left the caravan with our comrades while we went looking for camels and found the prices much higher in Aden. At the last place we stopped, the owner had a large pasture behind his stable with three dozen camels. I inquired why those camels weren't being sold, and he explained that they were camels that had gone "cold" in a caravan and were being sold for meat.

I remember my grandfather telling me that camels don't go cold. They just get tired of being abused and refuse to cooperate. I asked what the owner's price would be to sell them and was excited to discover that I had enough money to buy eight. Almuk was not excited about the idea of buying bad-tempered camels and started to tell me about all the problems we were going to have.

"Almuk, I disagree," I told him. "First, we have to gain the trust of the camels by treating them kindly. Once they understand things are different, they will perform." I sent Almuk immediately back to the market to buy some sugar cane and began my retraining. One week later my new "bad" camels were ready to pack.

We left Aden with a secure contract for the next two years to deliver myrrh and frankincense at 4½ denarii per kilo for this year and 5 denarii for next year. We also had a contract to deliver food, clothing, and other supplies to Wadi Dawan, Shibam, Seiyun, and Shabwah.

It was amazing how out of a bad situation a great door had opened with new and better opportunities. I continued each trip to buy more "bad" camels and bring them into my caravan. I started making new pack equipment from hides of old camels that had died rather than making them from coconut and flax fiber. The leather packs lasted longer, were easier to pack, and looked much better. It seemed like every new problem I encountered led to a new discovery.

My mother would have held my hand and said, "God has smiled on you. Your dream was bigger than you thought." I felt the warmth of her love as I thought about our conversation so many years ago. I knew she was watching, knowing that the dream of her small son had filled the heart of this man to overflowing.

Now, years later, gazing as far as the eye could see over the unending swells of sand in the midst of the most treacherous land known to man with over 300 camels and the men who rode them, I marveled at how my ultimate dream had been fulfilled as I again crossed the fierce Rub al Khali.

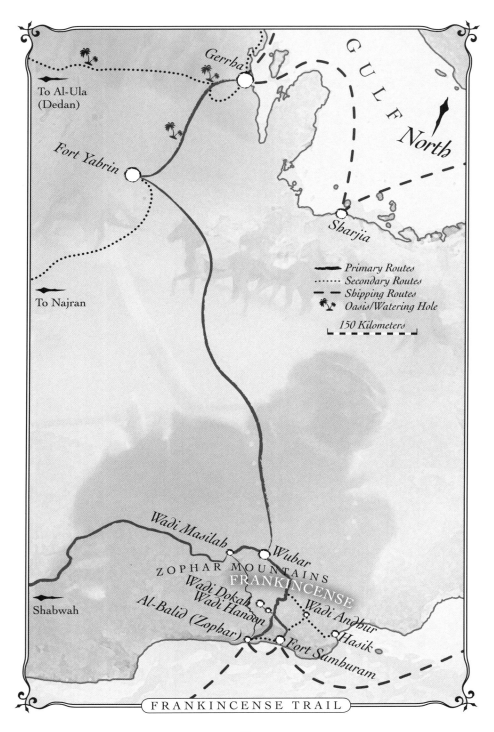

To Al-Ula
(Dedan)

Gerrha

G U L F

North

Fort Yabrin

Sharjia

To Najran

Primary Routes
Secondary Routes
Shipping Routes
Oasis/Watering Hole

150 Kilometers

Wadi Masilah

Wubar

Z O P H A R   M O U N T A I N S

FRANKINCENSE

Wadi Dokah

Wadi Handoon

Wadi Andhur

Al-Balid (Zophar)

Shabwah

Hasik

Fort Sumhuram

FRANKINCENSE TRAIL

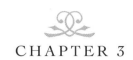

CHAPTER 3

The Sandstorm

The unknown of the changing desert always brought new challenges with each crossing. It never looked the same, except for the vastness of the sand and the intense heat of the day. Each caravan seemed to have its own personality, but the camels always had a keen sense of the journey. As the sun climbed higher in the sky, there was uneasiness in their movement. Something was coming. We could feel it in the air.

The breeze had turned into an unwanted wind and felt like a day in which we would face a lot more wind and very likely a sandstorm. The behavior of the camels was always the first sign of weather changes and indicated the direction from which the storm would come. This day it would come from the south.

The camels had picked up their pace and were moving so fast that the men were mounting them to ride because they couldn't walk and stay ahead. We could probably cover 45 to 55 kilometers today, depending on when the storm hit. How long it lasted would determine whether we gained or lost time.

I had my captains, who were each responsible for 50 camels, instruct the men to spread the caravan out abreast rather than in a train. This reduced the amount of dust the men would have to endure. As I topped out on a high dune and looked back over the caravan spreading half of a kilometer wide moving across the desert floor, I was in awe of the absolute beauty of such a breathtaking sight.

But yet at the same time, I felt a foreboding, knowing that so many men and their families depended on my decisions and the ability to execute them. It was of the utmost importance that these men have the greatest chance to survive the storm, to return, and to want to go with me on future crossings.

I was grateful for the things my father had taught me and the trust he put in me to make right decisions. Integrity and honesty were my father's foundation for all that he did and the example he lived. He often said, "If you don't do the right things, then you will never have the right relationship with your wife or God." He smiled and added, "With God, you might get away with it, but not with a good woman," and then laughed.

The thought of my beautiful Mirah's face filled my mind, causing a lump to come up in my throat. The longing for her is always really strong, even after being married for 15 years. She is more than just a good woman. She doesn't tell me things because that is what I want to hear. She talks to me straight up and tells me how she sees things. She is a good support and stands behind my decisions once they are made. She always poses questions about my ideas but never criticizes me. She just wishes that I wouldn't be such a risk taker.

She grew up in an affluent family whose father was a very successful merchant, trading resins and spices, and who is now the governor and chief accountant of the Fort Sumhuram Treasury House.

Contrary to her upbringing, I grew up in the mountains as a Bedouin, gathering the resins of frankincense and myrrh with my father. During most of my childhood, we lived like nomads, following the harvest from the Zophar Mountains to the Hadhramaut in Southern Arabia, living in tents and caves eight months of the year.

My thoughts came back full circle to Mirah, and I could see her sitting at the table teaching our children how to read and write—an opportunity that I did not have growing up. Mirah is a small, slender lady with a beauty that most women envy. The men would tease, "Shutran, what does such a beautiful woman see in such a plain, old, mountain man like you?" Each time I leave with another caravan, it becomes more difficult and she always cries, just like the first time.

We discovered that when I really begin missing her, the same feeling would come to her, so if we sit quietly, we can mentally see each other and communicate. This helps us stay close together. When we are facing danger, she immediately feels it and becomes concerned. She calls the children and together they ask God to send His protection. When the danger passes, I send her a mental message so that she can be at peace.

But now there were thick clouds of sand billowing on the south horizon, and I had to return my attention to the impending storm. No sand critters could be seen, which meant that this storm was building and heading our way. I gave Mirah a mental hug and kiss and headed for the caravan to make preparations.

Jona was riding towards me as I came down off the dune; we didn't have much time to plan our strategy. We had to spread the word that the sandstorm was likely to hit us about midday. We needed to keep the camels moving at a fast pace in order to make it to a place behind a ridge of dunes to help break the furious wind.

We pushed harder as the wind kicked the dust from under the camels' feet. With the sand churning around us, we covered our faces with barely a slight opening in the gutrah to be able to see. In the distance, we could hear the dull, faint roar of the storm—just enough that those of us who had lived through this kind of a storm knew that we didn't have a second to lose.

I rode ahead with my two Bedouin scouts, looking at our options to get 300 camels and 200 men ready for what was coming. This wasn't a normal storm, because the season for the big sandstorms had already passed. The roar was increasing as it continued its northward course straight towards us.

Several of the younger men and new recruits showed signs of nervousness, which could cause the camels to start running wildly. If this happened, we could have a major disaster, leaving many men and camels lost or dead. Everyone knew the storm was closing in on us as the wind was steadily increasing in strength.

The men had their gutrahs down over their faces, not wanting to breathe in any of the sand dust and trying to keep the blowing sand out of their eyes. At this moment, I gave the signal to run. My men who were experienced knew how critical it was to keep the camels as close together as possible, to not run over the slower ones, and yet to keep them from spreading out too far so that we didn't lose any camels or riders on the fringes. The anxiety was high and we knew the fear was mounting in those who had not experienced this kind of a storm.

An ancient wadi was about 2½ kilometers ahead and had been covered with sand for probably hundreds of years. The north face of the dunes was very sharp and would create a natural barrier if we could make it. This would give the protection that could make a difference in our survival.

I rode hard to stay to the east flank of the caravan, while Jona rode on the west flank with hopes of keeping everyone between us. My concern was that if we reached the top of the plateau and dropped off the north face at a run, we would roll both camels and riders. There was a notch that opened wide enough into the wadi, enabling us to run at full speed. The challenge was for the men to time themselves so that everyone could go through without piling up on each other.

The scouts gave the signal to start narrowing the formation to enter the notch. Jona rode to the west, directing the riders into a funnel formation, and I rode toward the east. The men had been briefed on what to do in an emergency. But talk is one thing and the fear of the moment could bring about a different outcome. When fear takes over, all reasoning and logic is forgotten, and good men's lives are put in jeopardy while trying to save themselves.

As we approached the notch, my two scouts rode on the outer flanks so that the riders would have a marker by which to judge their direction. The ever-increasing wind decreased our visibility from 30 to 20 percent, at best, for a short distance. Ibram, one of the captains, went through the notch and swung to the left along the foot of the sand bluffs. Dismounting quickly, he and his men started pulling packs, driving stakes into the ground to tether the camels, and systematically stacking packs to make a barricade, knowing that the eye of the storm was no more than 20 minutes away.

Three young men on their first caravan who were part of Seth's pack train of 50 camels were about two-thirds of the way back from the front of the caravan. Enos, who appeared to be the leader of the three, feared that by slowing down the camels to feed into the notch, they would not make it before the storm overtook them. The roar was deafening and young Enos' anxiety caused him to panic, and he yelled, "Come on, it's just a sand dune. Let's ride before we are buried alive," and broke from the caravan with his lifelong friends, Nahor and Salah, following him.

Seth yelled at them to stop but got no response. Jona saw the faint movement through the dust heading toward the crest of the ridge. He rode to intercept them before they went over the top but was not close enough to intercept them, and it was impossible for them to hear his cries.

Screams pierced through the roar of the storm as Enos, Nahor, and Salah rode swiftly up the dune, realizing they could not beat the ferociousness of the storm. Disappearing over the top, their camels lost footing on the steep north face and went end-over-end to the bottom 300 meters below.

When Seth reached them, one camel had a broken leg, one camel was dead from a broken neck, and one appeared to survive without injury.

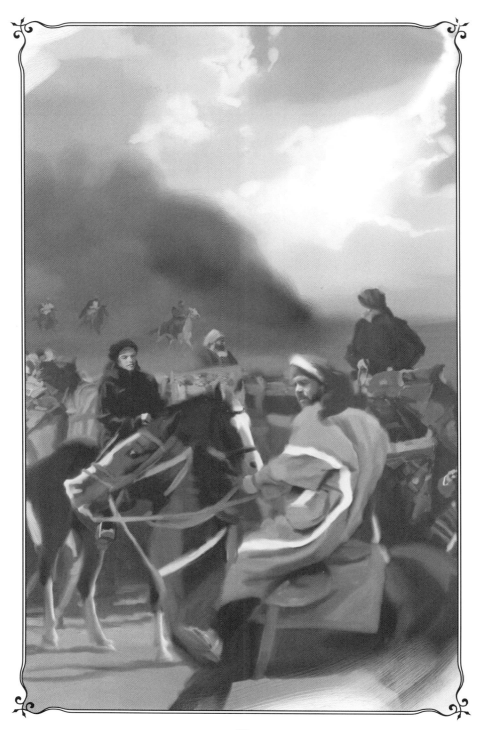

The pack saddles were all torn up, and the cargo was scattered in every direction down the bluff. Enos and Salah were found, but there was no sign of Nahor, and it was impossible to look for him during the storm. Seth yelled at them to grab the rope of the camel that was still alive and get over to the others to help unpack. When the camel and the packs were secured, he told them to get under their blankets before the storm completely engulfed them.

We managed to get all the camels through the notch and behind the sand bluff and were still pulling packs when the storm hit. The packs formed a circle on the inside, while the camels formed a circle as a barrier on the outside. The camels seemed instinctively to bury their heads underneath the packs and slow their breathing down to preserve what little air they had.

We dug in, covering ourselves as best we could with the pack rugs, blocking ourselves from the wind against the bodies of the camels. The bluffs broke the pounding force of the storm, dumping drifting sand on us a meter deep.

During the next three hours, the storm raged on, and we could periodically hear crying and whimpering. One man started screaming, "I'm gonna die!" until one of the other men hit him over the head with his sword handle, knocking him unconscious. I was always amazed to see who would break down first, and often it was the bigger and tougher-looking men.

One of my new men lying beside me asked, "Sir, how many storms have you been through?"

"Six, but only two others like this one, and it doesn't get any worse than this."

"Sir, have you seen men die in storms before?"

"Yes, and several who just disappeared."

"What do you mean?"

"Sometimes, men just panic and start running. Generally, they never get farther than just a few meters. Their lungs plug up with sand, they lose their eyesight, and they just go mad. Most of them we never find and never one alive! But this is not the time to talk. Get under your blanket and stay down until it's over."

We both became silent and not another word was spoken until the storm finished. The blowing sand was unrelenting and seemed to be piling heavier upon me, making it more difficult to breathe as the air under my rug diminished.

But finally, after what seemed like all day, the wind gradually dissipated as the storm passed. I shifted enough to move the sand so that I could stand up.

Not a single camel was visible — just mounds of sand that were starting to move. It was an eerie sight. Slowly their humps began shaking and popping up out of the sand. Then heads and long necks stretched for the blue sky, and within a short time it was completely clear as though there had never been a storm.

Jona and Seth had also come out from under the rugs and joined me to assess our condition, while the men started to unbury themselves and help each other. In some areas over ½ to 1 meter of sand was piled up around the camels, but around most of the men, no more than half a meter. When all of the camels and men were accounted for, we were relieved to see that all had survived, except for one slave whose heart had failed him because of the horrible fear he had of being buried alive.

When all of the pack saddles and bags were dug out and inventory was finished, I told the men to prepare camp for the night. We had only two hours of daylight left, and we had a camel with a broken leg that we had to put down, leaving us two camels to skin and butcher. We would make jerky out of the meat for traveling. The hides would make good sandals, pack rigging, and water bags for the next oasis. Enos and Salah were sent to search for the body of their friend, buried somewhere in the vastness of the sand.

Mohamed had the slaves start the cooking fires with some brush that they gathered on the edge of the bluffs and put the camel meat with some beans on to cook for the men. It was possible that these would be the last fires for the next three to four days because now there was almost no wood to find, only sand. By the time each man had taken a little meat and salted down the rest, only bones were left.

Enos avoided me and tried to busy himself, knowing that once the camp was in order and the camels and men had settled down, there would be a time of reckoning for him. When that time came, Seth, who was the captain over their caravan group, called the Council of Captains to determine the fate of these two young men.

Enos was asked to give an accounting for his actions — for disobeying direct orders. His voice was shaky and barely audible as he recounted how his fear overtook him, thinking that they would not make it to the wadi in time.

Salah explained that they were lifelong friends, and he was just following Enos and Nahor, as he always did. Enos had always had influence over his friends and had talked them into joining the caravan so that they could see the world. He had told enticing stories of his uncle, who had died on a caravan to Marib five years ago. Salah's voice broke, unable to continue. He looked down at the ground and never spoke a word after he had given his account of what happened.

The council felt that what Enos did was unforgivable and that he should be put to death by banishing him from the caravan without food or water. Salah was to receive 25 lashings with the camel whip. But the final decision was mine. In my wisdom I asked the council, "What would be accomplished by banishing him, since we are already shorthanded? His family would become very bitter towards all of us. If he had to live the rest of his life knowing that he caused Nahor's death and had to tell his family, they may want to put him to death, but it would not be on our heads. Maybe you should reconsider your decision before you make your final judgment."

Seth came to the fire a short time later and said that they had made their final decision. Enos was to receive 25 lashes with the camel whip and would walk the entire journey so that he could think about his mistake with every step he took. He would stand watch over the caravan every other night, and should he fail, he would be banished, receiving his original punishment. Salah would receive the same punishment.

A large Somalian slave was chosen to give the lashes. Enos was tied between two camels, and the whip cracked and tore at his flesh. He screamed and by the eighth lash had lost consciousness. When he was untied and laid on his rug, several men volunteered to care for him by boiling some cistus leaves and after allowing it to cool, pouring it over his back to stop the bleeding. They packed his wounds with cooked myrrh and camel fat and bound them with flax linen.

Salah took his lashes and never screamed or uttered a sound and stayed conscious to the final lash. Several men remarked how impressed they were, and although he had been the follower, in reality, he appeared to be the stronger. They cared for him in the same manner, easing the pain the best they could.

When the men bedded down for the night, I walked over to where Enos was lying on his stomach, carefully reached under his rug, and pulled his jambiyya out, keeping it safely from him. It was not uncommon for a man to take his own life when he became fully aware of the shame he had brought upon himself and his family.

Very early in the morning, the camp began to stir. The packs were being loaded and everyone was getting ready for an early start, wanting to make up for some of the time lost because of the storm. There was barely a hint of morning light before we were on the move again, and the two young men were struggling with pain but never said a word.

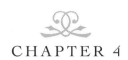

CHAPTER 4

Raiders in the Night

The day was difficult after such a dramatic event. Both men and animals were tired and still recovering from the exhaustion of the storm. We were glad to make our camp for the night, and soon a peaceful quietness blanketed the camp as sleep settled upon the weary caravaners.

I tried to sleep but the events of the day weighed heavily on my mind. I thought about my father and what he would have done. He always seemed to have the answer or at least a possible solution. I found myself reminiscing about many experiences I had had with my father that prepared me for the responsibility that I now carried. I loved the stillness of the night while I contemplated the movement of the caravan for the days ahead. At the moment all seemed calm, allowing me to drift into much needed sleep.

I don't know how long I had been asleep before I startled awake with a sharp gnawing in my gut. I wondered what that was all about as I lay quietly listening to the desert silence for any unusual sound. After a very long five minutes had passed, I hadn't detected anything out of the ordinary.

But this uneasy feeling that I had took me back several years when I was in the Al-Mawsaqah Mountains in the western Hadhramaut area with my father gathering myrrh. I had been awakened the same way from a deep sleep early in the morning with the same strange gnawing in my stomach. I remember pulling on my breeches, and without making a sound, I went out of the tent to settle my thoughts. My heart skipped a beat when I saw the silhouette of two Bedouins in the faint moonlight filling their bags with our food and other valuables they thought they could sell.

I quickly returned to the tent and with a whisper awakened my father. As I pulled my sword out from under my bedroll, my father came up out of his blanket like a puma springing for the kill. In an instant he arranged our bedrolls to look like we were still sleeping. Then we quietly slipped out of our tent. With swords in hand, we circled around the boulders behind our tent to intercept the robbers' escape.

We discovered that three men were holding our four camels, while two other men nervously gathered our possessions, not paying attention to anything else. Father eased in like a cat and handed me leather ropes to secure the front feet of the camels, after which he lay silently on the ground, waiting for our time of surprise. I drew back near the rocks where I could hide better and waited for instructions from my father. He was barely 3 meters away from the thieves, watching as their comrades raided our camp with great anticipation of the money they thought they would make in the marketplace.

The larger man of the three holding the camels seemed to be directing the raid as he gave an order to one he called Joab. "Go tell Momad and Laafi to bring what they've got, and let's get out of here. It will be daylight soon. Hand me the lead rope and go!" Father was still lying under one of the camels, quietly listening in the dark, as the big, gruff-looking man turned to the one standing near the camels and ordered, "Mulla, go check the tent and run your sword through the old man first. Then take the boy and we will sell him for a slave."

Mulla responded, "We agreed not to kill anyone, Abdul."

But Abdul was getting frustrated and said, "That was then; this is now. Do what I tell you." Mulla handed Abdul the two lead ropes and turned toward the tent, almost stepping on my father.

I knew in a split second what this meant, and I was the closest to the path to our tent. I knew from Father's position that he couldn't get there before Mulla discovered we weren't in the tent and would call out. Joab was crouched down over our fire telling the others that it was time to leave. Abdul was becoming uneasy and perhaps sensed something was going wrong.

Mulla was within 10 feet of me, and I knew Father could take on two or three men as he had in the past, but there were five. I had to make a choice fast. My stomach was churning with fear, and I thought I was going to vomit; yet I knew if I lost it, Father would be killed and I would never see my sister or brothers again.

I moved fast behind the rocks and thanked God for the soft sand

and dirt that allowed me to move without a sound. As I reached the tent and slipped inside, my heart was pounding so hard that I knew everyone could hear it. Every second counted as I anticipated what I had to do, knowing that if I froze, they would know we were not in the tent, and Father was under their feet. Even if he managed to kill Abdul, there were four others, and the Bedouins were fierce swordsmen.

The tent flap opened slowly as Mulla surveyed from the entrance, trying to determine in which bedroll Father was sleeping. Then making his move, he ran his sword through the one he had determined was Father's.

I was standing against the tent wall, and in the dark it looked like we were both still in our beds, as Father had planned. Mulla ran the sword a second time through Father's bedroll before he realized there wasn't anyone in it. He quickly reached down and pulled the blankets back and then recoiled with surprise. Mulla reached for my bedroll and threw back the blankets only to discover that it was also empty.

I could feel the panic race through him as he turned to run out of the tent and found himself slightly bent forward facing me directly. I drove my sword forward with all the force I had. It happened so fast that I could hardly believe what I had done as my victim staggered while trying to fight back. I was shaking hard with fear, my head was pounding, and I felt like my stomach was in my throat. Mulla let out a gasp of surprise and pain as he tried to swing his sword at me, but it caught the tent flap as he stumbled and collapsed outside.

At the same time Joab and the other two men reached Abdul and started to lead the camels away. But the camels came to an abrupt stop as the tethered ropes held them back. Abdul, realizing what had happened, called out to Mulla, "They are not in the tent. Come on; let's go! Run for the rocks and keep moving. They can't follow all of us," and swung his sword to cut the ropes.

Father ran him through and turned just in time to block the path of Joab and the other two thieves. They dropped their sacks of pillage, and in that second they realized that Mulla never answered Abdul nor returned when called. Although Abdul lay dead on the ground, the other three knew they had the advantage, and the four camels, food, myrrh, and camp goods would fetch a good price.

I was on my knees next to Mulla, vomiting and overwhelmed with the thought that I was just 16 years old and had killed a man for the first time. As I pulled my sword out of Mulla's limp body, I became conscious of men's voices and realized that my father was facing four men alone. I could not stay here on my knees. I had to face what was happening now and be a man. My father was at risk, and that thought pushed me beyond my fear.

I ran around the rocks, trying to make out the shadowy figures to determine which one was my father. I could see only four men, and three were moving in a circle around the fourth one. My father had taught me well the skill of the sword, but I had never been in combat, which was an overwhelming feeling.

In a split second I heard in my mind my father's voice speaking clearly, "Remember, Son, your enemy doesn't know what you don't know. Always act as though you are in charge and all knowing. Conduct yourself as a man until you are one, and the one you see yourself becoming."

"Yes, I always wanted to be the best swordsman," I said to myself. So with great determination and courage, I eased around the boulder to the right of my father as Joab was circling to position Father between the three of them.

When Joab came around the rock, our eyes met and he was taken completely by surprise. He swung in defense from his awkward stance, but I easily ducked, coming up with my sword, cutting him across the chest, and catching his chin while slicing up to the corner of his mouth to his nose and then to his right eye. He screamed and ran toward the other two men, who rushed my father, only to meet their fate.

Joab was still alive but bleeding badly. We carried him to our fire, and I started to retrieve our belongings while father tended to Joab's wounds. He put on a pot of water to boil some myrrh resin and then gathered some leaves of the terebinth tree to put into another pot of water on the fire.

He washed the wounds and then packed them with the oily gum of myrrh and balsam. It must have stung because Joab was biting on a stick that Father had put between his teeth to keep him from screaming, especially when Father started to pack the eye socket where the eyeball had been ruptured by the tip of my sword. Joab asked Father to end his life because he did not want to be disgraced, having lost his eye in battle to a mere boy.

I will never forget my father's reply when he said, "You didn't lose your eye to a boy. You lost your eye to a man—a swordsman—one of the best in all of Arabia, but you survived. That should be an honor to your family." Father gave this man a reason to live. Even though he was still a thief, he could go back and brag as a hero among his people, who wouldn't know the truth. With a larger mouth to brag, less of a nose to entice a woman, and only one eye to see, he could still have a life.

As we gathered our belongings and loaded the camels, Joab asked if we were going to leave him to the wild animals. Father replied, "You came to steal and kill, and you think you have a right to question me after I have saved your life? I could have just run you through."

Joab went silent as Father's words rang true. Then Father said, "I came here 40 years ago with my father to harvest myrrh. My mother's people are from Shabwah and never had a problem before. I spared your life in hopes that you will teach your sons to be better and more honest than you."

I can still remember my father's words to Joab as we were getting ready to leave him in the mountains. "My son, Shutran, will leave you enough water and food until someone finds you or you walk out on your own. The stench of your rotting comrades beside you should imprint upon your mind that stealing brings no blessing from God. Consider that He has smiled upon you this day for a reason that you must yet discover."

As we climbed upon our camels to leave the mountains, I broke out in a cold sweat and started shaking. I had just killed a man. How do I understand my feelings? How do I deal with it, and where do I go from here?

Father knew what I was feeling but rode in silence for a short time, allowing me to think and to try to understand those feelings. He knew that this was a life-changing experience for me. Finally, he broke the silence, "Shutran, all things happen for a reason. When you are faced with something difficult, know that there is a deeper purpose and start to look for the gift it brings. This will keep you from getting discouraged."

Father stopped, turned his camel around, and looking me in the eye said, "I know this experience was not what you wanted, Son. I want you to know that I am proud of you. You fought as a man and saved our lives. Every day will bring new challenges, and sometimes the solutions are not pleasant. Keep your heart close to God and pray always that He will give you strength and deliver you from the hand of evil." Father turned his camel back around, and we continued down the trail. His words brought comfort and gave me strength.

The light breeze rattling the tent snapped me back to reality. It seemed so long ago since I had been with my father gathering myrrh in the mountains. Yet the memory of that night when we were attacked and I had to kill a man for the first time seemed like yesterday. I missed those days with my father when we were alone in the mountains.

I thought about my son Kaleb, who was at home with Mirah. He was pressing me to take him with me on the next caravan. I felt a knot in my stomach, knowing that if I took him with me, he, too, could have a similar experience. Would he be strong and have the endurance and faith that life with the caravan demanded?

Kaleb seemed so young, and yet I was only five years old when I went with my father to harvest myrrh. It was seven years later when Father took me with him on my first caravan to Fort Sumhuram. What I learned in those early days of my youth set the foundation for what I have created today.

My thoughts wandered back to the sandstorm and the loss of Nahor. He wasn't much older than Kaleb, but because of his fear and lack of discipline in following orders, his life was now over. I felt so much pain for his family. He made his own choices, but it was still on my caravan.

My men had done well, except for Enos and Salah, whose lives would forever be marred by the loss of their friend. I wondered what my father would have done. Would he have let them live? He was a very powerful man who always tried to find something positive that could be learned from a bad or difficult situation. Surely two young men would have learned nothing if I had agreed with the council.

I continued to marvel at my father's wisdom as I grew in experience and understanding. He taught me a lot that helped me daily. The responsibility as the Commander demanded great discernment and calculated planning. My thoughts often went back to my father when I had to make difficult decisions. His words would come into my mind, and I seemed to know exactly what to do. It gave me great strength and determination to lead those who looked to me for their safety and protection.

We had made good distance that day in spite of the damaging effects of the storm. I felt peaceful as my thoughts wandered to my family.

I don't know how long I had been with them in a dreamy state, almost fading into sleep, with the moonlight illuminating the edges of the tent, when a strange feeling brought me more awake and took my thoughts outside the tent to the caravan. It wasn't a sound, but a feeling—perhaps a warning. I quickly grabbed my sword and whip, eased out of the tent, and quietly went through the camp, searching for anything unusual or missing. I checked the bedrolls as I passed and was not surprised to find one empty.

I went to the picket line where the camels were hitched. My father had taught me to never hitch more than 20 camels together per line because it was easier to count by 20's. My mind could identify 1 or 2 camels missing out of 20 but not 1 or 2 out of 50, 70, or 100 without taking time to count each one. As I walked past the picket line, I could see where one camel was missing. I ran up the sand dune behind the camels just in time to see someone in the moonlight disappear over another dune to the west about a fourth of a kilometer away.

We were headed northeast to Fort Yabrin. Although there were stories of an oasis to the west, it was still a two-day journey out of our way. Why would a man get up in the middle of the night, steal a camel, and travel in the opposite direction? It certainly wasn't because he had had a bad dream. This man definitely didn't have good intentions.

We were only four days from Fort Yabrin and one day to the next water hole for the camels. There was only one reason for this man's actions, and it could only mean one thing. We were carrying several tons of myrrh and frankincense resin; 450 kilos of pearls and 550 kilos of diamonds from Somaliland; and honey, dates, and bananas from Salalah. In addition, my sister and several of the women from the village had spent one year weaving beautiful rugs and blankets from camel and goat hair, which were highly prized in the markets.

Yes, we were heavily laden with expensive treasures and gifts that were destined for Gerrha and eventually on to be traded in Nineveh for cotton, embroidery work, brass, gold, ebony, sapphires, and rubies coming from China over the Silk Road. The entire livelihood of over 200 families depended on this caravan. Every man knew what we were carrying and knew the number of men who were guarding our payload. This information would be worth a lot to the right person and a band of desert pirates.

The camels were tired and the men were fatigued and anxious to reach Fort Yabrin, where they could rest before the final leg of the journey to Gerrha.

I started walking back and tried to calculate all the possibilities, knowing that the man who left had been planning this from the time we left Fort Sumhuram. It had to be someone who had traveled this route before and knew the distances between places and how many men and weapons it would take to overpower the caravan. As I reached the camp, I started to awaken the men. We had 300 camels to pack and 220 men to feed. The early morning was cold, about 18 degrees, as the men began moving about.

I called my six captains together and told them what had just happened. Jona said that one of his men was missing, a man by the name of Sabah. He went on to say how this man acted differently on this trip than on the other caravans. Jona also said that Sabah had always been the lively one around the campfire telling stories and talking about what he would do if he had a lot of money.

However, on this trip Sabah avoided the men, was very quiet, seemed withdrawn and preoccupied with himself, and wouldn't engage in conversation. We all assumed he had had a fight with his wife again, which was what usually happened, because he was always in the tavern laughing and having a good time with other women.

Mahedy, one of Jona's men who had made the journey several times, said that he had seen Sabah talking to some strangers down by the docks a few weeks ago who he had not seen in Fort Sumhuram before. When Mahedy asked Sabah who they were, he said that he had met them at a card game a few nights earlier.

The captains spread the word that we would move out in 45 minutes. There would be no fires, just camel jerky and water. The captains were to tell no one else what had happened, just in case we had another informant. Everyone was to act as though we hadn't noticed anyone missing.

We had to get to the next stop before the thieves did, water the camels, and move out before they arrived. Their plan would be to intercept us at the oasis, since we would be resting and unsuspecting. "Just make sure your swords and jambiyyas are out of sight but ready," I told them. "Watch your men to see if anyone acts differently and report." As we moved out, the men grumbled as usual about not having their hot tea and breakfast.

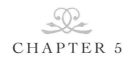

CHAPTER 5

Desert Pirates

We pushed the men hard and drove the camels as fast as possible, arriving at the oasis four hours ahead of schedule. I called all my captains together and explained our situation. We would probably be facing raiders in a few hours, so our plan had to be very clear to everyone. My captains understood what we had to do and spread the word to all the men so that they could be prepared. Jona was going to ride back to the west to watch for dust and to see if there were signs of anything unusual.

As soon as every camel and man had taken on sufficient water, we were moving on. In just two hours, pack saddles were retightened and packs secured, and we moved the caravan out toward Fort Yabrin. One hour later Jona caught up and reported that a large raiding party of probably 200 or more was closing in fast. They were about two hours behind us.

I sent Jona ahead to find places to off-load the myrrh, frankincense, pearls, diamonds, blankets, rugs, and other merchandise of value. We would bury them and act as though we were a food supply caravan going to Fort Yabrin and continuing on to Gerrha to pick up other merchandise with which we would return. In the worst case, if the odds were against us, we would be ready for a fight.

Jona returned shortly, reporting that he had found good locations to off-load. We sent each captain in a different direction to bury our cargo in different locations so that no captain's group would know the location of another's cargo.

We rearranged the food so that each camel was carrying no more than

40 kilos. Then as the raiders approached, we split, dividing the caravan into two groups just far enough apart that the raiders would ride up the middle, leaving us on each side of them.

The raiding party was closing in fast. They were so confident in the success of their attack that they never stopped for water. They thought they could close the distance, overtake and capture the caravan, and return to the oasis before the day's end.

Jona volunteered to be the decoy by pretending to hold back 15 camels that were either lame or sick. When the raiders approached, Jona and his men acted helpless and told them they were part of a food caravan headed to Fort Yabrin. The raiders dismounted their camels and searched the packs and to their dismay found nothing of importance. They were mad and when their leader, Abrassa, determined that the merchandise they wanted was with the main caravan, they headed out in pursuit, leaving Jona and his small caravan alone for the moment.

As soon as the raiders were over the crest of the hill, Jona and his men mounted their camels and rode fast, intending to catch the raiders by the time they reached the main caravan. Jona's camels were refreshed with water and lightly loaded, so they were able to move much faster. Because Abrassa didn't stop for water, he had put his raiders and their camels at a great disadvantage.

My men knew that this had to be close combat for survival. Once the raiders didn't find what they were after, they would kill each man until someone told them where we had hidden our cargo. Then they would kill every last man. This was kill or be killed. My captains had spread the word that every man was to tie his sword on the camel under the pack blanket, where he could pull it out instantly. Each man knew the plan and was ready to move quickly.

Abrassa and his men advanced swiftly, overtaking our "food" caravan. The raiders rode up the middle as we hoped with their swords raised to fight. Abrassa rode up next to me at the head of the caravan waving his sword in the air, demanding that I halt. Acting defenseless, I raised my arm to stop the caravan and gave the order to my captains to cooperate and spread the word. With that, Abrassa became less aggressive, thinking the caravan was his, and told the raiders to put their swords away.

I told Abrassa that we were just a food supply caravan going to Fort Yabrin and then to Gerrha to pick up merchandise for the return. He became furious to think that he had been made a fool of in front of his

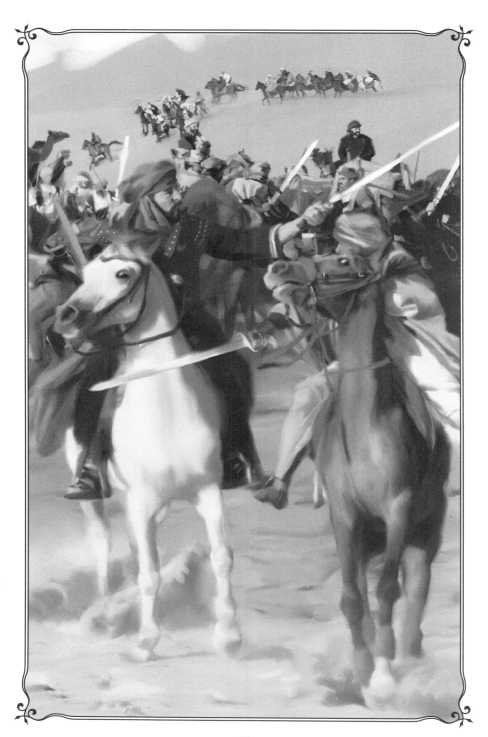

men. He immediately ordered them to search every pack. My men were spread apart as far as they could be without looking suspicious. It was just as I had planned. As each raider searched one camel, he was far enough away from the next one so that he would hopefully not notice what was happening to any of his comrades. I was sure a lot of dead raiders were going to fall to the ground almost at the same time.

I sat confident on my stallion, ready for battle. My men were intensely alert and ready for the kill at the right moment. As the raiders began searching the packs on one side and then on the other, my men showed no resistance and just asked simple questions, causing the raiders to drop their guard. As each thief turned to respond, he gasped as the sharp metal of a jambiyya was thrust into his gut just above the belt, and with a quick, upward pull, he was split open from navel to heart. As the thief staggered and collapsed to the ground, my man drew his sword, ready for the finish.

I continued my conversation with Abrassa to keep his attention focused away from the caravan. The attack was subtle and quiet as Abrassa's men collapsed in near silence until one of my men, out of fear, hesitated and didn't act fast enough, and the raider saw the intent and yelled, "Ambush!" But by this time over half of Abrassa's men lay dead on the ground. Shiric, the man who hesitated, also lay dead. At that moment it became man-to-man combat with sword and jambiyya. But now we outnumbered the raiders almost two to one.

Looking straight at Abrassa, I could see beyond him as Jona came over the dunes in a fury as the lightly packed camels closed the distance. Riding hard with swords drawn, they attacked the small number of Abrassa's men who were still mounted. I held my sword down to my left side out of Abrassa's sight, just waiting for him to make his move. Hearing the yelling and the commotion, Abrassa turned toward the caravan and saw Jona and his small group joining in the attack. At that moment Abrassa realized that he and his raiders were the ones who had been ambushed. He turned in a rage and pulled his sword on me.

Not expecting left-handed combat, he raised his arm to swing the death blow, leaving himself wide open. I recoiled backwards and with my left hand I crossed over, slicing his right upper arm to the bone, rendering it useless as it dropped to his side. He quickly grabbed his sword with his other hand and awkwardly charged again as our swords clashed overhead.

With the blood gushing down his arm, he weakened quickly, and only sheer adrenaline kept him fighting. We battled a few minutes longer, steel-to-steel, until my sword found its mark and pierced his heart. The battle was over almost as fast as it started. Abrassa and over 178 of his men lay dead, and another 53 were wounded.

When Jona and I finished counting our men, we had 3 dead and 14 wounded, and, unfortunately, we also had four dead camels that had been caught in the path of a swinging sword. Three of Abrassa's men escaped, but I figured there would be a time of reckoning with them later. In the taverns, they always talked too much and usually gave themselves away, but right now my men were more important. We gathered up our wounded and all of Abrassa's camels and returned to the oasis that evening, leaving the wounded raiders to care for each other. We left them water and food but took all of their weapons, camels, and provisions.

It was 20 kilometers back to the oasis, and by morning 24 of the 53 wounded walked into camp. Their chance of living was greater if they reached the oasis than waiting in the desert for the next caravan to come weeks or months later. Those who made it into camp were castrated and made into slaves. This way they would bring a better price in Gerrha because the new owner wouldn't have to worry about the slave lying with one of the concubines and getting her pregnant, which just brought more unwanted problems.

We stayed four days in the oasis, nursing our wounded and resting the men and camels. We retrieved our buried goods from their hiding places in the sand and reorganized the packs and camels. With 231 new camels and 24 more men who were now slaves to handle the additional camels, including packs and gear, the journey became even more challenging.

As the men healed from their wounds, their stories around the campfire grew bigger and bigger, creating a tremendous feeling of confidence about their success in battle. For many it was their first hand-to-hand combat. As I listened to them, I would have thought I was listening to seasoned fighters. Needless to say, they had reason enough to brag and spin their tales.

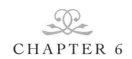

CHAPTER 6

My Cousin, The Thief

Three days later we reached Fort Yabrin and off-loaded one-third of our cargo. We met a small caravan that had come from Gerrha with 55 camels and 70 men. After they delivered some of their merchandise to Fort Yabrin, they were going on to Makka with spices and brass that they were carrying from India and the Persian Gulf. The men wanted to hear the stories of the great desert battle, and my men were only too happy to retell their stories, and, of course, encouraged by a little wine, their stories were even more colorful.

Not too many weeks passed before the news had spread from coast to coast of the great frankincense caravan raid that resulted in 207 pirates killed and 24 taken as slaves. Little did I know that the news had traveled to Marib, and even the Queen of Sheba had heard of our successful crossing of the Rub al Khali.

In the evening as we sat around the campfire, the slaves told stories about their homeland and how they became involved with Abrassa. One of them, who appeared to be near my age, said that he was from Shabwah. Jona came to my tent and said, "Shutran, you might want to hear this story. It could be of interest to you in your decision making when we reach Gerrha."

I walked over to where the men were sitting around the fire and talking. Without interrupting, I listened as this young man from Shabwah, whose name was Eeslum, told about his family.

My curiosity was piqued when he said his father's name was Joab. His mother's name is Sarah and she is still living. Then he said he had an aunt whose name was Armin, but she died many years ago. Armin had married some Bedouin from the mountains in the eastern territory near the Hadhramaut. Joab, Eeslum's father, never seemed to be able to find his place in life and couldn't make any money working the land, so he joined with some thieves led by a man named Abdul.

Abdul was a big man for a Bedouin. He measured 1¾ meters tall and weighed well over 100 kilos. He was mean and aggressive and always seemed to have whatever he wanted—money, women, camels, horses, etc. Abdul impressed Eeslum's father so much that Joab wanted to be just like him, not knowing that Abdul was nothing more than a bully and common thief. But by the time Joab found out, it was too late. Abdul told Joab that if he ever betrayed him, he would kill him, and because Joab was weak, he just went along with him.

The young man told how his family started to live well for the first time. They moved into a mud brick home, had nice things, and didn't have to live in a dirty shack built of sticks and mud any more. "My mother and sisters had nice hijab head scarves and dressed in beautiful abayas from the marketplace," Eeslum said.

"People respected my father for the first time because he had money, but we never knew where he worked. He would leave for two to three weeks at a time and always return with money and nice things for all of us. Then one day, when I was 17, Father didn't return home when he said he would.

"Two weeks later a Bedouin family brought him home all carved up with one eye missing. He said he and his partners were going over Mablaqah Pass to Bayhan to sell myrrh when a band of ten thieves attacked them. He was the only survivor and was left for dead when this family from the mountains found him and took care of him, or he would have died."

Eeslum went on to tell how his father became a tiller of the fields and worked the land like his brothers, but he always wanted money and finer things in life. His father died poor but Eeslum was determined he wasn't going to die the same way. Joining Abrassa's band of raiders was the first chance that came along for Eeslum to fulfill his dream for riches. With Abrassa he was able to provide better for his mother and sisters, while his brother and other family members worked the land, just surviving.

Eeslum had come to believe that if you wanted to get ahead in life, you had to take from whoever had it. As we listened, Jona turned to me inquiring, "Wasn't your mother's name Armin?"

I responded, "Yes, Jona, and my mother's sister, Sarah, lives in Shabwah. This man is my kin, and I just castrated him."

Jona questioned, "What are you going to do? Shutran, he is your family."

I quivered as I responded, "He may be family by birth, but he is not family by action, and I shall deal with him accordingly. It is good to know that his father did try to do what was right in his last years, but Eeslum does not need to know anything else."

I wasn't going to say anything but kept having the feeling that I needed to talk to him. I watched him as he kept talking for a minute, trying to see if I could recognize anything that might show me we were of the same family. "Yes!" His face had a familiar look, but that caused a feeling of anger to come up inside me.

As I walked toward him, I called out, "Eeslum, I need to set the record straight with you. I want you to know that I am the man who carved your father's face. I was gathering myrrh with my father when Joab, your father, and his comrades, Abdul, Mulla, Laafi, and Momad, tried to rob us.

"My father treated your father's wounds and saved his life and hoped that your father would change his destiny and raise his sons to be honest. Your mother's sister, Armin, was my mother, and you are my kin. Now you will go to your grave knowing that you will not pass your thieving genes on to any offspring. Your life could have been different if you had not chosen the dark way." With a pain in my heart, I turned and walked away before he could respond. He was my blood, but I would not take responsibility for his choices nor feel guilty, either.

Morning came quickly and the commotion of preparation could be heard from all directions of the camp. The sun was rising and we would soon feel the heat of the trail. When the caravan was ready, I gave the signal to move out as usual, but there was a different feeling in the air. We were 20 days northeast of Fort Yabrin and just four days out of Gerrha when the wind current shifted. The camels started to act up and seemed a bit unsettled.

I rode along with the caravan, watching for signs and trying to determine the problem so that I could be ready for anything that might happen. Jona, Seth, and Ibram were trying to assess the situation as well, as they could see the changes in the camels. We were out of the desert, and a storm wasn't likely, since the temperatures hadn't changed and the sky seemed peaceful.

"There is only one other thing to consider," I said.

"What's that?" Ibram questioned.

"Water! They can smell it a day away."

"You're right, Shutran," Seth answered, "but we are at best three days from water."

"That's true," I replied. "This doesn't make sense. Something has them stirred. Ride back and tell the men to have their swords ready and be alert. Have every man fill his bag with fresh water and mount his camel. No one is to be on the ground walking."

"And Enos and Salah?" Seth asked.

"Except them," I answered.

About 5 kilometers later, the camels seemed to settle down and ignore whatever it was that was bothering them. I rode ahead and stopped on top of a ridge running parallel to the caravan where I could see into the far distance all around me. I sat quietly watching the behavior of the camels, trying to figure out why they were nervous and why they had now calmed down just a few kilometers later. Jona rode up to where I was watching, and together we quietly surveyed the vastness in front of us, wondering about the strangeness of the situation.

"Shutran, what do you make of it? It is as though whatever it was that disturbed them has gone away," Jona surmised.

"You're right. The wind has already shifted and is blowing to the north rather than to the west as it was a few hours ago. But I still think that there is trouble ahead. You keep the caravan moving steadily but slow them down and conserve their energy. I am going to ride ahead with the scouts to see if I can discover anything."

Jona returned to the caravan to keep them moving in the same easterly direction. Due to the shallow canyon, the camels had to travel two and three abreast, stretching over 4 kilometers, which would certainly put us at a disadvantage if we were attacked.

My scouts, Musilum and Hussin, were riding points north and south about a kilometer ahead of the caravan. As I reached Musilum, I waved Hussin over to us so that we could talk together. I decided to leave Musilum in charge and took Hussin with me, since he was the better swordsman of the two, if the need should arise, and rode on ahead to our next stop for the night. As we crossed over a small range of foothills and dropped down into the valley below, a feeling of anxiety began building inside me.

Hussin was 100 meters to the south of me. From his posture I could see that he was not as relaxed as before, and his countenance was that of a warrior ready to fight. "He's sensing something's wrong," I thought to myself. Just then the breeze shifted, and for a brief moment, the smell of death came from the east.

Hussin waved and started riding towards me. "Captain," he yelled,

"Did you smell it?"

"Yes, I did before the wind changed."

We picked up our pace as we reached the top of a small hill 10 kilometers farther east. It was then that we could see desert vultures circling overhead. We swung south, turning down off the butte into the valley, and were shocked to see the remains of a small caravan that had been attacked.

As we rode through the carnage, it appeared that all the caravaners and camels were dead. It looked like this was an Ishmaelite caravan coming from Selah headed to Gerrha. We counted 57 men and 8 camels dead. I dismounted and told Hussin to circle the valley to see if he could find any clues that might help us discover the rest of the story.

It didn't make sense that an eastbound Ishmaelite caravan would be attacked, since all they would have been transporting was merchandise like wheat, honey, olive oil, wine, embroidery work, and perhaps blue and purple dyes from Israel, Syria, and Egypt. The things that were left would not have been worth killing for like this. It was very strange and right then I didn't have an explanation.

As I checked some of the wounds, it seemed obvious that the raiders expected something else to be in the caravan. It appeared that most of the men were not killed in battle. We could see evidence that many had been wounded and wanted to surrender or tried to escape but were then brutally murdered. It was one thing to rob a caravan, but to kill wounded caravaners was a horrible act of violence.

As I looked at the situation, I realized that it could only mean one thing—and that was that this was not the caravan they were expecting. The caravan they were looking for was ahead or behind, but one way or another, they were going to find it. The raiders did not want any survivors to later tell what had happened, which explained the brutal death of all these men. It became clear to me that surely they would be looking and waiting for the caravan that they thought they had attacked—and we were likely that caravan.

How would a band of raiders this far north and east know about our caravan and the time we would be coming through? Whoever was leading this raid was very calculating. I stood over one of the camel packs, poking through it with my sword and looking at the contents. There were bags of wheat, embroidered linens from Egypt, some cassia from the Hadhramaut, honeycomb from Israel, and dried meat for the food supply. Obviously, the raiders weren't concerned about food.

There was something strange about this pack load in front of me. It didn't appear as though there was anything of importance to the raiders, and yet something seemed wrong. When I opened the packs, I could see that the merchandise in two of them would not have weighed more than 40 kilos, and this camel could carry at least 220. This didn't make sense.

I started to pull the rugs and pack saddles apart, which had been piled together to create a barrier for defense, and uncovered two more bodies. I kept probing and felt what seemed to be a rug about three inches deep in the sand. I started to pull it back over something that seemed hidden and to my surprise found a man barely alive. He had lost a lot of blood from a chest wound. Apparently, the other men had covered him up during the battle and given him the water bags, hoping he would survive as they met their deaths.

I called Hussin over to help me dig him out. "I don't believe he is still alive," Hussin expressed in a surprised voice.

"Yes, he is, but he won't be for long if he doesn't get some help. We must keep him alive," I said. "He is the only one who can tell us what happened and, more importantly, tell us who the raiders were."

"You're right, Shutran, but this man hasn't had any water or food for probably two or three days."

"I know, but the lack of food slowed down his body, and that's why he's still alive." The man was too weak to drink, so we started very slowly just putting a few drops of water in his mouth at a time. I said to Hussin, "Keep digging through the other packs to see what else you can find. Bring me some honey to put in the water as it will help him."

Three hours later Jona pulled in with the caravan. He came over immediately so we could discuss what to do. "Jona, it will be dark in just a few minutes, so have the men start setting up camp and then come with the others, so we can talk." I cleaned and dressed the man's wounds and for over two hours continued to drip water and honey in his mouth. This man was probably in his mid-thirties. He appeared strong in stature and seemed to have a good constitution, and I needed him alive.

After the men were fed and the animals bedded down, Jona, Seth, Ibram, and my other captains came over to discuss our situation. Jona asked, "Shutran, when was the last time you had any food?"

"This morning," I answered. Jona called to Salah to bring some jerky and soup. Then Jona's thoughts returned to our wounded caravaner, and he asked, "Shutran, do you think you can revive him?"

"Jona, I've got to keep him alive."

"Well, if anyone can, it will be you," Ibram declared. "But I don't think he'll live. He looks dead already."

Jona spoke up, "As long as the Captain is taking care of him, he will surely live. You'll see."

I continued, "Listen, men, this has been a rugged trip, and we have just three more days to go. I have a feeling that we will still see another battle. Tomorrow we reach the last water stop before Gerrha. If Hussin and I hadn't ridden to scout the area, we would have missed this place by 2 kilometers. I would have kept the caravan farther north, since it is a little easier to travel. This obviously was the first trip for this caravan, as they didn't pick the best way. The raiders were following them and anticipated that they would be coming through on the old trail.

"Spread the word. We are going to load and move out at full moon. We'll swing to the south of the water by two days, which will put us at a great disadvantage. The country is rougher and slower to travel, and there is no water. This will delay our arrival into Gerrha two to four days more."

Alimud interrupted, "Sir, the men are tired and anxious to get to Gerrha. Adding two more days and no water is something I don't think the men will accept. Some might split from the caravan and continue on our route to Gerrha. Some will follow you, but not all of them."

Jona spoke before I could respond, "Alimud, you have been a good captain, but I have to ask you, how many trips have you made with Captain Shutran?"

Alimud replied, "This trip makes four."

"And how many have you made on your own or with someone else?"

"Jona, you know, none," he retorted.

"Alimud, you are alive because of Captain Shutran. Every trip you have made has been successful because of his decisions. Now, after four good trips, you are questioning the Captain and think you know more. You would still be herding goats in the mountains if the Captain hadn't taken you with him and taught you what you know. If it were my decision, I would say, 'Go,' and I would guarantee that you wouldn't live to see home again."

"Jona, that's enough. I said it was okay to let him express his feelings." Alimud turned and walked back to his men as Jona and I continued our discussion.

"Shutran, he watches you and you make it look easy, so he thinks he can do the same thing and better."

"Jona, you're right. You watch and when the next monsoon season is over, he will have talked people into backing him to start his own caravan.

He will undercut the prices and promise a shorter delivery time. Jona, there isn't the loyalty and respect like in the days of our fathers."

"Shutran, how old were you when you went with your father on your first caravan?"

"I was 12 years of age when I left with my father, and it broke my mother's heart. Now, with the experience of over 40 caravans behind me, I have to listen to this young know-it-all, who one day soon will cost good men their lives. Jona, I didn't expect to have this problem. He's like so many. He thinks he has the right to make these kinds of decisions without the years of experience in the desert. I was 13 when my father found the route from Wubar to what is now Fort Yabrin. I was very afraid but my father never knew it. That was the first time I saw my father kill one of his own men who went mad during a sandstorm. Those were hard times."

"Shutran," Jona surmised, "If Alimud starts to stir up the men, I won't tolerate it. I'll lower his lip with my jambiyya."

"Jona, you are a good man and a good friend. My grandfather once said, 'You can brag about your camels, you can be proud of your women and children, but you can count your blessings for every true friend you have.' I count my blessings, Jona, knowing that you are a true friend. We had better get some sleep, since we'll be moving out in four hours."

"What about the wounded caravaner?"

"I thought I would have Salah and Enos stay behind with two camels and watch him until he recovers enough to follow the original trail. They would catch up to us in Gerrha. What do you think?"

"Yes, that would work," Jona replied.

Three hours later the men were out of bed and packing, and the slaves were making a good breakfast of camel milk, meat, and beans. It could be two days before we would eat again. I walked over to check on Enos and Salah where they were taking care of the Ishmaelite. To my surprise, he was conscious and speaking.

His name was Micah and was from the land of Gilead just north of Selah. This was his first caravan, and he and the others were excited to be going to a big trade city to see the ocean and experience all the excitement they knew they would find there. He asked about the other members of his caravan. When I told him that he was the only survivor, he broke down and cried. He looked at me painfully and whispered, "My brother and three cousins?"

"No one else survived. No one! Someone covered you up after you were wounded."

"That was probably my older brother. He was beside me when the attack came."

"Tell us what you can," I asked.

"We were just making camp before dark when they rode in fast without warning."

"Do you know who they were and from where they came?"

"No," Micah replied. "I could hear someone yelling, 'Find the luban, the luban. It has to be here. Maybe they buried it.' That is all I heard, but I do remember that they tied their gutrahs differently."

"Micah, do you feel you can ride?" I asked.

"Yes, Sir, I can!"

"Enos, Salah, find a camel that is lightly packed so that Micah can ride. Let's get ready and move out." I called Musilum and Hussin over to make plans. "I want you scouts to ride north and intercept the raiders' trail and follow it until you are confident you know the direction in which they are traveling and then ride back."

Alimud's group came over and asked if they could talk. I said, "Yes," and asked what was on their minds.

"Well, Sir, we don't feel it is necessary to swing south by two days and bypass the water, delaying us another four days from reaching Gerrha. If we miss the trade ships, we will have to stay in Gerrha much longer to wait for other ships."

I listened as they each expressed their opinion. Then I asked, "Are you not concerned about the raiders?"

"No, Sir, they got what they wanted and left."

"Not according to Micah, the only survivor."

Alimud responded, "They are probably already in Gerrha."

"That is a possibility," I replied. "But what if they are not, and they realized that they robbed the wrong caravan and decided to wait for us at the next watering stop?"

"Well, Sir, we defeated Abrassa's raiders, and we can do it again."

"That's also a possibility," I said, "but are you willing to take that chance?"

Alimud argued, "We have 23 more men than last time who can fight."

"Yes, you're right about that, too," I answered. "But what makes you think they will fight to defend you or any of us? A thief is a thief and he will look out for himself and his own interests, and if the opportunity arises to put a jambiyya in your ribs standing beside you in battle, he'll do it. All right, I've heard you out, so fall back in your place, and let's move out."

"But, Sir, we are going to take the original trail," Alimud retorted defiantly. I spun on my heel, striking him squarely on the side of his jaw with my fist gripped around my jambiyya. Two of Alimud's teeth broke as he hit the ground.

I growled as I stood directly over him, "You joined this caravan and committed to see it through to Gerrha under my command. When we get to Gerrha, you are free to do what you want. But neither you nor anyone in your command is going to jeopardize the other 220 men and this caravan. If you want to follow the old trail, then you do it on foot with no food and no water, and so help me, if I ever see you again, I'll run you through. And if I hear one word of contention before we reach Gerrha, you will feel the wrath of my sword. Now follow orders and get those camels moving."

I followed Alimud to where he was packing his camel. Then I called out loudly so that most of the men could hear me. "Alimud, you are finished and removed from your responsibilities. Jona, appoint another captain over Alimud's command." As I finished speaking, Alimud started to protest again. Jona, Seth, and Ibram were now at my side.

Jona drew his sword so fast that Alimud never even saw it but felt the sharp tip like a needle against his throat as a small trickle of blood started to drip down his neck. Jona spoke with a very deep, cold tone of voice, "Alimud, if you had done this ten years ago with the Captain, you would be lying in the sand dead. I suggest that you listen and live." Alimud retreated with his comrades and went back to his camp. Jona slowly turned and faced me, "His blood has gone bad, so watch your back."

We moved out, traveling south by southeast. The countryside was becoming steeper and more rugged, slowing the caravan down considerably. On the third day Musilum rode into camp at daylight just as the caravan started moving. "Captain, the raiding party is hiding about a kilometer north of the oasis, and there are over 200 in their camp.

"Where is Hussin?" I asked.

"He will join us tomorrow. He wanted to watch and make sure they are still waiting. They have scouts watching the water hole. They would have ambushed us if we had gone in, without any warning." Alimud was within hearing distance with some of the men who had wanted to split off, and not a single complaint was heard during the remaining few days that it took us to reach Gerrha.

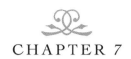

CHAPTER 7

Alimud's Betrayal

here was great excitement and relief as the skyline of the city came into view. Everyone was anxious for the rest and to see the big city with all that it had to offer. We soon found a suitable place to stop the caravan and set up camp. We had our merchandise to off-load for the market and packs and pack saddles to repair that would carry new merchandise back home.

Gerrha was a busy city of trade with so many beautiful things we had never seen before such as embroidered tapestries, silk cloth, brass figurines, tools, and housewares. We spent several days selling, trading, and bartering until all of our merchandise was gone. We sold the slaves, along with the rest of the frankincense and myrrh, to a Chinese trader going back to the Emperor.

The trading had been good and Gerrha had held the interest of my men for these few days. They had bought many wonderful gifts to take back to their families and had enjoyed themselves in the frivolity of the night life. But now thoughts were turning to the preparation of the return journey ahead, and we were all feeling the anticipation of going home.

While I was tending to my camels, the Chinese trader came to me about one of the slaves who kept speaking of my family and me, begging for a few words. I had a strange feeling of resistance and yet felt compelled to go with him, even though I did not want to speak with Eeslum again.

The merchant was soon going to sail to Nineveh and then travel east by camel caravan on the Silk Road to China. As we neared the vessel, I felt a hesitation as I boarded. I knew Eeslum was in the hold of the ship with the other slaves. When I saw him already chained to the floor, a feeling of despair came over me, knowing I could do nothing for him.

As he saw me approaching, he begged me to tell his family that he was alive and would return home to them some day. With great pain I sadly told him, "Eeslum, it would be better for me to tell your family that you died in battle because you will never see your home again. You died the day you joined Abrassa and his bandits."

There was nothing more I could say, and not wanting to feel any more pain, I turned and quickly left. I felt such sadness to think that one of my kin had brought such a miserable fate upon himself. I returned to my camp to continue preparations for our journey homeward. I was deep in thought when Jona came walking up to me and with a look of disbelief said, "You won't believe who I just saw in the marketplace down by the boats."

"Who, Jona?"

"Sabah," Jona blurted out.

"Sabah who?" I asked.

"You know, the man who deserted us before the raid."

"Are you sure, Jona?"

"Yes, no doubt. I've known him for several years."

"Did he see you?"

"Yes, when I drew my sword and challenged him to fight."

"What! You took him on in the street?"

"Yes, of course, Shutran. He's a deserter and traitor."

"So, what happened?"

"Well, the last I saw of him, he was running and screaming, minus his two ears. I marked him for life. People watching asked why we were fighting, and now the whole city of Gerrha knows about Sabah. Shutran, he had money and was spending it like water running through his fingers."

"Jona, what do you think he will do?"

"I personally don't think he'll go back to his people because there would be too much shame. He will hire on with a westbound caravan, most likely."

"Jona, do you think he had anything to do with that raiding party?"

"Yes, now that you mention it, I am sure he was paid for selling us out in Fort Sumhuram. Then he went on to Fort Yabrin to wait and see what happened with Abrassa. When Abrassa didn't show up, he went to another raiding party and sold us out for the second time. He collected money twice for the same information. Shutran, if I had put that together before I saw him, I would have killed him, not just cut off his ears!"

"Jona, you may still get your chance, but as long as we are in Gerrha, don't walk alone. Enemies have friends of their own kind. Watch your back."

"Good advice, Shutran."

"Sabah is a coward but he won't forget what you did, and every day his hatred for you will grow."

Changing the subject, Jona asked, "Have you decided exactly when you want the caravan to leave? We have a couple of unexpected requests. Micah wants to return with us."

"And what about Enos and Salah?"

"They want to go as well," Jona answered. "Shutran, you're a wise man. I was ready to kill them both, but you saw something that I didn't, and they both proved themselves. They walked every step of the way and never complained. They are grateful for their lives and have no resentment. It did not matter what I asked them to do. They did it. The care they gave Micah is the reason he is alive. You made men out of boys. They will follow you for life."

"Well, Jona, life is a long time, yet has a short memory. But listen! There is also something else. Something new! I have made a fantastic deal."

"What's that?"

"I bought the first silk woven cloth and skeins of silk yarn to take back to our country for the first time. Look at this jade that came with the caravans over the Silk Road from Hotan, the rubies and lapis from Upper Mesopotamia, and the turquoise from Persia. Don't you think Mirah will like this silk hijab with the way it wraps around the head and the rubies and lapis with the gold to wear around her neck? Look at these jambiyyas. I am having jade stones put in the handles with silver studs for each of the boys, and look at this silky abaya for my little princess. Don't you think they will like these things?"

"Shutran, my heart is beating faster just from the way you talk about your family. Now I am really missing my wife and children, too. You are making me feel guilty. How can I go home without something for my family? I was going to keep my money to buy more camels for our next journey."

"Ah, Jona, you can always do that, but don't miss the opportunity to make your sweetheart cry when you give her a little gift. She will hit you on the chest and say, 'Jona, you shouldn't have done that. We needed the money for other things.' She will hug and kiss you until you can't breathe, and then when the little ones are asleep, the great reward comes."

Jona turned a little red and in a teasing tone asked, "Shutran, at your age, you devil you; you still think about that?"

"Jona, the day I quit thinking about that will be the day they plant me!"

"Your beautiful wife will still be making your temperature rise when she's in her sixties," I said. "When you lavish a few gifts on her and she doesn't give you a few special nights that will keep you out of the camel stable, I'll pay you twice the cost of those gifts. You watch; she will think of all kinds of reasons the children need to go to bed early. Just make sure you bathe-up and put on some of that sweet smelling myrrh and cistus oil. Just add a drop of cassia to ignite her."

"Shutran, I don't believe what I'm hearing. I didn't think you thought of anything except work and the next trek."

"Jona, how many hours a day can a man think about work? Why do you think you don't see me for a week after we arrive home? Take care of your precious wife. Let her know that when you are gone, all you think about is her, and believe me, she will take care of you."

"Shutran, now you have my mind racing with thoughts that aren't about camels. I'm going to the market to buy some special gifts for Salmah and the children. Thanks, I've not thought about that before. So you really will pay me double if—you know—if she . . . ?"

"Jona, of course, I'll pay you double. Get going. We leave tomorrow. Pass the word to the men."

"Yes, Sir. By the way, did you know that Alimud and four of his comrades won't be returning with us?"

"Sure, Jona, that was an easy assumption. Let them go. I don't need my focus fractured because of their small minds and big egos. Our trip home will be more peaceful."

"You were right about Alimud. He has already bought 12 camels and is leading a caravan out of Gerrha but is only going to Najran and then on to Shabwah. The other night he was in the tavern bragging about how he could make the trip a week faster than you and that you took more time just so you could charge more."

"That doesn't surprise me."

"He was telling everyone that the men were given little to eat, that you pushed them at night, and gave them no water. He said you even whipped them into an unconscious state and then made them walk. He never said a word about why some received such punishment.

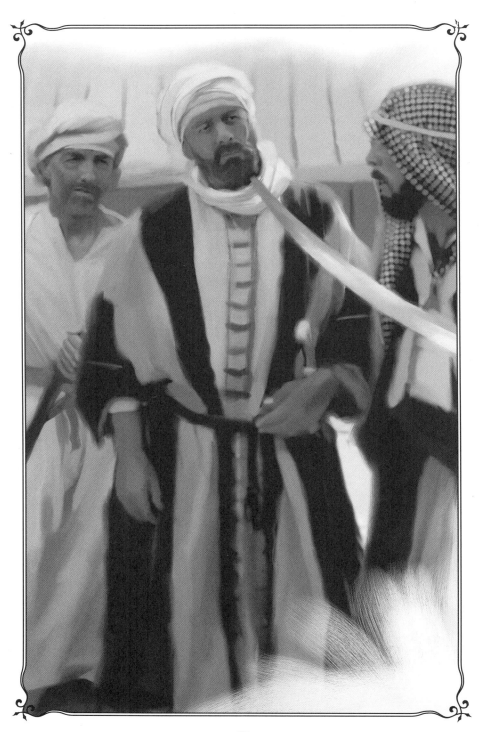

"He tried to make you look so bad that even those who know you just listened and said nothing. I was so mad that I called him outside and told everyone that he was lying. I told them that I have been with you for over 20 years, and if they want to know the truth, they could ask anyone who has been with you as long as I have, if they didn't have a hidden plan. Some of our merchants are going to send their merchandise with him. It made me so mad that I wanted to run him through."

"Jona, people like that have no integrity. They try to make others look bad so that they can feel important. The world is full of people who are so puffed up in their pride and self-importance that in their twisted minds they lose all sense of reality. Life has taught me that these kinds of people always fail when they start down that path. Just walk away from them. Leeches feed on leeches, and when the blood stops, they drop like flies."

"But some of the merchants who always brought their Persian rugs for us to carry have signed on with Alimud."

"Jona, it doesn't matter. For every merchant who signs on with Alimud, we will pick up two new merchants and more cargo. One day they'll come back if their businesses haven't been lost. You'll see."

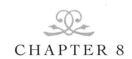

CHAPTER 8

Return to Al-Balid

As we prepared for our return to Fort Sumhuram and Al-Balid, we heard many stories in the city about a great King of Israel named Solomon. This new king had conquered many lands and was a man with a thousand wives. He desired to add the Queen of Sheba from Marib to his harem and had extended her an invitation to visit him. At the same time, in the year 967, a mighty Pharaoh from Egypt was raiding Israel and had become a great threat to King Solomon's army during the time that he was building the new temple in Jerusalem to house the Ark of the Covenant.

On every street corner, different stories of new things in the world were being told. The Chinese had discovered a way to keep meat fresh in the heat of the summer using something called ice, whatever that was. There were stories in Hebrew—a song of Deborah—and musicians singing and playing at religious ceremonies in Israel. Tales of Greek gods like Hercules, Zeus, Aphrodite, and others promoted the belief in multiple gods, which certainly was changing the thought and attitude of the time.

We sold our extra camels to caravaners going west, fetching a handsome price, which allowed each of my men to have one of the captive camels to keep or sell as a reward for his loyalty and bravery in achieving victory in the great desert battle. The men bought their women fine linens, robes, and ceramic dishes from China and other gifts and surprises for their children. I kept 13 of Abrassa's camels to carry our personal purchases home and things that I thought would be good for the village. It was exciting as everyone repacked and prepared to leave.

The market was in a frenzy bartering for the frankincense and myrrh. The prices had doubled as the demands in the Indus Valley and China were growing. The monks in the Hemis Temple, the Jagannath Puri, Temple of Krishna, and the Emperor of China were all demanding more resin. Before leaving, I had received enough orders to make up a caravan of 1,000 camels, which was more than I wanted.

Every merchant on the street was burning frankincense and talking about how it would cure all their diseases and ailments. Traditionally, myrrh had been in demand for protection during the lotus birthing of royalty. But now it was sought after by all the people because they believed that the smoke purified the mother and prevented evil demons from possessing the infant.

I watched the bidding for the myrrh exceed that of the frankincense and recognized that the increased demand would increase the harvest and the need for bigger caravans. Already Egypt was demanding more and more for its rituals and mummification ceremonies. I needed to think this through. I didn't want to expand my caravan, but neither did I want to lose the business to others like Alimud, who had no concern for putting men's lives at risk. I really wanted to slow down, but this was also a great opportunity to make a good life for my family so that my boys wouldn't have to work like this. I would certainly have a lot to think about on this homeward journey.

That evening as I was repairing the last two pack saddles, a young Persian lady came into our camp. She was the most striking beauty I had seen besides my beloved Mirah. She had large, dark, round eyes that sparkled as she swirled her raven black hair back behind her ears. It fell to her waist and shimmered against a body that had not seen the labor of childbearing and would twist a young man's neck if she walked by him. Her skin was a silky, olive color, and she smelled of jasmine oil from the Indus Valley. When she walked by, just about every man in Gerrha stared with lust in his eyes.

I pretended not to notice her while occasionally glancing up from my work. She came close and called out, "Captain."

"Yes," I replied.

"My name is Jasmine and I am looking for a caravan that I can travel with to Wubar. I hear it is a rich city with a lot of work and single men."

I kept working and glanced up as I responded. "Yes, it is a rich city, but I am not sure what kind of work you are looking for there."

"Well, I want to make money that I can send to my family so that one day we can move to Al-Balid."

"Do you have a husband?" I asked.

"No, there is no time for that now," she replied. "I was told in the marketplace that you have the greatest caravan in the world and that I would be safe traveling with you," she explained.

"Do you have money to pay?"

"No, but I can be of special service to you on the trip."

"Oh, can you cook?" I asked.

"That is not my specialty, but I'm sure I can heat you up."

"Jasmine, that is not of interest to me, thank you. I suggest you go with another caravan. I am sorry."

In a voice of indignation, she said, "I'll find someone who will appreciate my services."

"Yes, I am sure you will; but if he is a married man, you won't be able to trust him, so be careful."

While this conversation was taking place, Jona was standing back in the shadows listening. He stepped up and said, "Well, Shutran, how do you feel? Every man in Gerrha has his tongue hanging out, and you are the only one she offers herself to, and you insult her."

I looked up at Jona, almost laughing, and said, "Well, would you have taken her offer?"

Immediately he started to grin and said, "I couldn't do that to Salmah."

"Jona, I know that. You're a good man and I'm proud of you and Salmah is, too. When we're married to the most beautiful women in the world, no one else is of interest. Come on and help me finish these packs. I want to be on the trail tomorrow."

"Sure thing, Shutran. I am longing for my family and anxious to get going as well. By the way, look what I found for Salmah. She will look beautiful in this silk abaya, and she will love these tin pots for cooking."

"Jona, you did it! What a wonderful surprise for Salmah. You'll enjoy watching the expression on her face."

Morning came very early. The men were eating and preparing the camels, and two hours later we headed out for Fort Yabrin. We had acquired 20 more camels and 10 more men, and even though Alimud and his comrades left the caravan, the journey back was still faster. The camel packs were much lighter, making it possible for every man to ride most of the time, enabling us to make about 65 kilometers each day, besides the fact that everyone was excited about returning home.

We stopped in Fort Yabrin for only one day and one night. A few of the men were leaving the caravan and not continuing on with us, so we off-loaded food supplies for them and their families. We bid them fare-well and continued on to Wubar, about three weeks to the south. Most of the men didn't want to stop in Wubar, but the camels needed to rest, so we stayed for one day. As we pushed on and came closer to the Zophar Mountains, the more excited the men and camels became. By the time we reached the crest looking down into Al-Balid, I thought the men were going to outrun the camels the last 15 kilometers.

As we came across the desert floor into the village, the streets were lined with all the family members, friends, and even some strangers to watch the parade of 325 camels and 240 men enter the city. We stopped at the central courtyard to unload at the Treasury House, inventory our merchandise, and put it into the storehouse rooms for those who would start receiving their goods after our Sabbath, once all the accounting was completed.

Oh, how my heart swelled with joy as we rode in and I heard my name called over and over mixed with the sound of "Papa, Papa," as the children called to their fathers. We were all anxious to get to our families. I looked though the crowd and saw Kaleb and Joshua running alongside the camels, trying to get closer while hanging onto Mirah's robe.

The boys were trying to run faster and were practically pulling her over as she held onto little Armin, who couldn't keep up with them. A giant lump came in my throat, which I tried to keep down, but it wouldn't move. It was stuck! Tears welled up in my eyes as Enos rode up and said, "Sir, let me take your stallion so that you can go to your family. I'll bring him to your house with your belongings."

"Enos, thank you."

"No, Sir, it is the least that I can do for you."

The boys finally let go of their mother to run, and as I stepped down out of the saddle, I had two boys jumping on me just seconds before Mirah and Armin reached me. They smothered me with hugs and kisses until I could hardly breathe. I looked over my shoulder and saw Salah holding the reins of Jona's horse while his family smothered him as well. As the men were dismounting, their families were rushing to greet them.

The dancers were already celebrating in the square as the musicians played. Fires were starting to blaze and the smell of good food was in the air. Yes, it was a celebration after being gone for five and a half months.

I was stunned to see how much my children had grown. Kaleb was soon turning 14 and desperately wanting to go on his first caravan, as Mirah dreaded the day, holding out as long as possible.

As I started to walk with my family to find Enos to retrieve my horse, I saw that he was with his family engaged in conversation with Nahor's family. I slowed down to listen to the conversation, wondering how he would explain what happened and why Nahor didn't return.

I was impressed with how much Enos had grown up, taking full responsibility as he told Nahor's parents how he panicked during the storm and beckoned Salah and Nahor to follow him against the orders given. Salah was now standing with his parents engaged in the conversation as well. Nahor's mother, Samira, was crying uncontrollably as her husband, Ahsein, tried to comfort her. The horrible fear that she had felt for the last few months had now become a reality.

I could feel the pain and anguish that enveloped her heart and even more so when Enos told her that they could not find his body buried in the sand. I approached the family and offered my sympathy and sorrow for what had happened.

Nahor's father was angry but controlled himself with quiet solemnity. He looked sternly at Enos and said, "You always thought that you were so smart getting the boys to follow you. You had to show off and be the center of attention, which has now cost us the life of our son. When our time of mourning is over, we will see how you like the attention when I come for you." Enos' father stood still, knowing it was something that Enos had to face—it was the tribal law!

There was much excitement as we sat by the fire telling stories about our journey, the raid, and the new discoveries in the market. There was more talk about King Solomon, the new temple he was building, and his interest in the Queen of Sheba. There was talk of strange markings on a stone from India that was called Sanskrit, a form of storytelling by marking special colored stones. We had so much to share, and everyone sat with fascinated interest.

We talked about the amazing water vessels that came down from Nineveh loaded heavily with merchandise and news of a new caravan route from China and India called the Silk Road. Mirah wanted to know about Wubar. I told how it had become very rich and beautiful, and that the bigger it grew, the more wicked it became. The people were flocking to the city for all kinds of fun and ungodly activities. We had stayed only

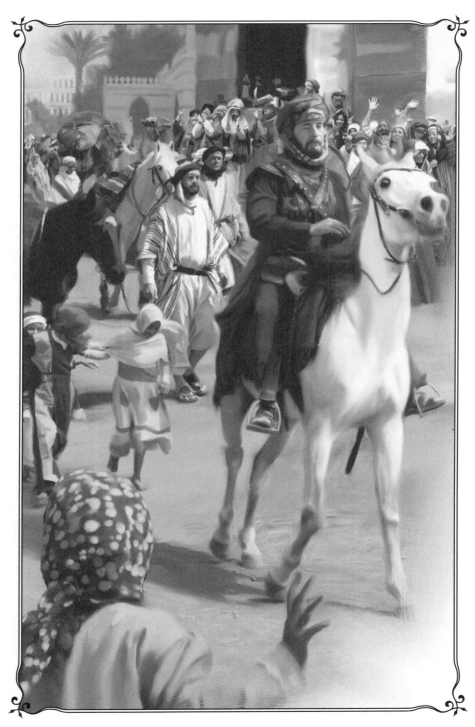

one night to off-load merchandise as none of us wanted to stay any longer. She thought for a moment and then responded, "Someday God will destroy Wubar if it doesn't change."

"Let's go home," I said. "I have many other things that I want to share with you." As we walked, the air was filled with, "Good night, sleep well, I love you," which brought that warm feeling of being home again. Enos had taken my horse to our stable and unsaddled him. Then he put the rest of my things at the entrance to the house.

Salmah came walking towards me with teary eyes. She put her arms around me, gave me a big hug, kissed me on the cheek, and said, "Shutran, thank you for bringing my man home safely again."

"Salmah, your man brought me home, too. You are blessed, as are we."

"I know," she said. "I just wish you didn't have to be gone for so long."

Mirah nodded her head and added, "That is our greatest trial and for the children especially. I have thought so much about it and wondered if there is a way that you two could start another business."

Jona, who had just joined us, responded, "Shutran, maybe we should think about it. We are not as young as we used to be, and we are missing out on seeing our children grow."

"Jona, you are so right. Let's talk more in these next few days." With that, we bid each other a peaceful good night.

I enjoyed watching Kaleb and Joshua, who were waving their new, stone-studded jambiyyas engraved with their names. It made me happy as they strutted around pretending to be such ferocious caravaners with their new knives. Armin, who was named after my mother, was twirling around in her new abaya, vying for everyone's attention. Mirah was more beautiful than ever in her new burka and hijab with the stone jewelry in gold around her neck. Yes, it was a wonderful homecoming.

"Children," Mirah called, "father is very tired and needs to rest. Let's retire early. Tomorrow will be another exciting day." I smiled with such pride and gratitude for the happiness I felt with my little family. Then I thought about Jona and Salmah and couldn't help but smile to myself and wished I could hear their conversation.

A couple of days later, I saw Jona and he was smiling from ear to ear. Chuckling, I asked, "Do I owe you any money?"

"No, Sir, not 1 denarii! Shutran, I will never spend my money on camels again when I am returning home. No, Sir, never. Your idea for my investment was the best one I have ever made." Salmah walked into hearing distance and curiously asked what the two of us were talking about. Jona smiled, "Oh, we're just talking about a business investment."

She looked at me curiously and asked, "How long are you going to be home this time?"

"Well, other than a few supply trips to Wubar, Fort Sumhuram, and maybe Marib, we should be around until the season of khorf, when the monsoons come. Then it will be time to move with the big caravan again."

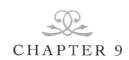

CHAPTER 9

The Parting— Kaleb's First Caravan

We had been home for two months when one day a messenger arrived at the door with a message for me. I was tending to my camels, so the message was given to Mirah. When I walked into the house, I knew something was troubling her because of her quietness. As I looked at her curiously, she finally spoke. "Shutran, a messenger came today with a message from the Queen of Sheba requesting that you bring 30 tons of frankincense, 10 tons of myrrh, and 1 ton of balsam from Fort Sumhuram to Marib. When you arrive in Marib, the Queen would like to meet with you. She wants to talk to you about taking her caravan to Jerusalem."

Kaleb quickly interrupted, "Papa, may I go with you on this trip? You always said the west route was not so dangerous. Mama, please, may I go with Papa?"

"Well, your papa has not yet said that he would go."

"Mirah, with this caravan I could make enough money so that I wouldn't have to be gone all the time. I really want to breed horses because I believe the time will soon come when horses will be worth as much as camels. I also have been thinking about putting money into some ships."

In a disbelieving tone, Mirah questioned, "Ships? What do you mean, 'putting money into some ships'? Is that a new business idea?"

"Listen, Mirah, times are changing. The Egyptians are demanding more and more resins for their burial ceremonies. I've been told that the Emperors of China and India are burning frankincense in their temples and are paying a lot of money for the resins. With a ship I could replace

100 camels and 100 men and with the monsoon winds deliver my cargo three to four times faster."

"Shutran, are you going to the sea now? Whatever are you thinking?"

"Mirah, someone has to do the buying and preparing of the shipments. It could all be done at home. I have good men now who could run the caravan from the mountains of the Hadhramaut and bring the resin to the Treasury House to stockpile it for the ships until we get the order to go to Gerrha. I wouldn't have to go since Jona, Seth, Ibram, Ahmad, and Mohamed know the trail, and they could take the caravan."

"Do you think they would go without you?" Mirah asked.

"Sure they would. It's in their blood and you know that Salmah can only put up with Jona for a short time at home. Micah told us that when they were in Egypt last year with their caravan, there was a lot of talk that Shishak may take over the throne in another ten years or so. When he does, he will lead his army against Israel and try to take the throne from Solomon. If that happens, the overland caravan won't be traveling, because there won't be an army to guard the way, and it will be too dangerous. The waterways would then offer the safest transportation and would become very busy with many new shipping routes."

"Why do you think this is going to happen, Shutran?"

"Solomon has been raising the taxes, and the people are getting angry. The talk is that he has changed with his riches and power. They say he has over 700 wives and 300 concubines. He recently married one of the daughters of the Egyptian Pharaoh, Siamun, turning all of Egypt against him.

"Solomon is claiming to be one of the gods and is now building idols. It seems he wants to appease his foreign wives. Micah said the rumor is that Solomon has an eye for the Queen of Sheba. Things could get rough over the next ten years. Mirah, just give it some thought. Did you say the messenger is coming back today?"

"He said tonight. He has to take your answer back to the Queen."

"Well, what should I do?"

"Shutran, you know that I don't want you to go, but the money would help with the expenses now that you're breeding and raising horses. Besides, you're always making new pack gear for your camels. Couldn't you stay just two more weeks?"

"Mirah, I think I'll have the messenger tell the Queen when I can be there and see what happens."

The time flew by very quickly, and I knew that I had to go. That night, lying beside Mirah, I turned towards her to speak, "Mirah, my beloved, it has been two weeks today since you asked me if I would stay home a little longer."

"I know," she replied. "I know that tomorrow you must prepare for your journey." She turned into my arms and gave me a gentle kiss, and with longing eyes she softly said, "Just hold me all night and don't let go."

"Mirah, Kaleb is going to ask again in the morning if he can go. What do you think?"

"You know how I feel."

"Yes, I do, but that doesn't change how he feels and what he desires to do. You know that boys his age are joining caravans all the time. I was 5 when I went the first time with my father to the mountains to gather myrrh, and then when I was 12, I went with him on my first caravan to Fort Sumhuram."

"I know," she responded quietly with a pain in her voice that overflowed from her heart swelling into tears that ran down her cheeks. "Shutran, I couldn't bear it if something happened to him."

"I know; I couldn't either. Let's not talk about it any more tonight. Tomorrow is another day. Sleep well, my precious wife."

While Mirah was making breakfast, I was sitting with Jona, Seth, Ibram, Ahmad, and Mohamed organizing our caravan to Marib. Jona looked up at me and inquired, "Are we not short someone to take Alimud's place? You know he never returned to Al-Balid and is probably staying in Marib or Najran."

"What about Micah?" I questioned. "What do you think?"

"Shutran, it might work and he would be getting back closer to home."

"Will one of you men go and ask him, and let's find out if we need anyone else."

At that moment someone knocked on the door. Joshua answered and called out, "Papa, Enos is here to see you."

"Invite him to come in and speak with me." Seth stood up and said that he would go find Micah.

I turned to greet Enos, who was looking very downcast and appeared to be struggling as he began to speak. "Captain, I heard that you are leading a caravan to Marib and perhaps traveling on to Jerusalem."

"Yes, that is possible."

"I would like to go with you, and if you don't hire me, may I go in exchange for work?"

"Sit down, Enos, and tell me what is troubling you."

"Nahor's father, Ahsein, has been telling people that he is going to kill me. My mother is crying day and night, and my father says that I have to accept what comes. It would help my mother to know that I wasn't just sitting around waiting for it to happen. I made a terrible mistake that will haunt me for life. I have learned a lot and offered to work in Nahor's place, but his father refuses."

"Enos, you have done all that you can do. Nahor's father must work that out and must also accept the fact that Nahor received the same orders as everyone else and had the choice to follow orders or go his own way. He paid the price of disobedience, which resulted in his own death."

"But his father chooses not to look at that. He is angry and wants others to hurt the same as he is hurting."

"Enos, my question to you is, can you face this or are you just running away? Ahsein's anger will consume him and your guilt will consume you. You are young and have your life ahead of you. Find a way to let it go and put it in the past, or it will destroy you until you can no longer think and make the right decisions. Your soul will no longer be able to carry the burdens of your physical life. Have you been burning frankincense and praying?"

"No, Captain, I haven't."

"Have you forgotten that the white smoke purifies the soul and mind and becomes the wings that carry your prayers to heaven? Give it some thought; it could help you a lot, and the answer is, yes. I need help. Go to the corral, take one of the red geldings, and ride to Fort Sumhuram to check with the dispatch to see if they are ready for loading tomorrow."

"Yes, Captain."

As Enos turned to leave, there was a heavy banging on the door that forced it open before Joshua got to it. Ahsein came through the door yelling, "Shutran, you can't hide that boy! I want him now! My time of mourning is over, and Enos cannot think he can run and hide in one of your caravans!"

I turned toward Ahsein's loud voice and said, "You are in my house, uninvited, and you are yelling and insulting one of my guests. Now, silence your mouth, turn around, and go back out through the door."

"Shutran, we have been friends our entire lives. Don't tell me to leave your house."

"I just did, Ahsein. You have crossed over our line of friendship by coming into my house yelling, regardless of your reason."

With a threatening stance, he yelled again, "Don't you try to hide that boy!" At that moment I hit him with my left fist with all my strength, forcing the weight of my body against him as he lunged forward to grab Enos. My fist landed directly on his mouth, splitting his lips over his parted teeth and breaking his nose. I then hit him with my right fist on the chin, causing him to stumble backwards, falling to the floor.

Mirah, hearing the yelling, came running into the house from where she had been hanging laundry just as Ahsein, covered with blood, hit the floor. "Shutran, what are you doing?" she cried.

"He was out of control and insulted our guest, but not now," I said, grabbing his wrists and dragging him outside. "Mirah, please bring a bucket of water. Joshua, would you please clean the blood off of the floor!"

"Yes, Papa."

Enos stood frozen in disbelief to think that I would defend him when his own father wouldn't do anything. Mirah brought some water, which I slowly poured over Ahsein's face until he regained consciousness. As he became aware of his plight and felt the pain in his face, he started wiping the blood. I knelt down and said with a penetrating look into his eyes, "Ahsein, you have a choice. You can get up and walk away and never come near me or my house again, or you can get up and knock on my door again, apologize, and start over," and with that I took Mirah by the arm and walked back into the house and closed the door.

Enos stammered for words. "Sir, I don't know what to say."

"Enos, you don't need to say anything. I didn't do it for you. I did it for Ahsein. He is my friend. Enos, just trust that everything is in God's hands." I reached up and touched his shoulder and said, "You can go now." I looked at Jona, Ibram, and Mohamed and motioned for them to sit down so that we could return to our planning. Kaleb, as my scribe, was listening and writing intensely when a knock came at the door again. Joshua called out, "I'll get it," but Mirah stopped him and said, "No, Joshua, I need to answer the door this time."

As she opened the door, Ahsein, covered with blood, stood there in what seemed like a dazed state. His nose and cut lips were swollen so much that it was difficult for him to speak. Acknowledging Mirah, he begged for her forgiveness and asked if he could speak to me. Jona, Ibram, and Mohamed came to their feet when I did as I invited him to enter. Ahsein, a larger man in stature than me, stood near my side trembling, almost in tears. In a barely audible voice, he said, "Shutran, I was wrong. I am sorry. I miss my son so much that my pain has caused me to lose all reason and common sense."

I knew that if Ahsein ever needed a friend, it was now. I motioned to the pillow on the floor and invited him to sit down. Turning to the men, I rolled my eyes toward the door, indicating that they should leave. "You men have plenty to do; check back after you have eaten. Kaleb, go to Ahsein's house and ask Samira to please come with you to our house. Tell her that Ahsein is here."

"Yes, Papa."

Ahsein was sitting on the floor attempting to compose himself. Finally he said, "Shutran, you really hit me hard."

"Yes, Ahsein, I did. You insulted me and you needed to be hit hard." Ahsein winced with only a faint smile, since his mouth hurt so much.

At that moment, Samira came in with Kaleb. She kissed me on each cheek as I welcomed her into our home. But as her eyes moved to her husband, she gasped in shock, realizing who it was with blood all over his swollen face and crooked nose. "Ahsein, what happened?" she asked as she moved towards him.

He reached his arm out to her as she embraced him, surveying his injuries. He blurted out, "Oh, I said something I shouldn't have and got kicked in the face by a mule. Thank goodness I was close and Shutran and Mirah came to my aid."

Mirah brought tea for everyone and more wet cloth for Ahsein with drops of cistus and balsam to help ease the swelling. Samira looked at me and quietly uttered, "I understand." I returned her acknowledgment with a wink. While Mirah gave Ahsein a little more to drink, Samira tried to hide her pain as she looked quizzically at me with her deep-set, raven eyes that were puffy and swollen from crying. She whispered to me, "Our pain has kept us from asking you about Nahor, and Ahsein is so eaten inside with the desire for revenge that we are hardly talking to each other any more."

"Yes, I understand," I replied. I turned and spoke so Ahsein could hear as well. "I have not personally suffered a loss like this, but any loss of a loved one is hard. Let me tell you about Nahor and the other two as well. Nahor was a good, young man. He worked hard, getting up very early in the morning to start loading the camels and never once did anyone have to wake him, unlike some of my seasoned men. He learned fast and was always willing to do whatever he was asked. He was good with the camels, and all the men liked him. He was a son that you could be proud of, and you can carry that in your heart.

"But there is something that I would like you to think about. Nahor had been given the same orders as Enos and Salah but chose to disregard them as well. If he had obeyed the orders, regardless of what anyone else said, he would be alive today. He made a choice and paid the price for that choice.

"The council decided the punishment for Enos and Salah, and they each took 25 lashings with the camel whip. They are scarred for life. They walked every step to Gerrha, even when the other men rode, and many times had to run to keep up. They alternated standing watch every night after walking all day. They spent three hours digging in the dunes in a weakened state the morning after their lashing, looking for Nahor's body. There is no question that it was one of the worst storms I have seen on any of my caravans.

"Later we came upon an Ishmaelite caravan coming from Selah that had been raided and found only one survivor, who the others had hidden under many blankets after he had been severely wounded. I assigned Enos and Salah the responsibility to nurse him and see if they could save his life, and they did.

"The boys have paid a heavy price and will for a long time to come. With all that they were told to do, they never uttered a complaining word. However, they also knew that if they didn't keep up or if they fell asleep on watch, the punishment was death. I believe that Enos has died many times over in his mind. Now, my question to you is, can you leave Nahor in the grave, let the dead take care of the dead, and live for your other children, who do live and need you?"

Ahsein stood up and looked directly into my eyes, as tears swelled and began running off his cheeks. "Shutran, you are a true friend. I needed to hear that."

Samira spoke up, "Ahsein, the other children are hurting twice as much as you. They lost their brother and their father because you have shut them out of your life in your anger and your need for revenge."

Ahsein, looking down into the eyes of his wife, took her into his arms and begged for forgiveness as he sobbed, letting the pain turn into tears that ran forth from his heart until they fell to the ground where he stood. Wiping away the tears, he looked up, trying to regain his composure. He looked over to me, barely able to speak, and uttered, "Thank you, my friend."

Seth came back with Micah a short time later, joined by Jona and the others so that we could finish planning. Depending on how long we would stay in Marib, we could be gone close to a year. Looking over at Kaleb, I said, "You really want to be gone that long away from your mother, brother, sister, and friends?"

"Papa, I wouldn't choose to be gone from them that long, but I have dreamed of this time since I was very small. Yes, Papa, I want to go."

"Then I want to say this in front of these men and your mother. If you choose to go, you go with the responsibility of a man and not as my son or my friend. That means you will be expected to pull your weight with the others. You will get up when the others get up, as I will not come to wake you. You will be treated as a man, and everyone will expect you to act like one. You will take full responsibility for your choices, whether good or bad.

"There will be days that you will be so tired that you will want to cry, but you won't. You will keep moving forward and doing what has to be done. If something happens to me, you must see me as another man. If you don't, you might not be able to think clearly and could make a decision that could cost the life of another man or even risk the entire caravan. Do you understand that?"

"Yes, Papa."

"No! Try it again."

"Yes, Captain."

"That's right. Now I think you understand. Go and check on the horses and pick out the one you want to ride while we finish here."

When Kaleb went out the door, I turned to the men and asked, "Does anyone here have anything to say? If so, I want to hear it now and not on the trail. Jona?"

"No, Sir, I have nothing to say."

"Anyone else?"

Each man responded with a strong, "No."

"I expect you to treat him the same as the others—no different than the other men.

"Jona, do you have the camel count?"

"Yes, 325."

"Seth, the packs and saddles?"

"Yes, 325."

"Mohamed, food?"

"Yes, three weeks for 65 men."

"Ibram, camp supplies, tents, and water?"

"Yes, it is all ready."

"Ahmad, do you have all the men lined up, and are they ready?"

"Yes, all 65."

"We will be taking slaves on to go to Marib, probably 75 to 100, and also another 75 camels. Micah, what about the horses?"

"We have six scouts on horses, you, Kaleb, and the six of us. We also have the 45 horses you requested for market, including the 18 to switch out at midday with the horses being ridden."

"Jona remains second-in-command and the rest of you in the following order: third, Seth; fourth, Ibram; fifth, Ahmad; sixth, Mohamed; and seventh, Micah. I'll meet you all here at four in the morning for final orders if we need to change anything else. I want you to be at Fort Sumhuram to start loading at six and be finished and ready to move out by nine, unless they do not have our dispatch ready. If we have to wait, Jona, send Kaleb back with a message.

"You know that the feed is in the canyon for the camels, so they can be left there; we will load the next morning. Since we may be going into Jerusalem, you'll want to take a change of your best clothing. Now, go home and make the evening the best you have ever had with your families in case you don't come back, because some of you might not." As I looked at each man, Seth turned white, and I felt a heaviness come over me.

Kaleb returned as the men embraced just before leaving. It was easy to see his excitement. "Papa, I would like to ride Spirit, the big, red gelding. May I?"

"Yes, you may. Did you select your saddle pads and bridle, and do you have all of your personal things ready?"

"Yes, Sir, I do. Papa, are you riding your white stallion this time?"

"Yes, I am. And I'll take the black stallion as well." As Kaleb looked at his mother as if to say goodbye, I put my arm around Mirah's shoulder and pulled her to me. "Mirah, let's all go for a walk on the beach and eat a little dinner over the fire. I'll help you gather some things. Kaleb, go and get Joshua and Armin to help. We are going to have a great time for what is left of this day, playing, eating, and just being together."

As we played and wrestled in the sand and ate over the fire, the pain that I felt was like a jambiyya in my heart, knowing that this would be the longest trip that I would probably ever make. There were so many things to think about, and so many things could happen while I was gone that it was difficult to be playful and pretend to be happy for the children. I kept reminding myself that it was my quest to provide a better life for my family. But it was a haunting success, knowing that I had such little time to enjoy it. "Yes," I said to myself, "this will be my last great caravan that takes me away for such a long time."

Mirah must have read my thoughts as she took my hand in hers while we walked back to our house. "Shutran, my heart is joyful to think that this will be your last big caravan."

"Yes, and with these new things coming to our world, there will be a need for new merchants to sell and trade these different goods. Perhaps there could be something new that you and Armin could do together as she grows up, if you have an interest."

"Shutran, what are you saying?"

"Think about it. You already make the clothes for our children. What if you were the first to make new clothes with silk from China and cotton from India? It may take a little time to get started, but I think it could become something huge."

"Shutran?"

"Yes, Mirah?"

"Will you ever stop creating new things? Last week you told me you want to start breeding and racing horses, warehousing, and even get into the shipping business and charting new shipping routes. Now you are making clothing."

"Well, my dearest, I am just looking at all the possibilities so that I do not have to lead the caravans and be gone for such a long time."

The next morning after the final planning with the men and while the camels were being loaded, I bid goodbye to my family. Little Armin was crying aloud while Mirah cried silently, but undoubtedly the hardest. Joshua was quiet as tears rolled down his cheeks. We all embraced and even though Kaleb's heart was pounding with excitement for his first caravan, his eyes were swollen with tears as he realized that this was all very real and that he wouldn't see his mother, Joshua, or Armin for close to a year.

He had no real idea what that meant, but there was no doubt in my mind that he had a lot of thoughts, and some were not the most pleasant. Mirah was going to have a difficult time without Kaleb. He carried a big responsibility at home, taking care of the horses and camels and milking the goats. That responsibility now fell to Joshua and, of course, to Mirah.

The trek to Jerusalem was to be the longest journey I had taken in my life with my camels. I choked back the tears as I thought about the three celebrations of birth that I would miss as well as the celebration of the day that Mirah and I joined our lives together. Part of their growing up years would disappear before me in the hundreds of sand dunes that I would cross, never to be experienced again. I wouldn't be a part of their little hurts and injuries, and I wouldn't be able to comfort them in my arms or give them their father's reassuring love. The mere thought of leaving them again intensified my pain, and I wanted to turn back and say, "No, no more will I go."

But my commitment was made and the day was ahead of me. I moved forward, knowing that every new day would bring me one day closer to my return. My heart swelled with pride to see my son riding with the men, knowing that even though I would feel homesick, Kaleb's presence would bring me a great deal of happiness. It was a double-edged sword because I knew that having him with me put his life at risk, and it weighed heavily on my mind. I must watch him and make sure that he returns safely to Mirah.

I sat tall in the saddle as my eyes scanned the immensity of my caravan, and I thought about the journey ahead of us. It would be a tremendous accomplishment and a great reward for everyone who did the work and made the sacrifice for the success of the immense trek ahead.

I felt a twinge of excitement, as I knew we were heading into a new country that I had never seen before. I bowed my head in silence for a moment and gave thanks to God for all things to come, the protection of my family, and our safe return. Then with the power of my stallion that I felt beneath the saddle, I turned to take my place as the Commander of this great caravan.

As I rode up the hill, I wanted so much to turn and look back, but the pain was too great, and I didn't want Mirah and Joshua to see the tears streaming down my face. But suddenly it seemed that my heart would split open as the silence was broken with the cry of, "Papa, Papa, wait!" I turned my stallion around to see Joshua and Armin running after me as Mirah was running to catch them. I stepped down out of the saddle, dropping the reins as the children ran towards me. I knelt down in the sand, scooping them into my arms, just holding them, never wanting to let go.

As Mirah reached us, the tears were pouring off her cheeks, and we all embraced. "Papa, Papa, please don't go," cried Joshua and Armin as though in a chant.

Mirah was trying to comfort the children as she said, "Papa has to go one more time, and then we will never be apart again." She held me tightly and whispered in my ear, "Shutran, my dearest, promise that you will come back home to me with Kaleb."

Choking back the tears, I spoke with total conviction, "Mirah, my love, I promise."

I knelt down and looked my children in the eyes. "I promise that Papa will never leave you again to take another long caravan after this trip. This will be Papa's last big one. Help each other and help Mama with all the chores, and when you go to bed at night, pray to God and ask Him to let you see me in your dreams, and I will be there. Papa will always be with you. Do you understand?" The children tearfully nodded. "Mirah, I will talk to you every night."

Mirah spoke gently, "We will be waiting for your return, and I will be in your dreams." She passionately kissed me goodbye again and called to the children, "Come now; Papa must ride."

As I swung up in the saddle, it seemed harder than ever before to leave, and the pain felt more intense. I thought to myself, "Shutran, you must be getting old." I leaned forward in the saddle as my stallion bolted into a full run to catch the caravan. As I topped the hill, I turned to see Mirah and the children waving. I waved back and blew them kisses and then turned to disappear over the hill and down into the wadi with the caravan.

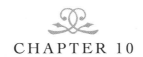

CHAPTER 10

The Night Storm

hile we were preparing to leave Fort Sumhuram, an eastbound caravan of 63 camels came in from the western Hadhramaut, loaded with frankincense. There was a lot of talk about Sheba, the Desert Queen, possibly joining with the Pharaoh of Egypt to raise an army to conquer Solomon, the King who believes in One God. That seemed strange to me, since Sheba wanted me to take her and her caravan with gifts to Solomon.

I wondered if this could be a peace mission, or did she have a hidden motive? The caravaners from the Shabwah region talked about Solomon's brother, one of Israel's military captains, who marched his army to the south to war against the Pharaoh while the Pharaoh's army was marching north to do battle with Israel.

Yet, everyone was saying that Solomon was peaceful and wondered why they wanted to fight. It seemed to me that both Solomon and the Pharaoh would have great interest in the Hadhramaut because of its vast abundance of resin. Perhaps they both thought they could take it away from Sheba and were trying to keep each other from knowing their hidden plans of conquest over her. I thought to myself, "It's going to be most interesting to meet this Queen of Sheba."

Jona walked over, "Shutran, have you heard what the men are saying?"

"Yes, and it is most intriguing. Where is Kaleb?" I inquired.

"He is with his grandfather at the Treasury House going over the weights and measures. He is doing a good job and is very accurate."

That night we camped at Wadi Hanoon just long enough to rest, water the animals, and have some food. I had Jona pass the word that we were going north through the Wadi Dokah Mountains to Wadi Masilah, which meant that we would be bypassing Wubar. I knew that the men would be disappointed, but we would cut three days off our trip. Besides, Wubar was a busy city of entertainment with lavish spending and decadent, immoral behavior that I didn't want Kaleb to see.

"I'll pass the word, Shutran. I didn't think we were going to make Jerusalem in a week," Jona said with a chuckle as he rode back down the trail.

I turned to Kaleb and said, "Go with Jona and listen to what the men are saying. "We have many new recruits and I want to know before we get to Shabwah if we are going to have trouble."

"Yes, Sir," he eagerly responded. I felt a sense of pride as I watched him ride to catch Jona. I thought about how he had matured since the caravan started. It seemed as though he had become a man overnight.

It was dark when we made camp. The men were tired and some were disappointed that we bypassed Wubar. But with five camels per man, we would spend one more hour at the beginning and end of each day, making the nights even shorter, besides the time we would be saving.

The next morning we took the trail to the head of Wadi Mitan and followed it through the Hadhramaut Valley. We spent just one night in Seiyun, and then from there we crossed the head of the Wadi Dawan and Wadi Doan and continued west to Shabwah, the taxation port.

It was hard to tell which was larger, the eyes or mouths of the men as we came in view of the immense stone gates at the south entrance into Shabwah. The welcome message was carved in a large stone on the left side of the gate. It was written in the Shahri language from 1,000 years ago and was believed to be the first language of the Hadhramaut.

As the caravan passed through the gates and headed towards the marketplace, the massive, white limestone construction of the Queen's palace was on the right side. We stopped in front of the Treasury House and off-loaded and weighed our goods. All merchandise coming into the city had to be recorded and then taxed, but because our goods were for Sheba, we didn't have to pay the taxes.

Beautiful Shabwah was home for over 1,000 people, but only 120 families lived within the protective walls of the palace grounds. The lifestyle of these families seemed very luxurious, with many servants to tend to their needs. The gardens were lavish with exotic flowers and shrubs as well as beautifully sculptured marble fountains. Numerous animals were cared for outside the 2½-kilometer walled city believed to have been the location of Sodom and Gomorrah 2,000 years earlier.

Shabwah was a rich trading city that saw many caravans coming and going weekly. Before moving to Marib, this was the Queen's first palace and the first taxation port. Anything new that was carried by the trade ships could be found in Shabwah. World news was a topic of conversation heard in the taverns that served the rich date wine.

Everyone talked about the famous, fermented goat milk mixed with honey and date wine, and the apothecary was known for the oils that were extracted there to make exotic perfumes and lotions.

We stayed for three days, taking care of the needs of the caravan, the animals, and visiting the city. While we were getting ready to leave, Seth asked in a rather curious tone, "Captain, what is our next stop?"

"We need to go to the salt mine and load 5 tons to take to Marib. Then we will meet up with a small caravan coming from the west through Mablaqah Pass to Bayhan bringing 2 tons of myrrh that we will load."

"Will we stop in Timna?" Seth asked.

"No, I don't think it will be necessary. Why?"

"Well, there is a young woman who lives there, who I met some time ago, and I would like to see her, if possible."

Ibram spoke up, "Oh, is there a possible romance in the air?"

"Seth, we will stay in Bayhan for three days, and it is only a one-day ride to Timna. You could take the trail from the salt mine that goes northwest from Nisab to Timna and then travel back south to Bayhan."

Jona protested, "But Captain Shutran, I don't think we could load the myrrh without Seth," and then he laughed. The others joined in the laughter as Seth just looked at us trying to keep a straight face.

We arrived at the salt mine in good time and had all of the salt loaded before dark. Seth left early the next morning for Timna, while the rest of the caravan headed towards the flood bed of the Wadi Markhah to follow it from Nisab west to Bayhan.

Three days later Seth arrived with quite a happy look on his face. I grinned at him, wondering if he was going to tell us what happened, but he just grinned back at me and said nothing. I raised a questioning eyebrow at Seth while I gave the order for the caravan to start moving. My plan was to travel west through the Mawsaqah Mountains and join the Qana caravan route that turns and goes northwest to Marib.

Everyone was ready for camp that night, as traveling through the mountains was always more tiring. The night seemed short when I awoke three hours before daylight. I turned on my side and reached over to Kaleb but found his blanket empty. I came straight up out of my bedroll, wondering where he was. I was amazed when I saw that he had the fire going and breakfast ready. My horse was saddled and as he started to ride away, I heard him say to Seth, "I'll wake up the others."

As Jona gathered his blankets, he looked up at me, chuckling, and said, "It looks like he knows his papa is getting old and thought he would let you sleep in a bit."

I smiled as I proudly acknowledged Jona with a laugh, "He certainly never got up like this at home. I would practically have to drag him out of bed with a camel."

"Yes," Jona laughed, "that was when he was a boy. Now he is a man and really wants to make his father proud."

"Jona, you are right, but his challenge will be to see if he can do it every morning for the duration of the journey."

"Shutran, don't be disappointed if he doesn't. After all, he is only 14."

"Now you sound like his mother."

One night, as we were all sitting around the camp fire eating, I said to Kaleb, "The land of the Masaquah Mountains is where I grew up harvesting myrrh. This is the land of your grandfather. His family belonged to a tribe of people who broke away from the Edomites, migrated north to the land of Moab, and started to carve their homes out of the multicolored sandstone rock."

"Papa, what were they like?"

"They were a very smart and industrious people. Their culture was built around the incense and spice trade hundreds of years ago when donkeys and mules were used to transport goods."

"Papa," Kaleb asked, "Where did your family come from?"

"As near as we have been able to determine, we are from Mesopotamia. We are Ishmaelites. My father's people were herdsmen of sheep and goats. That is how we arrived in the Hadhramaut. Many years ago after the great flood, there was a drought throughout all the land for several years, and the whole face of the land started changing.

"A group of Ishmaelites had intermarried with people from Gerrha, who were farmers who tilled the soil and planted crops. Their animals grazed along the coast where the fields were lush and the nearby mountains offered caves in which to dwell. As the drought gradually moved south, so did our people, until they came to the Hadhramaut, where they worked hard, and became a prosperous people."

"Papa, why were they called Ishmaelites?"

"Well, there is this story about a very faithful man named Abram who talked with God and guided his people as God directed. At 80 years of age, Sarai, his wife, had not borne him any children, so she gave him Hagar, her handmaid, who was an Egyptian slave, as a wife to bear him an heir. She bore him a son, who was named Ishmael.

"When Ishmael married, he had 12 sons, and all of their families became known as Ishmaelites. We are the descendants of Ishmael and of our great ancestor Abram, who lived 500 years ago. Many years later God changed his name to Abraham, and we have followed his same belief since then that has always made us a little different."

"Papa, do you really . . . I mean, I know we pray and you and Mama talk about God, but do you really believe in the One God? Most of my friends believe in many gods."

"Kaleb, let me tell you a story about something that happened when I was a young boy, perhaps ten years old. My father and I were high up in the mountains not far from here, near Bayhan, gathering myrrh. We had two days more to collect enough to fill all the packs on our eight camels when a storm moved in with heavy rain.

The wind was blowing hard and driving the rain sideways. The temperature had dropped considerably and it was very cold. I could tell that my father was concerned that we could be trapped in the mountains with the rain washing out the trail, making it impossible to get the camels out, so we hurriedly loaded our packs and started down the trail.

"Darkness came earlier because of the black clouds. Father was riding in front and leading a pack of six camels. We wound our way down the steep, rocky, mountain face with its deep darkness invading every open space between the trees. With every second the rain was coming down harder, making channels of water that were washing the mud off the side of the mountain, covering the trail.

"Through the chilling darkness and the cloudbursts of pounding rain, I heard Father yell out, 'Shutran, stop!' Then I heard a horrible grunting and braying sound from the camels. I called to Father but there was no response. I stopped my camel, Mulik, and got down and secured him to a nearby tree. I grabbed a stick caught in the mud and started probing ahead like a blind man looking for the first step into his house.

"The lightning ripped sharply and the thunder cracked and roared with a deafening echo in the steep canyon, almost shattering my eardrums. Then the lightning flashed through the darkness with such brilliance that it lit up the canyon like noonday, firing in rapid succession as though God was providing me with enough light to stop me from taking the next step that would have thrown me into a ravine that had been carved out by the rain.

"I continued calling out to Father—but still no response. Fear gripped every part of me as the realization came that Father and the seven camels were somewhere below in that deep gorge. I started down the foreboding gorge where the trail was now gone. To my relief, the lightning continued to light up the whole sky so that I could see.

"I slid and stumbled to the bottom of the chasm some 40 meters below. In a flash of lightning, I saw the camels lying in a heap, all entangled. The three above Father were grunting and spitting as they struggled to regain their footing. The lightning continued to show me the way as I climbed over rocks and camels until I saw my father's head and arms sticking out from underneath Suca, Father's camel. Two other camels that had partially landed on Suca were moving but seemed disoriented.

"I let out a bloodcurdling scream, as I thought my heart would be wrenched from my chest. Sliding down over the pack on Suca, I landed in the mud next to my father. I cried aloud until I felt my lungs would split. There was no movement. I knelt down beside him and touching his face sobbed, 'Father, Father, oh, Father, please be alive.'

"Then Father's words resounded in my head, 'Remember, Son, when you're in the mountains and if anything should ever happen to me, you must take the responsibility of a man in that very moment. Keep yourself calm and your head clear so that you can think, and then ask God Almighty to give you strength, and He will if you trust and don't question. If you doubt, you or someone else might die.'

"Choking between sobs, I lifted my head towards heaven and called out to God to please help me. As I gathered my thoughts, trying to take control of the situation, I pulled my thobe up over my head and rolled it up like a pillow to keep Father's head out of the mud.

"I climbed around Suca, only to discover that another camel was right below us and was trying to get up. The two that had been lying on Suca were now standing and shaking with their packs that were hanging

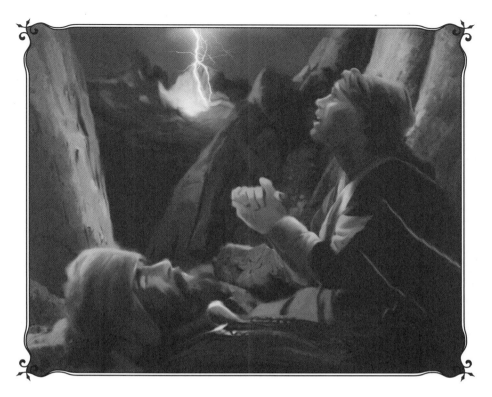

almost to the ground, but Suca was dead.

"The rain and mud were filling the basin little by little where Father was lying trapped underneath Suca. It was easy to see that if I didn't get him out, he would drown. I cried out to God with all the strength I had, 'God, stop the rain now and let Father live!' At that moment the lightning and thunder stopped. Then one minute later the clouds parted, and a giant, full moon replaced the lightning so that I could see.

"I knew that somehow I had to move her off of Father. I looked around and saw the halter rope lying in the mud. I quickly grabbed it and tied one end around her legs and then the other end to Doka's pack saddle. Doka was still shaking as I led her away, pulling Suca off of Father.

"With Suca's weight gone, I felt Father's faint breath, so I rubbed his chest and face until his breathing became stronger and he slowly regained consciousness. Father tried to turn over but couldn't move his legs or even feel them. As I tried to lift Father's arms to help him stand, he whispered, 'Shutran, my back is broken.'

"I felt such despair as I dropped on my knees, sobbing, 'Father, I am not going to leave you.'

He reached out to me and touching my arm said, 'Shutran, I am not asking you to leave me here. Listen to me! You prayed for God to stop the rain, and He did and even gave you light. Now we are going to pray together for God to heal my back so that I may stand and walk. And, Son, we must know without any doubt that God will heal me. Allow no other thoughts to enter your mind. Can you do it, Son?'

"With the intensity of *knowing*, I said, 'Yes, Father, I can.'

"I will never forget the words he uttered, 'Father, God of the universe. You said that if we ask You with absolute knowing, You will hear and answer our prayer. Father, my back is broken. My son cannot help me. Only You, Father, can heal me so that I may stand and walk now. In Your holy name, God, amen.' Then Father just said, 'It is time for me to get up,' and he did!"

I looked deep into Kaleb's eyes and said, "Yes, my son, I know there is a God and that He stopped the rain. Your grandfather would have drowned in that very spot in less than 15 minutes, but I watched God heal his back instantly, and I have never questioned God from that moment. Don't ever question if there is a God. Just get to know Him."

"But, Papa, how do I do that?"

"Talk to Him all the time—aloud and in your mind."

"Yes, Papa, I will."

"Morning is coming quickly so let's get some sleep."

Jona never said a word during that time. Then as the quietness of the night replaced our talking, he spoke up, "Shutran, I never knew that about your father, but as I listened, I had such an overwhelming feeling of the truth. I think now I understand how it is that you always seem to know things long before the rest of us. I too, want to know God."

"Jona, your ancestry teaches you to believe in many gods, and I believe in the One God. We have been friends for many years and have always shared that difference, but I believe when we open our hearts to God, this same God will answer us when we call upon Him.

"When you joined me to help lead the caravans many years ago, I knew God was blessing me with someone who would become a great friend. God is with us, Jona, regardless of our different beliefs."

"Shutran, my heart is so full that I just want to go home to my family and put my arms around them and tell them what I feel."

"Yes, Jona, it fills the soul."

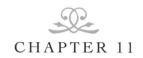

CHAPTER 11

Meeting Balkis, Queen of Sheba

Four days later we arrived in Marib, a bustling place filled with beauty in motion like the breeze moving through the hectares of date palms, flowers, frankincense, myrrh, balsam, cistus, and cassia trees, filling the air with a most intoxicating fragrance. The Queen's guards met us as we entered the city and guided us through the streets to the palace gates. We unloaded the camels and put them with the horses into pastures filled with lush, green grass surrounded by a border of billowing date palms.

"Papa, did the Garden of Eden look like this?" Kaleb questioned. Then thinking for a moment, he curiously asked, "Papa, where was the Garden of Eden?"

"Well, Son, all I can tell you is what has been written in the records of the prophets, and that is that it was the land east of Ethiopia towards the Euphrates River."

We enjoyed walking the streets and marveling at the grandeur of Sheba's city. I thought Kaleb's eyes were going to pop out. That evening the Queen's guards came to escort us to the palace. Jona, Kaleb, and I walked through the central courtyard that was lined with gentle, cascading waterfalls. From there we entered the garden with its beautiful flowers, trees, shrubs, and elegant statues of indescribable magnificence. The beauty of Marib and the Queen's palace were beyond anything we could have imagined.

We were invited to sit down at a marble table beside a rock wall where the water gently rippled down into a colorful, mosaic pond where little fish curiously swam back and forth.

Jona spoke quizzically, "Shutran, could you ever have imagined something like this?"

"No, I could not create this picture in my mind."

Just then we heard voices that seemed to be coming from behind a nearby, large rock. Two guards appeared, followed by two servants, who heralded the entrance of Queen Balkis and eight other servants. Next to the Queen was a very proud, muscular, young man, maybe half my age, who stood about 2 meters in height. He carried a rather arrogant air of ownership as he walked with the Queen, which seemed quite unusual. His clothes did not indicate that he was military or her personal guard.

Queen Balkis walked gracefully towards us in a smooth, alluring way. She was taller than the native women, with soft, refined features. Her eyes were large and round, giving her a seductive look that validated the rumors about her beauty. She carried herself with a look of authority and was obviously impressed with her superiority.

Jona and I were not prepared to see a Queen of the Hadhramaut who was black. We could easily see that she was not a Sabaean. She walked with very seductive body movements. Her gown was very formfitting and accented her youthful curves. Her long, wavy hair hung down over her shoulders, and its thickness framed her face like a beautiful painting, bringing our eyes directly to hers in amazed wonder. Her voluptuous, full, bottom lip with her concise, thin, upper lip indicated that this woman was not one to have on your bad side.

She seemed to be a no-nonsense person and not one to talk a lot but would get directly to the point. We had no question about who was in charge. Her features indicated that she was Egyptian of Ethiopian descent, and whoever mixed her gene pool was a master craftsman.

She stopped in front of me, looking directly into my eyes, and said, "You are Shutran, I assume, Captain Shutran from Al-Balid."

"Yes, Your Highness. You sent a messenger requesting that I bring to you frankincense, myrrh, and balsam. That I have done. Do you wish anything more?"

She introduced me to Captain Tamrin, her caravan captain, who seemed to feel a bit threatened by my presence. Queen Balkis spoke again, "Shutran, I have heard that you are the first caravaner to cross the Empty Quarter to Gerrha. I have also heard that you have never been defeated in battle and that you have the largest single caravan in all the Hadhramaut. But I have also heard that you are hard on your men."

I could feel Jona swelling for a response, but before he could speak, I quickly spoke, interrupting his growing anger. "For what reason have you requested my presence? If you have heard all these things, surely you have drawn your own conclusion."

"Yes, Shutran, I have, and that is why I have asked you to come, so I could see for myself this legend of the Empty Quarter. I have found that men are virtually lazy and often do only enough to get by, and most of the time they will betray you for money and power if they have the chance."

"Queen Balkis, forgive me if I disagree with you. I find that all people in the human race have weaknesses, and they will act as you described if they have the innate characteristic in their blood. However, what I find more often is that man is a creature who prefers to do the right thing and will do more if one shows a little appreciation."

"Oh, Shutran, I detect a little weakness in you."

"So be it, Queen Balkis. Perhaps another person, even a woman, should lead your caravan. I thank you for this time to speak with you and now bid you well."

As I turned to leave, the sound of the Queen's voice stopped me. "Shutran, may I ask you a question?" Turning around to face her, I answered, "Yes, please ask."

"You see, Shutran, I am impressed by intellect and wisdom, and I wish to see yours. I have traveled to many places and have seen many things, and you impress me. Perhaps you might solve my riddle. What is it that has many heads and in a storm at sea raises a loud, bitter wailing and moaning? It bends its head like a reed and is glory to the rich and shame to the poor. It honors the dead and dishonors the living. It is a delight to the birds but a sorrow to the fish. Shutran, what is it?"

After she had finished the riddle, I looked at Jona and he looked at me and raised his eyebrows as if to say, "Sorry, I cannot understand this." Rubbing my forehead and looking away from the Queen for a moment, I thought how clever she must be. She knows I am a caravaner and that I have spent no time at sea. She hopes to embarrass me in front of her servants and Tamrin. I could see a smile breaking out on her face as I looked down at Kaleb, who was anxiously waiting for me to prove myself.

At that moment the thought of a story my grandfather once told me flashed through my mind. It was about the reed boat of Queen Hatshepsut. A faint smile came on my face as I turned back towards the Queen, anticipating her surprise as I solved her riddle. I looked straight into her eyes and said, "Flax, for it makes sails for ships that rise above the water and moan in the wind. It provides fine linen for the rich and rags for the poor, a burial shroud for the dead, and a rope for hanging the living. As a seed, it nourishes the birds and as a net, traps the fish."

She was shocked with almost a look of disbelief, and then slowly a smile broke out on her face as she looked into my eyes and said, "You are right. You are the first to know the answer. You are the wisest in my entire kingdom." I saw the red flush in Tamrin's face as his jealousy overflowed almost to the point of losing control. "Shutran, I want you to lead my caravan. Tamrin has found many families that want to go and have their own camels. In my own pasture, I have over 200 camels, and the rest are at my command after it is determined how many are needed."

A bit reluctant, I carefully responded, "We will start organizing tomorrow."

Queen Balkis invited us to have some fresh wine sweetened with honey, as we conversed about her desire to make this great 3,500 kilometer journey. Tamrin never spoke but we could feel his anger and his feeling of possibly being replaced. He was not someone I felt I could trust, and if my gut instinct was correct, before the caravan reached Jerusalem, there would be a showdown between the two of us. He would push it until it happened. Obviously, even as strong and powerful as he was as the caravan captain for the Queen, it wasn't enough. He wanted more!

As we listened to Queen Balkis express her desires, I felt the first challenge coming with Tamrin. Kaleb sat very quietly, just taking it all in with total amazement as she talked about the silk, flax linen, gemstones, ivory, and incense that we would be transporting. Kaleb was writing as fast as he could to get her every word, when in the middle of the conversation, she stopped abruptly and said to Kaleb, "Are you writing down all that I am saying?"

He looked up very matter-of-factly and said, "Yes, Your Highness. We will need to calculate how many camels, possibly mules, horses, animal feed, men, archers, sentries, scouts, food, and water, along with the many other details that have to be considered."

She then inquired, "How many camels will we need?"

"I have calculated that we will need 789 camels."

Then she asked, "And how many men?"

Again Kaleb responded, "1,624 men, plus servants."

Tamrin squirmed as Queen Balkis asked, "And how do you figure that?"

"Your Highness, through my observation of your servants who have been with you this evening, attending to your care for special meals and clothing as well as for morning and evening preparation, I can calculate your needs in order to keep the caravan moving in a timely manner."

It was easy to see that the Queen was impressed but also very indignant and a little humiliated by the fact that this young man could have figured her out so quickly. She snapped back, "Be more specific."

"You see, Your Highness, if Captain Shutran moves the caravan at first light or even earlier, as he often does, in order for you to be ready, you will need two cooks to prepare your food, three servants to prepare your clothing, three to prepare your morning bath, two to do your hair, and four to bring your food and then clean up.

"You will need five men to take down your tents, ten men just to prepare your personal camels and chariot, and five men to attend to your horses. If all of your servants work together packing and loading, along with the six bodyguards, we would not need more men. The cooks could start packing the food when they finished cooking. The other servants who pack your clothing could do the same with your tents. Once the horses and camels are saddled, the men could start loading them and your wagons. None of this includes Captain Tamrin and his men, who must also be added. Queen Balkis, you will need to be ready to travel no later than first light."

Captain Tamrin spoke in an angry voice, "Who do you think you are to tell the Queen when she must be ready to ride?"

Kaleb looked at Tamrin as if he didn't have any concern about his attitude or position and simply said, "With permission, Queen Balkis, I will answer Captain Tamrin's question."

Now the Queen was somewhat amused with the young man's unwavering confidence and obvious intellect and wanted to entertain herself a little. She smiled at Kaleb, nodding her head, and simply said, "Please."

Kaleb continued, "You see, Sir," addressing Tamrin, "the Queen asked me to be specific. Captain Shutran has his highly respected reputation because he runs a very punctual and orderly caravan company. His men are well trained and very efficient. Is that not why the Queen sent for him? In order for the Queen to make decisions, she needs information. If she does not know when the caravan moves out in the morning and she wishes to sleep longer, then it will take more servants to prepare for her. So I gave her the information she needed."

Tamrin bristled and snapped back with anger, "You have no idea when the Queen wants to get up. Who do you think you are? And don't you dare look me in the eye when I talk to you. I am the captain and you had better show me some respect, boy!"

Kaleb glanced at me, and I nodded with approval of his position. His eyes went back to Tamrin, and without a blink, he rose to his feet. Looking Tamrin in the eyes, he said, "When I see a captain to respect, I will."

Tamrin started for his sword in his anger towards Kaleb and said, "I'll teach you some respect!" At the same moment I watched the Queen nod to her guard, and in a flash he had his sword at Tamrin's throat.

Without hesitating, the Queen spoke very matter-of-factly, "Tamrin, you are out of place, and this young man is right. If you ever speak to him in that way again, you will not be a part of this caravan. Now you are dismissed to your quarters."

"Yes, my Queen." As Tamrin bowed, he said, "I beg your forgiveness" and then turned to leave.

I spoke up boldly, "Queen Balkis, before Tamrin retires, with your permission, I would like to address some concerns."

"Yes, Shutran, go ahead."

"I have been leading caravans for 25 years. I have engaged in 11 caravan raids and survived. I have fought in three military campaigns, but I do not have a need to lead your caravan. Your Captain Tamrin appears to be very capable and willing but resentful of our very presence."

"Yes," she answered. "You are right! However, I requested you because of your reputation, and Tamrin does not have the experience or ability to command such an undertaking as this. So what else do you wish to say?"

"Queen Balkis, Kaleb gave you information so that you could make choices. First, if I become the commander of your caravan, then it must be without interference. Second, if you wish to see the caravan move smoothly and with supreme organization, then again, I must be the only commander, and everyone will follow my orders, including your Captain Tamrin. Third, if Tamrin ever speaks to one of my men or anyone in the caravan as he spoke to Kaleb, I will kill him. Is that clear?"

Tamrin's spine stiffened and I could feel him wanting to reach for his sword, but he cautiously restrained himself. The Queen looked up at me challengingly and responded, "Shutran, that is a strong statement. Do you think you can back it up? Tamrin has 20 years or more of youth than you and is a great swordsman."

Turning and looking Tamrin in the eye, without a flinch I emphatically responded, "Without a doubt, Queen Balkis," as I watched the blood drain from Tamrin's face. "And, Queen Balkis, that also includes you. You will be under my command, and I will be responsible for the lives of everyone in the caravan. If I give the order that we travel all night, I cannot have you, as the Queen, countermand my order. If I call for the caravan to move out at two in the morning, I must know now that you will follow my command and not countermand any order that I give."

"And what if I say no to this request, what will you do?"

"Then I shall take my caravan and leave."

"But you have no merchandise with which to return."

"That is true but I would go to the old salt mine near Shabwah, load my caravan, go to Qana to trade for merchandise to take to Wubar, and then return home."

"I see," she replied. "Do you always have an alternate plan?"

"Always," I answered.

"What if I refuse your conditions and yet made you lead my caravan?"

"Queen Balkis, you can refuse my conditions, but you cannot make me lead your caravan. I will not put the lives of others at risk because of someone else's decision."

Queen Balkis stared at the ground, and then slowly raising her eyes to mine, she said, "Shutran, you are a stubborn man. I could have you put in prison, take your caravan and men, and you would have nothing!"

As I nodded in acknowledgment, Jona spoke up and said, "Queen Balkis, forgive me for speaking, but I have to tell you that all of the men would go to prison with Shutran before they would betray him, and I would be the first. We know that he would give his life for us, and we feel the same for him. You could take the caravan, but not one man would go with you."

Kaleb then spoke, "That is true. I would die before I would leave the Captain."

Queen Balkis thought for a moment and then said, "The loyalty of your men speaks of your success. I admire a man who can create such allegiance. As you have spoken, I accept your request. However, I also have a request. I want to hire this young Kaleb, and I will make him the overseer of all my servants and will pay him three times whatever you are paying him." She looked straight at Kaleb, awaiting his reply.

Kaleb responded with certainty, "Queen Balkis, please forgive me for not accepting such an honorable request, but I wish to stay with Captain

Shutran. With the Captain I can learn much. I can learn to be like him one day and perhaps lead a great caravan, and that is what I want."

The Queen nodded her head. "I see," she said. "Then I will dismiss you this night and bid you well. You have had a long day, and we will meet in the morning to finalize the plans and your payment."

That night as Kaleb and I were lying in our beds, Kaleb asked curiously, "Papa, will Tamrin not want to save face?"

"Yes, Kaleb. His ego will not see it any other way."

"Papa, what if he is faster than you?"

"Faster does not make him better, my son. A man driven out of resentment and hate will always make a mistake, and that is what I look for day and night. I already know his style, but he knows nothing of mine, so do not worry, Son. Better men than Tamrin have tried."

At the breakfast fires the talk was all about how I caused Tamrin to back down. Obviously, the Queen's guards who had been there were quick to tell stories. It was interesting how the news spread throughout the day.

That night as we were eating, Seth came over and sat down beside us to tell us that Alimud was in town. Seth explained, "Alimud lost his whole caravan that included 48 men in the desert one month ago to a raiding party. Only he and two others survived and were luckily found by a southbound caravan. Alimud asked if there was any chance he could come back to our caravan. I told him that he would have to ask you."

"Seth, gather the men after breakfast at my tent."

As the men gathered, I told them that we were going to Jerusalem and that this would be one of the longest caravans we had yet experienced. Most likely we would end up having two enemies to watch as Alimud would certainly join with Tamrin. I emphasized that we needed to be alert, watching and listening, because the two would try to sabotage us, causing loss of time, loss of merchandise, and death to the camels. I warned all of the men to keep their eyes on their cinches and ropes, as this would be the first place where they would try to cause trouble.

The second thing was to watch for thorns in the pack pads that create sores that cause the animals to start bucking and throwing off the merchandise. Third, it would also be critical to watch for holes in the water bags; and, fourth, our enemies would try to feed the camels the qat plant, which would drug them into such a deep sleep that they would not be able to get up. And if they were given enough of the weed, it could cause a heart attack in some of the older camels. Our enemies might also stick cistus thorns in the camels' feet that could make them really lame. I was adamant that the men check everything each morning at first dawn. The last step Tamrin and Alimud would take would be to provoke a fight between different caravan chiefs or family groups.

"Tamrin will find Alimud or others like him to support his cause in taking over the caravan. Some of you might be led into such deception because of their slick tongues, and even after ten years of being with me, you might find yourself going another way. When you realize what has happened, you will spend the rest of your life trying to convince yourself and others that you were right in your betrayal and speak falsely to support your actions, trying to cover up your own guilt. Eventually, that guilt will cause your guts to rot, and everything you eat will turn to burning acid.

"Today carefully go through every pack and pack saddle, check every camel, and watch to see if they have more feed than you gave them. Watch to see who is new in the marketplace and taverns and then later shows up on the caravan."

Micah spoke up, "Captain, a man in town came to me and asked about a job and said he worked for you before moving to Marib. Could this be the Alimud you have been talking about? What should I tell him?"

"Micah, tell him to come and see me tonight."

Jona then spoke, "Shutran, you are not serious, are you?"

"Jona, listen. If we hire him, we can watch him. If Tamrin hires him, we cannot. Know your friends and keep them close. Know your enemies and keep them closer."

"We know he is our enemy, and the men won't be happy about this, Shutran."

"I know and that is good. They will be watching his every move."

"Jona, a small caravan will be arriving from the Al-Marwaza Mountains in the next day or so with about 110 camels carrying sweet myrrh. The caravaners want to travel with us, so we will need a captain over that caravan. We have some men who I feel are ready for a new position and greater responsibility. Let me know who you choose. I am leaving now with Kaleb to finalize things with the Queen."

"Now, Shutran, don't go taking a fancy for the Queen just because you've been gone for two months. Her beauty is tantalizing."

"You are right about that, Jona, but I'll bet she sleeps with a jambiyya."

When the planning was completed with Queen Balkis and her scribe had finished writing, we had 789 camels with an estimated 220 kilos of merchandise for each camel, plus a water supply for each one. Queen Balkis had been planning this journey for about four years, gathering her gifts of dried flax linen, silks, gemstones, ivory, spices, dried dates, honey, cistus, luban, myrrh, sweet myrrh, diamonds, and copper. She was also taking Cassia, her most prized, black Arabian stallion, as a gift. There were two dozen sentries, chariots, and, of course, the Queen's wagon pulled by six Arabian stallions and ten mule-drawn wagons carrying the Queen's food, tents, gifts, and personal belongings.

As I reviewed everything, I thought that this was not going to be a normal caravan. I could see that the Queen was going to travel with the grandeur of her court for all to see the beauty of her riches, which meant absolutely nothing to me or anyone else in the caravan. She wasn't going just to meet the great and wise King Solomon. She had a hidden plan.

I felt a twinge of pain in my heart, knowing that we would not be back in one year, as I had told my family. Kaleb saw the tears in my eyes and asked, "Papa, is something wrong?"

"No, my son, I just got some sand in my eyes."

What Balkis had offered me to lead the caravan was more than I could make in five years, but was it going to be worth the risk and the separation from my Mirah and the children? I knew that I had to discuss this with Kaleb. I said to him, "Son, this is the biggest caravan I have ever commanded, and there is something I need to tell you so that you can make a decision. This is going to take longer than we had planned. It could take a lot longer than a year to return home."

"Papa, you mean we could be gone for two years?"

"Yes, Kaleb, it is possible. If you want to go home, I will arrange for you to go with a food caravan to Shabwah, with a salt caravan to Qana, and then with a trade ship from Qana to Al-Balid. You could be home in four to six weeks."

The tears welled up in Kaleb's eyes as he turned so I wouldn't see. Then he asked, "Papa, may I have a little time? I would like to pray about this."

"Yes, take whatever time you need."

I could feel Mirah's presence. I could feel her holding me and the warm tears rolling down her cheek against mine. Her heart was beating hard as she tried to choke back her deep sobs. I could hear Joshua and Armin running to me crying, "Papa, Papa, please come home. We need you. We miss you. Please, Papa, come home." My heart was tearing with pain. I called to Kaleb, "I am going for a walk up in the mountain for a while to talk to Father. Do you want to come?"

"No," he replied, "I am going to lie down and sleep a little."

As I reached a quiet place in the rocks on the mountain, I knelt and pleaded with Father to help me — to let me know what I should do. Then I heard His voice saying, "Son, I will not make the choice for you or tell you what to do, because that would take away your freedom. But as you believe in me, I will fill your heart with understanding and the knowledge to make the right decisions. However, if you choose to go, your family would be safe, and although your journey would be hard, you would be able to teach and help many. Trust in yourself and know that I am with you. Trust in that *knowing* and as you decide what is best for you and your family's future, my blessings will be upon you."

From this I learned that what we resist the most often yields the greatest blessings. In my meditation, I hugged and kissed my young Joshua and Armin and my beautiful Mirah and bid them farewell for the moment. With a sigh of sadness, I looked around me, but at the same time, I felt the strength of conviction in my legs as I walked off the mountain.

As I entered the city and looked around, I found myself pondering about how many people really seek to have a relationship with God or think they do because they believe in what someone told them and then wonder why their lives never get better or why they can't heal.

When I entered the tent, Kaleb greeted me with happy eyes and a big hug. "Papa, I talked with Mama, Joshua, and Armin, just like you said, and they said their prayers would go with me as I continue on my journey with you. Mama said that when I think about her, I will always be able to feel her near me, and that although our separation will be a little longer, she knows that God's protection will be upon us. Papa, it is just as you said."

We walked out to the fire where dinner had been prepared. As the men gathered to eat, Seth came over with Alimud, who was not as arrogant as the last time I saw him in Gerrha. "Captain," he said, "could I talk to you for a moment?" We walked away from the men towards the camels grazing nearby and stopped near a rock. Alimud was the first to speak, "Captain, I made a big mistake. Because of my pride and arrogance, I lost 48 men and my entire caravan. I am hated by 48 families and have nothing. I cannot go back to Al-Balid and face the humiliation of my family. I will work hard if you will allow me to go with the caravan.

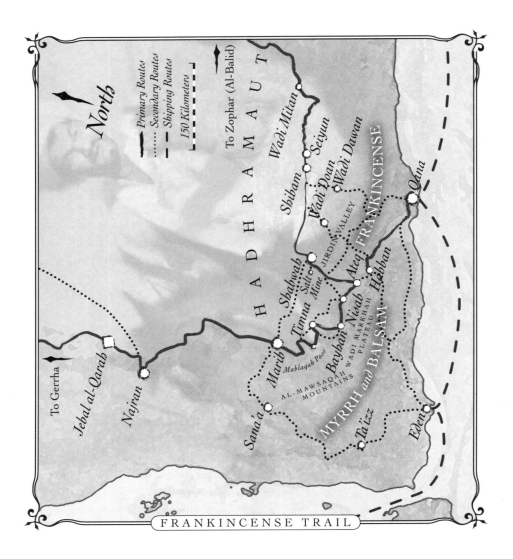

North

Primary Routes
Secondary Routes
Shipping Routes

150 Kilometers

To Zophar (Al-Balid)

H A D H R A M A U T

Wadi Mitan

Shibam
Seiyun

Wadi Doan
Wadi Dawan

JIRDIN VALLEY

FRANKINCENSE

Qana

Shabwah
Salt
Tinna Mine

Ateq
Habban
Nisab

Marib
Mablaqah Pass
Bayhan

WADI MARKHAH
PLATEAU

AL-MAWSAQAH
MOUNTAINS

MYRRH and BALSAM

To Gerrha

Jebal al-Qarab

Najran

Sana'a

Ta'izz

Eden

FRANKINCENSE TRAIL

Hopefully, I can make my way to Damascus and start over."

"Alimud, the men hate you for your betrayal, and they will never trust you, nor will I. I cannot say that before we reach Jerusalem that someone will not stick a jambiyya in you while you sleep."

Alimud, with a beaten and broken spirit, said, "It would be welcome."

"All right, I will let you come. Report to Jona for your assignment."

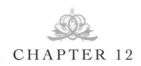

CHAPTER 12

Tamrin's Deception

e took five days to organize everything before the caravan left Marib and headed to Najran. It was a grand moment when the caravan and all of the wagons, chariots, soldiers, and horses started the journey. Tamrin was in charge of the Queen's personal caravan but was ultimately under my command, and every time I gave him an order, I could feel his resentment building. After four days of traveling, Tamrin rode up and said, "The Queen wishes to stop for the day and have a bath and rest."

I said, "No, we must keep moving. There will be times ahead when we have to stop, but we will not stop when there is no need."

He responded, "But the Queen said. . . ."

I abruptly cut him off and reminded him of our agreement and gave the order to keep moving. I rode forward to the Queen's wagon and asked her why she wanted to stop.

She said, "Tamrin said we had come a good distance and that this would be a good place to stop for the day."

"Queen Balkis, may I remind you that Tamrin is not giving the orders, and the water here is not good water. We will keep moving."

Each camel carried 20 gallons of water with its regular load so that we would have enough water for the men, mules, and horses. Two water holes were dry where I had watered in the past, so the water had to be rationed. The men were edgy and tempers flared. My captains had to continually be on guard to prevent fighting from erupting among the men. Thirty days after leaving Marib, we reached Najran, and what a celebration there was when the word went out that we would be here for four days, allowing the camels to feed and replenish their energy reserves, to repair packs and gear, and replenish our food supply. Until now the journey had been fairly uneventful, but little did I know that was soon to change.

Three days on the trail out of Najran, we came to the ridge of a steep dune. We had to use four camels roped to the back of one wagon to ease it down slowly. Shortly after we started the descent, a cinch strap on one of the camels snapped. The weight was too much for the other three camels to hold the wagon. As the momentum increased, the wagon dragged the camels 300 meters as it rolled, scattering the Queen's personal things along the face of the dune, breaking an axle, and coming to a halt upside down at the bottom.

As Seth and I were assessing the damages, I looked up to the top of the ridge in time to see Tamrin turn and ride away. Micah came riding up and handed me the cinch strap, and sure enough, it had been cut very cleverly so as to look like a natural tear, but the cut was much too uniform. Micah was mad as he spoke, "Captain, I checked the cinches this morning."

"Micah, be on notice! Tamrin has just started. He created this mess and he can clean it up; however, we are not stopping the caravan for him. He can catch up to us later. Send the word throughout the caravan to keep moving. Kaleb, ride up and notify the Queen that we are continuing, and I will meet with her when we make camp. Tamrin will be looking for me as soon as he gets the word. We were fortunate to come out of this without any injuries to any of the men or camels, but next time may prove to be a different story."

While the Queen's servants were gathering the merchandise and her personal belongings, others were addressing the repair needs. Tamrin came riding up, just as I had expected. Looking at me, he said, "Shutran, you have to stop the caravan so that we can repair the wagon."

I looked over my shoulder towards him and then slowly turned my horse to face him. With great sternness I said, "I am Captain to you, Tamrin, and don't you ever address me by my name again; furthermore, the caravan is not stopping. You caused this problem and you can fix it. We are traveling to the oasis 20 more kilometers ahead before we stop."

Tamrin angrily blurted out, "Are you accusing me?"

"Is a chariot wheel round?" I retorted. "That wagon was under your command. Yes, I am accusing you and the report I give to the Queen will be such, or you bring me the man who did it." I abruptly turned my back to him and rode away, knowing that the first confrontation was coming soon. You don't insult a man of Tamrin's stature and walk away without a fight, and I had now insulted him twice, due to his insolence.

However, Tamrin was easy to read. He was a big man, extremely muscular, and as the Queen's commander was very arrogant and impressed with himself. He bullied the servants and exerted his power over anyone who crossed his path. The Queen watched with amusement as she, herself, enjoyed wielding her power. She, too, was obsessed with the need to be in command.

Tamrin, according to the Queen, was a great swordsman, and although 23 years younger than me, he had never served in the military. I was very doubtful that he had really fought anyone with any ability other than Bedouin bushmen or servants; otherwise, he wouldn't have backed down from our little encounter at the Queen's palace. He was very courageous with an audience and guards to back him up, but on his own, he was a coward. This kind of a man was dangerous. The first time I laid eyes on him, I knew I would have to watch out for him.

Kaleb came riding up to me with a message, "Captain, the Queen wishes to speak with you as soon as she can after we reach our camp, as your time allows. She asked about the wagon rollover, and I assured her that no one was hurt and everything is under control."

"Thanks, Kaleb, I want you to stay close to me, Jona, or Seth at all times. Do not ride out of sight. Do you understand?"

We arrived at the water hole just before dark. The men were busy pulling packs and pack saddles, making picket lines, watering the donkeys, mules, horses, and, lastly, the camels. Dinner fires were burning while others pitched tents. Queen Balkis remained in her enclosed wagon until her tent and quarters were ready, while her servants scurried like work ants. I was somewhat amused to watch her chief servants bark orders while directing the show. They all carried out their duties very carefully, knowing that to displease the Queen was not something they wanted to do for fear of their life and well being.

Riding on my stallion, taking it all in, I circled her camp, making a mental assessment of the tents, picket lines, campfires, and guards. Evidently, the Queen had never camped with the thought of defending herself against an assault of desert pirates. The most valuable treasures of the caravan that the common thieves of the night could steal were the camels and horses, then the food, the merchandise, men, mules, donkey carts, and, lastly, the wagons. When making a line of defense, the men should set up camp in such a way that the attackers could approach from only one strategic point, not leaving it vulnerable to four or five different possibilities.

Tamrin had instructed his captains to make camp in the open flat. The tent of Queen Balkis was in the center surrounded by servants' tents and then the wagons with food. The camels were on one side of the camp, and the mules, horses, and donkeys were picketed on the other side. The donkeys and mules made a good line of distraction, making it easy for thieves to steal the camels. I rode up to the Queen's wagon as she was getting out. "Queen Balkis, Kaleb said that you wish to speak with me."

Turning on her heels abruptly, she looked angrily at me and without taking a single breath demanded, "What is it that makes you feel you need to prove your superiority by making us travel another half of the day when we were tired and could have stopped when the wagon rolled over?"

I listened quietly and looked her right in the eye and without flinching said, "Queen Balkis, when you regain control of your temper, come and find me and we will talk," then turned abruptly and rode away.

Enraged, she yelled and ordered me to stop, or she would have me arrested and flogged like a slave. I never looked back.

Jona, Seth, Enos, Micah, Kaleb, and some of my other men had just finished eating when Tamrin rode up behind me and stopped a bit of a distance from our cook fire. As I was still squatting, finishing my meal, I raised my left elbow slightly and looked under my arm to see how close Tamrin had actually come behind me. Hardly moving, I raised my voice just enough to make sure Tamrin heard me and said, "Tamrin, don't you ever ride up to my camp again without asking permission."

Ignoring me, he just barked an order, "Shutran, the Queen wants to see you now!"

I reached to my side as he spoke and untied the leather thong securing my whip. I grabbed the shaft as I came to my feet and brought the whip around as I spun on my heels. The whip coiled around his throat as I jerked him out of the saddle, landing him on his back. Before he could catch his breath, my sword was at his throat drawing a bit more blood than my whip. "Tamrin, you will address me as Captain Shutran. I warned you once and if I have one more encounter with you before we reach Jerusalem, I will kill you. If you want a fight, save it until then and I will gladly give it to you."

As I withdrew my sword and stepped back so he could get up, I looked squarely at him and the three guards who had accompanied him and said, "You go back and tell the Queen that I will not be insulted again. Tell her that she had better never again send a boy to do a man's job." As Tamrin stood up, he glanced around and saw 30 to 40 sets of eyes staring at him. He tried to speak but nothing came out. His throat was bruised, and it would be days before his voice returned. I nodded to Tamrin to get out of my camp. "As long as you live, do not ever enter my camp again without permission."

As they rode away, Kaleb was at my side. "Papa, I have never seen you move like that. You were so fast."

Jona spoke, "Kaleb, few people know your father as I do. Every journey we have made has been successful because of him, and what he can do, no man can. If you walk in your father's footsteps, even half of them, you will be a great man."

"Jona, that's enough," I said as I coiled my whip while we walked back to the fire.

Kaleb asked, "Papa, can you teach me how to use the whip?"

"Of course, Son, but you have to learn to respect it. I've never laid a whip to a camel, horse, mule, or donkey. It seems that only a few of the two-legged kind provoke the whip."

Seth spoke up and asked, "Captain, what do you think will happen when Tamrin returns?"

Looking down at the fire that needed more wood, I responded, "Before you put another log on the fire, the Queen's chariot will arrive. She will be boiling mad like a trapped cobra ready to strike but will remain in control. She will have 20 to 25 of her military riding with her, so let the rest of the men know and have them in a circle of defense. You men know what to do." Turning to Micah, I said, "You and Kaleb take two men and go check on the guards on the picket lines and tell them to be prepared tonight."

"Captain, what shall I tell them if they ask?"

"Micah, we will have visitors tonight. They have been following us for three days."

"Did you or one of the scouts see them?"

"No! They have been very careful not to be seen."

"But, Captain?"

Jona interrupted, "Kaleb, the Captain can feel it, and when he does, don't question, just do what he asks. He is never wrong." No sooner had we finished our conversation when we heard the sound of an approaching chariot.

I knelt down at the fire with my face to the tents to adjust my eyes to the night. Jona and Seth knelt beside me. I heard the chariot stop and then a voice called out, "Captain Shutran, may we come in?"

I stood up and moved out of the light of the fire and responded into the darkness, "Yes, enter."

The Queen's chariot came up slowly with guards flanking both sides. Tamrin was behind her chariot.

The Queen spoke, "Captain Shutran, we must talk."

"Step down, Queen Balkis. Welcome to my tent. Please, come."

Two of her guards helped her down and escorted her to the open face of the tent. Seth brought a rug and pillows. I invited her to sit down and offered her some wine, which she cordially accepted. I waited for her to speak.

She took a deep breath and said, "Captain, you are a difficult man to read."

"I am sorry, Queen Balkis; I didn't think you needed a man to read. I thought you needed someone who could take you to Jerusalem and return you safely to your home."

This helped to break the icy feeling she brought with her, and she chuckled, "Captain, you are absolutely right. Now, may I ask you a question?"

"Yes," I replied.

"Why did you make us travel another half day when we could have stayed where the wagon rolled over?"

"Queen Balkis, that is a fair question. But let me first ask you a question. Why did Tamrin send that wagon down the dune and not around it as he did yours? And who cut the cinch on your camel's saddle?"

"Tamrin thinks your men did it to make him look bad," she said. I responded, "That could be, but how would my men know which camels he would use and which wagon he would send down?"

"That is a good question, Captain. I didn't think about that."

"Queen Balkis, your Captain Tamrin has been like a myrrh thorn in a camel's foot ever since we left Marib. Why?"

She was quiet and then looked up and said, "Captain Tamrin is angry. You have insulted him and challenged him, and he won't be satisfied until he does battle with you. I agree that what he received at your hand, he deserved. However, this behavior is affecting all of my command."

"Maybe you should consider replacing him with someone more mature and skilled."

"That is my second reason for coming. After what happened tonight, my military has lost all respect for him, and his humiliation is too much. The only way for him to regain face will be for him to kill you. However, I will not allow a fight to happen until we reach Jerusalem. I'll talk to my guards and make sure that is understood."

I was silent for a moment and then resumed speaking, "Now to answer your first question. Why didn't I stop? May we go for a ride in your chariot?"

"Of course," she said, nodding her head and motioning towards her chariot.

I helped her up, took the reins, and said, "Queen Balkis, I wish to show you something." The moon was climbing high in the desert sky, illuminating the landscape as though it were late afternoon. "Do you see your men sitting with their horses?"

"Yes," she answered.

"Now watch." I made a whippoorwill chirp and instantly my men were at the side of her soldiers with a sword in their sides before she could blink. Then I dismissed them.

She looked at me a bit embarrassed and whispered, "Captain, I get the message."

"Yes, but there is something more I want to show you. Tell your men to wait here." I pointed to the oasis and asked her to look beyond the water and trees. "Now, what do you see?"

"A rock cliff," she replied.

"Yes, and look how far it stretches to the north and south. Now tell me, what do you see to the south?"

"I see a large sand dune perhaps 120 meters high."

"Yes," I answered, "and to the north?"

"Open desert."

"Yes, and the position of the great light in the sky to the south shining north, illuminating the skyline of the dune, makes it easy to see thieves approaching in the night, and it is impossible to come over the cliffs behind them.

"Now, let's look at the camp. The camels and horses are the closest to the water, and next to the tents with the food and packs are the wagons with the mules and donkeys. The donkeys are as good as dogs and should be put on the outside of the picket line on the outer perimeter with the guards. If raiders come to steal, they have to pass the donkeys, guards, dogs, wagons, men sleeping, food, merchandise, and finally the camels and horses. There is no pass through and so the route of escape is the same as the way they entered. Now, let's look at how Tamrin has prepared your camp."

As we rode around her encampment, she could see how vulnerable she was in the bad way her camp had been set up. "Now, Queen Balkis," I said as we rode back to my camp, "I shall answer your question. Where the wagon rolled over, there was no water and no suitable campsite."

"Now I understand," she said, releasing the anger she had displayed earlier. "Captain Shutran, I shall never question you again," she sighed with a rather seductive tone in her voice as she reached over and placed her hand on my arm, giving me a gentle squeeze. "I feel so secure knowing that every moment you are thinking of my well-being. Captain, how can I repay you?"

The bumping of the chariot over the sand mounds gave her the excuse to move closer and the opportunity to put her other arm around my waist, hanging on tightly as if there were a need for her safety.

"Queen Balkis, you are paying me very well, and my responsibility is to care for you and everyone else as well in the caravan."

"Captain, could you drive me to my tent?"

"Of course, Queen Balkis," I responded as I turned the chariot around and headed for her tent. When we stopped at the entrance, four guards and four servants were there to greet her.

As she stepped down, she turned to me invitingly and said, "The least you could do is let me offer you a glass of wine."

"Thank you, I would be most honored to share a glass of wine with you, but perhaps another time would be more suitable. Right now I think you need to reorganize your camp. From now on, until we reach Selah, we could encounter desert raiders. Let us be careful. I bid you good night until the morrow."

As I drove up to my camp, Tamrin and the Queen's guards were still in the same place, waiting for my return. Stepping out of the chariot, I passed the reins to the driver without any verbal exchange, and they returned to their camp.

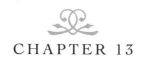

CHAPTER 13

Theft in the Queen's Camp

I was startled awake early in the morning with a strange sound that brought me to my feet. As I stepped out of the tent to determine what it was, the stars were still bright in the sky. I scanned the skyline to look for any unusual movement but could detect nothing. I grabbed my bow and quiver of arrows just inside the tent while securing my whip and sword.

I nudged Jona awake, who came to his feet like a mountain lion springing for the kill. I told him to circle south past the picket line to the sand dune while I went to the Queen's picket line. Jona nodded as he clenched his sword in one hand and reached for his bow and quiver with the other. Kaleb was still sleeping and didn't wake up as we left in silence, not knowing what to expect.

The night cook fires had burned down to smoldering ashes, and a few glowing embers barely gave any light. I crossed the camp to the Queen's line. As I had expected, I saw that she had not moved the camels or resecured her line of defense, and there seemed to be no guard moving about. An eerie quietness gave a hint of trouble. With one glance toward the line where the horses were tethered, I could see that Tamrin's red stallion was missing, as well as the grey horse belonging to Nadab, who was Tamrin's second-in-command.

As I circled to the east under the light of the stars and approached the camel line, I could see that some of the camels were missing. Staying low, I moved carefully, not wanting to alert the raiders if they were still present, and crawled under one of the wagons. As I raised my head to stand up, right in front of me on the ground was one of the guards with his throat cut. From his position, I could see that he had obviously sat down with his back to the wheel and had fallen asleep. The blood running down his chest was still warm and told me that it had happened only a few minutes ago, probably about the time I was awakened.

I turned and ran across the camp to Tamrin's tent, and stepping inside, I pulled my sword and stuck it under his chin. The cold steel brought him fully awake but so terrified him that he was unable to speak or move. I knelt down and wiped my hand on his face so that he could smell the blood and then withdrew my sword and moved back, allowing him to come to his feet. I retreated from his tent while motioning him to follow. I then informed him of his dead guard and the horses and camels that were gone.

Before he could call out to his soldiers, I jammed my sword handle into his gut, stifling his attempt to speak and signaling him to be still. I whispered, "Stay quiet and get your men. They've been gone only a few minutes. If you ride now, you will overtake them. You have an advantage because the horses they took will slow them down in the desert. You can easily pick up their trail, but once they reach the mountains, they will move fast and you won't catch them. The caravan will keep moving. Now go!"

One of the guards returned to report that six camels and three horses were gone and that two guards were killed. By now the entire camp was stirring. Balkis came out of her tent and demanded to know what all the noise and commotion was about. Jona informed us that the raiders had six camels and seven horses and that their trail headed south. I quickly explained to the Queen what had happened and headed back to camp.

The men were busily putting pack saddles and packs on the camels, while the breakfast fires burned brightly as the sun began to crest over the mountains. The smell of goat and camel fat frying signaled that breakfast was ready. The caravan was soon loaded and ready to move out.

The second night after the raid, Tamrin and his two comrades rode into camp, and by the sound of the Queen's voice, they undoubtedly had returned without the camels and horses. Seth, looking across the cook fire, spoke, "Captain, you didn't really think they would catch them, did you?"

"No! I knew they wouldn't."

"Why?" he questioned.

"It's simple. Tamrin has nothing to lose. It wasn't his stock and it doesn't affect him one bit.

"He never followed them the first night, and the thieves counted on that. If Tamrin had wanted, he could have caught them. His story will be that they lost the trail because of a sandstorm."

"Why does the Queen keep him in charge?"

"Simply because she likes to make men her slaves, and Tamrin is big, muscular, good looking, and in love with her, and she has complete control over him. She loves the power."

"Well, Captain, she sure has eyes for you," Jona teased, keeping a serious look on his face.

Trying not to laugh, I responded, "If I let her have her way with me, afterwards she would discard me like an old camel blanket. But watch, by the time we return from Jerusalem, she'll hate me. Those who she can't control or manipulate become her enemy."

Ibram spoke up, "Captain, why are we taking all of this merchandise to Solomon? Does she think she can buy him and take over his whole kingdom?"

"Well, I think that is what she wants everyone, including Solomon, to believe. However, she is underestimating him. He already has some 700 wives and 300 concubines. I personally think it is a smoke screen for another reason. If she doesn't get what she wants, she will seduce him in the end. Mark my words, she is Ethiopian and he is Hebrew—and they don't mix."

Alimud walked up to the fire to talk with me. "Captain, tomorrow we will be in Tathlith. May I stay with the caravan and not go into the village? These people know me and the humiliation is too great."

"Yes, if you would like. We have enough men to trade for the supplies we need. Alimud, you take ten men and do an inventory of our pack gear and see if anything needs to be repaired. Most of the day will be spent trading for food and supplies and repacking to leave the next day. Get some sleep; tomorrow will be a long day."

Queen Balkis was dressed "for the kill" as she rode into the village in her gold-plated chariot with Tamrin at her side. The two of them made a very impressive picture, and heads turned as they drove through the streets. The Queen was in top form, knowing that all eyes were on her and Tamrin. Her servants were busy in the marketplace buying fabric, linen, vegetables, and goat milk. Everyone enjoyed the day visiting and bartering in the market and swapping colorful stories with the desert Bedouins.

The news had already reached Tathlith about the robbery and the thieves getting away with it. As the rumors spread throughout the village, they eventually landed on Tamrin's ears. He became very angry as he realized they were making fun of him and how these desert raiders had outsmarted him. He was even more humiliated when he had to buy six more camels and pay double the price.

The Queen was not happy now that the word was out that it was her camels that were stolen. That made them worth a lot more, if someone were foolish enough to buy them and stay in the village. These camels would likely be sold to an eastbound caravan, never to be seen again.

I sent Jona and Micah to the livery stable to see when the next eastbound caravan was scheduled to arrive. The caretaker was very talkative and anxious to have some news to pass along the trail. He informed Jona that two days earlier two men had come by to sell one horse and two camels, but he wouldn't pay their price, so they headed to Thumala, a larger trading post 120 kilometers up the trail. Obviously, these desert brigands were trying to unload the stolen livestock as quickly as possible.

When Jona and Micah returned with their report, I wasn't surprised with the information they received. It sounded like the caretaker was trying to mislead them so that we would all leave without asking further questions. I asked Jona, "Was the man at the stable talking fast, and did he seem nervous?"

"Well, as I think about it, yes, he was a little."

"Didn't Tamrin just buy six camels from him this morning? Why didn't he say something to him? Think about it!"

Jona spoke up as he analyzed what happened. "Captain, he said he knew of no caravan coming through for maybe three weeks, but the people in the marketplace said there is a caravan from Gerrha coming any day. They would rest for ten days, reload, and return. Did Nadab already pick up the six camels?"

"Yes, just before noon."

As we started to mount up and ride back to camp, I felt a gnawing feeling in my stomach. I turned to Kaleb and Ahmad and told them to take the supplies back. "I have a visit I need to make. Jona, you go ahead with Kaleb and Ahmad. Salah, you come with me." We rode back toward the stable and turned down the little dirt road just before reaching it. We circled around behind where there was a large adobe stable that was enclosed, creating a blind barrier from the front part of the livery stable.

A small pasture ran out into the rocks through some brush that provided a little feed for the stock. I handed Salah my reins as I stepped out of the saddle and walked to an old door about to fall off its wooden hinges. I stepped inside and as my eyes were adjusting to the dim light, I felt the railing where two of the Queen's camels and Nadab's grey horse were tied.

As I came out, Salah was anxiously awaiting my report. "Captain, did you find anything?"

"Yes, they're in there." We rode back to camp and over to the Queen's tent, where she was lying stretched out under the tent top having some wine and a foot bath with hot sandalwood oil while other servants were massaging her head and hair with rose oil. The aroma was so inviting. She turned as we rode up and spoke immediately, "Oh, Captain, have you come calling?"

"No, Queen Balkis, I have some information for Tamrin."

At the sound of his name, he came out of his tent next to the Queen's. "Tamrin, I have seen two of your camels and Nadab's grey horse tied up in a back room behind the stable where you bought the six camels this morning." With that we turned and rode back to our camp.

Queen Balkis came up off the bed immediately and turning to Tamrin asked quizzically, "How does he know?"

Tamrin snarled, "Maybe it's to make me look bad."

"Tamrin, you haven't learned anything yet, have you? Shutran doesn't have to make you look bad, but one thing is for sure, he will be watching to see what you do about it."

When Tamrin and Nadab rode up to the stable, the owner, a big, burly, muscular man greeted them. With a cynical smile and qat juice dripping from his bottom lip, he asked how he could be of help. He was 1½ times the weight of Tamrin and had a look of "mean" that went all the way to the bone. Tamrin said, "I understand you might have some of my stock here."

The stable owner asked, "And who might you be?"

"I am Tamrin, Commander and Chief for the caravan of Queen Balkis, and who might you be?"

"I am the owner of the livery stable, and you can call me Sleeman. Now again, what can I do for you?"

"I was told you have two of my camels and one horse here, and we would like to look to see if they are, indeed, here."

Sleeman, in a jeering voice, growled, "None of your stock is here, only mine and my customers' stock."

Tamrin snapped back, "Well, then, you won't mind if we have a look, will you?"

Sleeman planted his feet squarely in front of the door, and with a daring look barked, "I imagine I would!"

Tamrin bristled as he swiftly came out of the saddle. "In the name of the Queen, we will look," he commanded.

Sleeman never moved. He just responded boldly, "I don't care who your Queen is. She is nothing here, and I said no one is looking in my stable."

Tamrin reached for his sword but as his hand grabbed the handle, Sleeman's fist hit him squarely in the face. Tamrin went down with his hand still on the handle. Nadab pulled his sword while jumping down from the saddle, but as he came around in front of the horse, Sleeman's club caught him just above the ear, splitting his skull and leaving him unconscious on the ground beside Tamrin.

Back at camp, Queen Balkis was disturbed that Tamrin and Nadab had not yet returned, so she sent a servant to fetch me. I was with my captains reviewing our supplies, since Makka, our next stop for food, was 250 kilometers northwest, a journey of about 10 to 13 days. Her servant, Issa, found me, with Kaleb's direction. Approaching very respectfully, he called out, "Captain Shutran, the Queen has sent me to ask you if you would come. She fears something has gone wrong since Captain Tamrin has not returned."

"Please assure the Queen that I will be there shortly. I am almost finished."

When Issa returned, the Queen was pacing back and forth. "Where is Shutran?" she demanded.

"He said he will come shortly, after he finishes something he is working on."

"Did you tell him that I want him to come immediately?"

"Yes, my Queen. Please forgive me, but Captain Shutran is not going to hurry for a poor servant such as me."

"Oh, go back to work and don't come here again."

"Yes, my Queen."

I finished my conversation with my men, saddled my horse, and some minutes later rode to the Queen's quarters to be welcomed by her fit of rage.

"I sent my servant for you several minutes ago, Captain."

"That you did," I replied. "How may I help you?"

"Captain, when I send for you, I expect you to come immediately; do you understand?"

"Queen Balkis, may I remind you that you are under my command; I am not under yours."

"I am your Queen and I am paying you."

"Yes! You are paying me to lead this caravan, not to be your servant or guardian of your men, and, second, you are not my Queen. If you have time to stand and yell at me, you must not need me for anything too important, so I will return to my affairs."

Catching herself, she realized she was looking quite childish, although I doubted it bothered her. She wasn't getting anywhere with her ranting and raving, so she abruptly stopped. She blurted out, "Tamrin and Nadab haven't returned."

As I looked at the shadows falling from the Queen's tent, I realized that some time had passed. "Queen Balkis, I will take some men and go find them. Just calm down and remember that you never eat camel stew as hot as it is cooked!"

"What is that supposed to mean?" she snapped.

Looking over my shoulder, I said, "You are the one who likes a mental challenge. You figure it out." I turned and rode back to camp and called Mohamed, Ibram, and Ahmad to go with me as well as Jona, who fought as well with his fists as he fought with a jambiyya.

I explained to my men, "Tamrin and Nadab rode into the village to get their stock and haven't returned. I suppose they've met with a little opposition. The Queen is concerned about her pretty boy, so let's go rescue them." My men chuckled as they mounted.

Mohamed was large in stature and 30 kilos heavier than Jona. He and I loved close hand-to-hand combat, and he was wicked with a sword. I saw him one night in Wubar when some man hit him twice with a closed fist. He told the man to quit, but the man was mad because he thought that Mohamed had stolen his ugly girlfriend. He hit Mohamed a third time, so Mohamed hit him once and broke his neck. Ibram was slightly built but was the best with a sword and had never been beaten or even cut. Ahmad carried two swords and could carve a man's name in his chest so fast that he could be finished and have his swords sheathed before the blood started to run.

We rode swiftly from camp, not knowing what we would find. The village was not far and the sun was barely beginning to close the day, giving us plenty of light, so I figured it would be easy to find Tamrin and Nadab. With Tamrin's fighting attitude and lack of experience, I wondered if we would even find him alive. Nadab was easy prey. He just followed along and would get killed just because he was there.

Sleeman had grown impatient, waiting to have some fun with his new opponent, so he threw some water on Tamrin, expecting him to get up and try to fight again. When Tamrin and Nadab finally regained consciousness, they realized that their swords, jambiyyas, and horses were all gone, and they were facing Sleeman and two of his bullies, who were almost the same size. Sleeman held his club, the man on the right was carrying a sheathed sword, and the one on the left carried a whip. Sleeman spoke with anger and glee in his voice at the same time, "You come on my land and accuse me of stealing with no evidence. Do you want to walk away—or die?"

Now fully aware of what was happening, Tamrin snarled, "You won't insult the Queen and live. Let me fight you in sword combat."

"Sure," Sleeman said. "Comrades, stay out of this. This young whelp thinks he's a great swordsman."

Tamrin boldly stated, "If I best you, you give us back our animals."

Sleeman yelled, "If you kill me, you can have everything, providing my comrades agree."

"This is between you and me, Sleeman." At that moment, it could go no other way.

Nadab was barely conscious with his head pounding unmercifully and blood slowly coagulating on the side of his head as it ran down his neck onto the ground, turning the dirt to mud where he lay. Nadab posed no threat so Sleeman turned his attention to Tamrin. He circled awkwardly to the right with his heavy frame that outweighed Tamrin by 20 kilos and stood 10 centimeters taller.

Tamrin was confident as he moved to his left with his smooth, quick, cat-like moves. But he totally misjudged Sleeman when he advanced, swinging his sword. Tamrin was shocked by his opponent's military skills but was quick to block blow after blow, even though he was unable to strike back. His head was still pounding and he felt sick to his stomach as Sleeman advanced aggressively with quick over and under strikes to Tamrin's body. Tamrin took a cut across his bicep and chest, which opened his thobe and drew blood.

Fear was overtaking Tamrin quickly and Sleeman could see it in his eyes. Tamrin knew that he had to kill now or be killed. Tamrin was weakening from the constant blocking of Sleeman's blows, and Sleeman was becoming overconfident and egotistical, thinking he had Tamrin beaten, while he enjoyed playing with him like a cat plays with a mouse before the kill. He was milking all the pleasure he could out of carving up this arrogant, young commander of the rich and powerful Queen of Sheba.

Nadab was trying to get to his feet. With blurred vision partly from the blood in his eyes, he shook as he pulled himself together and stood. Sleeman's men were guarding him, which really wasn't necessary since he was in no condition to fight. Sleeman glanced for a moment to see Nadab stand, giving Tamrin his chance. With a right back swing, he dropped to one knee and came up, catching Sleeman across the thigh, drawing good blood. Sleeman stumbled but caught his balance and came again at Tamrin, who was now regaining confidence.

By now Sleeman was a raging bull, and Tamrin knew he had better stay out of reach until the heavy bleeding brought Sleeman down. As the blood gushed from Sleeman's leg, he became more aggressive and ready to kill. Tamrin could see only two ways to beat him. He had to outlast him and stay out of Sleeman's reach, or he had to keep Sleeman moving fast in order to weaken him quicker, even though he felt himself weakening as well.

As I rounded the street corner with my men, near the stable we saw that Sleeman and his men had Tamrin at sword point and were about to run him through. Nadab was on his knees, struggling to stay conscious. The moment I saw the situation, I gave Sultan the signal, and he bolted into a full gallop and plowed into Sleeman and both of his men, knocking them to the ground.

Jona, Ibram, and Ahmad dismounted and had their swords drawn and at the men's throats before I got out of the saddle. As I stepped down, Mohamed walked up to the men, and I could see the rage in his eyes. With his fists, he hit both of Sleeman's men on top of their heads like a sledge hammer, knocking them unconscious, and then with a flax cord, tied them up. Jona had his sword under Sleeman's chin, pinning him to the stable wall, so if he opened his mouth, blood would run.

"Ibram, Ahmad, come with me." As we walked back to the second stable, two men were running across the pasture in the opposite direction. Stepping inside we saw the two camels and Nadab's grey horse. Ahmad spoke, "Captain, we should take two more camels for the misery he caused."

"Yes, you're right, but we found what is rightfully ours. Now I'll deal with Sleeman." As we came out of the back stable and walked around with the camels and horse, I turned to Sleeman and said, "Hmm — so these are yours?"

"Yes, of course, I paid good money for them."

"Did you check to make sure they were unmarked?"

"Of course, I did."

"Then you saw the ear mark on these two camels that identifies them as the Queen's, right? And did you see the 'S' in the front hoof of the grey?"

"Well, uh, I didn't see that."

"But Sleeman, you lied when you were asked about the camels and the horse," Tamrin said. "You refused to let us look at the animals in your stable, and then you attacked us."

"Sleeman, you know that the punishment is death for a camel or horse thief." He just stood there and didn't say a word. "You appear to be good with a sword, so I will let you defend your life on one condition. I am going to ask you a question, and if you have the right answer, you can go free, but if you do not, then you will face the sword of Ahmad."

Sleeman growled, "Go ahead. Ask your question."

Looking Sleeman in the eye, I asked, "What is the greatest power within the body?"

Sleeman was staring at the ground, and then lifting his head and looking around, he answered with a question, "How do I know if the answer I give will be right or wrong?"

"That's a fair question. The answer is already written by a great and wise king, and King David is not the answer." Sleeman was really struggling now more than before. Then he spoke, "Your mouth," he said. "If you don't eat, you die. If you eat, you live."

"Wrong answer, Sleeman. The answer is the tongue because it has the power of death and life in the words that it utters! Jona, give him his sword. Ahmad, this one is all yours. Spare his life only if you feel so inclined, but he shall not negotiate with another thief, sign another bargain for stolen stock, or listen to another offer."

Sleeman, even though weakened from the loss of blood, was certain that he could beat Ahmad. Ahmad looked like a simple herdsman and nothing more, but when he picked up his sword, he transformed into a puma on two legs.

Within seconds Sleeman lost his left ear and then his right one, which made his will to fight even more ferocious. But Ahmad's skill with his sword was masterful and beyond anything Sleeman had experienced. Ahmad's sword cut across Sleeman's face to the back of his mouth and slit out his tongue. Sleeman screamed as Ahmad's two swords together like scissors cut off Sleeman's fingers on both hands, causing his sword to drop to the ground. He ran inside the stable to the water tub, babbling like a baby.

I turned to Sleeman's two comrades, who were standing in disbelief and begging for their lives. "The penalty for stealing a camel is death," I said. "Find the other four camels and six horses and return them, and you may live; if not, you will surely die. In 13 days we will be in Makka. If you don't show up with our animals by that day, Ahmad will come back for you." Jona handed the first sword to one comrade, and I handed the second sword to the other comrade. As the men reached out to take their swords, Ahmad and Ibram swung swiftly, severing the men's fingers and part of the thumb off of one hand, leaving them screaming as they grabbed the cut hand with the good hand that was left.

Tamrin watched white faced and trembled in shock as we mounted to ride. Ahmad asked, "Captain, how do you know they will bring back our animals?"

"Because they are part of the band of thieves who stole them."

"How do you know?"

"It's simple. A man will not defend another man's lie for his own life. He will only fight to defend his own lies."

On the ride back, Tamrin finally broke the silence and said, "Captain, I owe you my life."

Without looking back at him, I said, "Tamrin, you are a fool. I didn't do it for you. You are not worth it. You could have recovered those animals, and there wasn't any sandstorm that covered their tracks. You are a liar like them, and you know what else, Tamrin? When a man will lie, he will eventually steal, if he hasn't already. I didn't do it for you; be clear on that." Tamrin and Nadab never spoke the rest of the way back.

When we reached camp, Queen Balkis was a bit shocked by what she saw. But from the look on her face, the shock gradually turned to disgust as Tamrin told the story. She looked at me with a bit of awe in her eyes and asked, "Captain, when will we move out?"

"At first light," I responded.

But then she gasped as she saw the gravity of the injuries of her two men and immediately sent for the priest, who came and began examining their wounds. As he washed away the coagulated blood from Nadab's head with lemon juice and grape wine mixed with some herbs, we could see that the incision went from above the temple and extended back behind his ear into the skull, which was definitely cracked.

I sent for Kaleb and Enos to bring some myrrh and frankincense resins and some cistus leaves. When they arrived, I had them put two pots of water on the fire, one for the resins and one for the cistus leaves to make a tea. I'm sure the priest felt we were interfering with his work, but since I had saved their lives and brought them back to camp, he didn't say anything.

While waiting for the resins to come to a boil, the priest cleaned and soaked not only Nadab's wounds but Tamrin's cuts as well, which were already infected. I had Kaleb take some of the resin water and add a few drops of balsam oil to put on the cuts, knowing this would quickly kill any infection.

While the priest was finishing, Kaleb mixed the myrrh oil with the paste that he had made from the myrrh resin, wrapped it with flax linen, and placed it on Tamrin's wounds. Enos packed Nadab's cuts with a paste of myrrh and frankincense mixed with balsam oil to repair the skull fracture. After their wounds were taken care of, Kaleb gave each of them two liters of cistus water with honey to drink to prevent blood clotting. When there was nothing more we could do, we returned to our camp, exhausted.

Several of the men were waiting to hear what happened. I looked at Kaleb and said, "This is not a time to tell you how we cut up three men for stealing and that they should have been put to death." I looked at Jona and shook my head, "I must be getting old. I just couldn't do it."

Jona put his hand on my shoulder, "No, my friend, you just let the human side of you come out this time. Letting them live will be a reminder for the rest of their lives of what they did."

"Jona, you're right. They were too slick for this to be the first time that they had stolen. They had a pretty good thing going."

Ahmad spoke, "Captain, do you think Sleeman will live?"

"Yes, unless he ends his own life." I instructed Kaleb to go and get a white goatskin and write on it 'Sleeman and his fingerless friends were caught stealing camels and horses.' "Tomorrow we will hang it on the tavern door as we go though. Sign it 'Captain Shutran, Commander of the Caravan of the Queen of Sheba.'"

Morning came quickly and I did not want to delay any longer. I sent Kaleb to check on our two wounded warriors. When he returned, I was pleased to hear that they were recovering well. Nadab never even had a headache, his vision was clear, and he was able to ride. Breakfast was finished, the campfires were out, and the camels were packed and ready. My heart swelled with gratitude for the outcome of the past event and for the dawning of a new day as I gave the order to move out.

While our caravan went through the village, the people were cheering, as everyone had already heard the story. The two men we had seen running away earlier had circled back, watched what had happened, and told the whole story to the villagers.

Four days later, in Thumala, we learned that for quite some time Sleeman and his gang of thieves had been stealing camels, horses, cows, goats, and anything else they could take and sell. No one could prove it and everyone in the village was scared because of his bullying threats and the beatings that some of the young men received who worked for him. Sleeman was never heard of again. The story went out that he was last seen wandering into the desert.

The first night out of Thumala as we were pulling packs and making fires, two of our scouts rode in with Sleeman's comrades leading the Queen's four camels and six horses. I sent Kaleb to get the Queen, who returned in her chariot with Nadab and her new commander, Ayaar. She had demoted Tamrin to be the personal attendant of her horses and chariot, which seemed to suit him well. She looked at me and asked, "What will be their punishment?"

"Queen Balkis, they stole your animals and were going to kill your men. Their fingers are severed on one hand, and they have returned the stolen animals. It is your decision."

"Put them to death," she yelled.

"Queen Balkis, may I offer one thought? It is true that the punishment for stealing a camel is death; however, in one moon no one will remember the deed or their deaths. But as long as they are alive, they will remind everyone not to steal from the Queen, and the young men will talk about that day at the stable in Tathlith for many years to come. Would that not have more meaning?"

Balkis turned to Ayaar and said, "Shutran is getting old and weak. What would you do, Ayaar?"

"I do not think Shutran is old and weak, perhaps just wiser from many years of experience. It is easy to kill a man for stealing, but it is not so easy to let him live. I agree with the Captain."

"So be it," she said as she turned and climbed into her chariot. "But I want them flogged for the pain they caused me. Bring them."

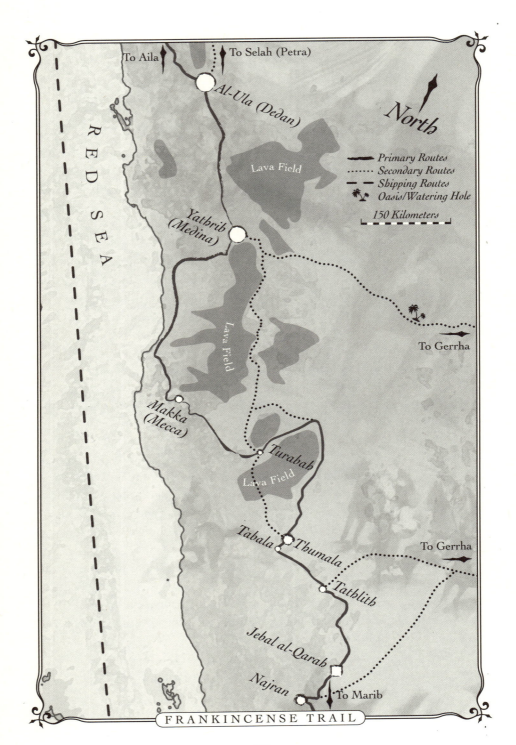

To Aila

To Selah (Petra)

Al-Ula (Dedan)

RED SEA

Lava Field

North

Primary Routes
Secondary Routes
Shipping Routes
Oasis/Watering Hole

150 Kilometers

Yatbrib
(Medina)

Lava Field

To Gerrha

Makka
(Mecca)

Turabah

Lava Field

Tabala Thumala

To Gerrha

Tathlith

Jebal al-Qarah

Najran

To Marib

FRANKINCENSE TRAIL

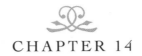

CHAPTER 14

Taming The Camel

When we reached the outskirts of Makka, we rested our caravan for four days to replenish our supplies and make any repairs needed for the next leg of the journey to Yathrib. While the caravan was circling and preparing to make camp, I rode up on a small hill to view our surroundings. I sat on Sultan, looking over the vastness of the valley as it sloped down from the mountains and out to the sea.

Kaleb came riding up and asked, "Papa, what are you doing?"

"Oh," I responded, a little startled, realizing that Kaleb had caught me daydreaming. "Son, is everything all right with the camp?"

"Yes, Papa." Again Kaleb questioned, "What are you doing?"

"Kaleb, the great prophet Abraham blessed this land and built the Ka'aba sanctuary in the village here, knowing that it would grow and become a great and rich city of the desert where millions of people would come and worship. The great Zamzam well could supply water to millions of people and irrigation for their crops.

The people would prosper and build a great city that would become a major crossroad for caravans coming in and out of Gerrha going to Marib, north to Jerusalem, east to Damascus, or even into Egypt. This growth will bring many changes that may or may not be for the better. It is sad when wealth and prosperity bring unhappiness and the downfall of a people."

"Why do you say that, Papa?"

"Time changes people and cultures, and the negative forces around us would have you fall away from God. You need discipline and commitment to stay your paths, but when you know in your heart what is right, then you must stand strong like the mighty cedars of Lebanon and not blow in the wind like the dust of the earth."

I was sure Kaleb was thinking about some of the things that he had seen since he had been with me. He had already experienced both the negative and positive at work on the caravan that would certainly help shape his destiny. Looking into the distance straight ahead as if to tell the whole world, I said, "Kaleb, I'm proud of you."

"Papa," Kaleb began.

"Yes," I said as I turned to look at him.

"Thank you for letting me come with you. I love the desert and the caravan, and I love being with you."

His words gave me such joy that I could hardly speak. We just sat there on our horses looking into the horizon as the light of the sun was gradually going out. I gave Sultan a gentle nudge, which was his signal to move, but before we headed down the hill, I smiled at Kaleb and said, "I love being with you, too. Let's ride to camp."

Not much was said around the fire as we were all eating. The fight with the camel thieves had been a terrible ordeal for those who had been there and had seen what happened. We all just wanted to put it behind us. The night was hot and we could feel the heat waves dancing out of the sand around us as we finished eating. The night was quiet except for the crackling of the fire. Suddenly, the braying of some of the camels broke the desert silence.

The sound must have triggered something with Kaleb as he had an inquisitive look on his face. Finally he asked, "Papa, are you ready to go to bed?"

"Well, that's a good thought. Why?"

"Well, I was wondering, when did they pack the first camel, and how did it start?"

"That question has a very interesting answer. There is a legend that has been passed down through our family for many generations about one of our great ancestors who packed the first camel. As I remember the story, it happened with a donkey train going from Marib to Makka."

"Papa, tell me the story."

"Well, let me think."

By now Jona and several of the men had gathered around and were eagerly waiting to hear, while my mind started meandering through the

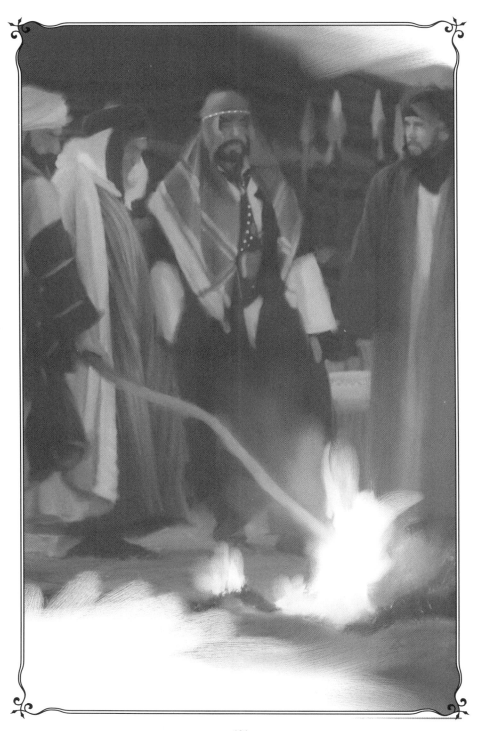

maze of stories told around the campfire in the evenings by my father. "Long before my time, maybe 1,400 years ago, our great ancestor, who we call Great-grandfather Abdul, was said to have been the first caravaner to pack the camel.

"My Grandfather Shutran, after whom I was named, had been a great caravaner for 50 years and had told many astounding stories about life on the caravans. My father grew up traveling with him and heard the stories many times. As my father, your Grandfather Shudulla, told the stories, the desire to be a caravaner like him was buried in my heart forever. I clung to his every word, not wanting to miss anything.

"Grandfather Shudulla said that for hundreds of years, the people believed the Rub al Khali was the home of a 'sand devil' that ate people, or that there was a vast, dark hole that swallowed up both camels and men alike who ventured to cross it, since no one ever returned. Yet, they believed the land of wealth lay beyond the treacherous Rub al Khali—the barrier that stopped civilization from entering our country. Except for a few small reed vessels driven by trade winds that landed on our shores more by accident than by purpose, we had little, if any, awareness of the world beyond.

"My father often heard Grandfather Shutran talk of the attempts he and several of his comrades had made to try to find enough water to make the crossing after the sandstorms were over. With the donkeys and mules, water was needed two to three times daily, forcing a small donkey caravan to travel along the shoreline, leaving them vulnerable to pirates.

"One of his greatest discussions around the campfire at night was the possibility of journeying several days without water, like a camel. They had heard about the new world beyond and thought about how much more a camel could carry than a donkey or mule. Then the story took on a new meaning when they started calculating the cost difference and the possibilities of earning more revenue from a larger payload. Even the unschooled could calculate denarii.

"Great-grandfather Abdul was resting his caravan for two days at a desert oasis to repair packs and pack saddles. While they were eating breakfast, the discussion came up again about the possibility of packing a camel. Great-grandfather Abdul always laughed, but this time when challenged by Fedaht, his second-in-command, he decided to try it.

"They were not going to travel until the next morning, so this was a good time. Nuka, one of the milking camels that was almost to the end of her producing years and would soon be table meat, seemed like a good camel for the experiment. Since she was an older milking camel, Great-grandfather felt she could probably stand long enough to have a pack saddle from a mule put on her back. She stood patiently as though she knew this was more her destiny than to be made into camel jerky for hungry caravaners.

"Everyone was curious and several of the men joined in on the experiment. The question was how to put a pack on, even if they succeeded in getting the saddle on her. The idea of standing on rocks seemed easy enough, except that she kept moving. Soon all the men in camp were getting involved with their different ideas. They started betting, which turned into an all-morning rival of wit versus camel intellect. After they discussed many ideas, it was decided to dig a pit for her to stand in, so part of the day was spent digging a trench so that she would be low enough for them to reach up and put on the pack—a feat achieved with great excitement and anticipation.

"Nuka walked down into the trench-like hole without any nudging. Everyone was very proud of their success, unsuspecting of what was about to happen. She seemed to almost enjoy the attention as two men on each side of her began to put the carpets on her back, trying to build a platform around the hump for the saddle. With the saddle and cinches on and tightened, every man cheered as the packs were fastened into place.

"Great-grandfather Abdul was proud of his masterful accomplishment and proclaimed to everyone that this would change the world and the way we lived. Little could anyone imagine the magnitude of what he was saying.

"The very accomplishment of putting a pack saddle on a camel with a pack weighing two to three times more than a pack put on a donkey or mule meant that now caravans could travel for three days in the intense heat of the summer and seven days when it was a bit cooler in the winter without stopping for water, opening the future to a vast new frontier.

"The next question was to find out if the camel could be led like the donkeys and mules. Even though Nuka had been milked for years and would follow them around like a wet-nursed calf, the answer to this question was yet unknown.

"Great-grandfather told Fedaht to lead her out of the pit, so he put a rope around her neck and looping it around her nose started to coach her forward out of the trench. She stood frozen in place, not sure how to respond to this unfamiliar feeling on her back. Some of the men moved up along her side and started pushing and encouraging her to walk forward.

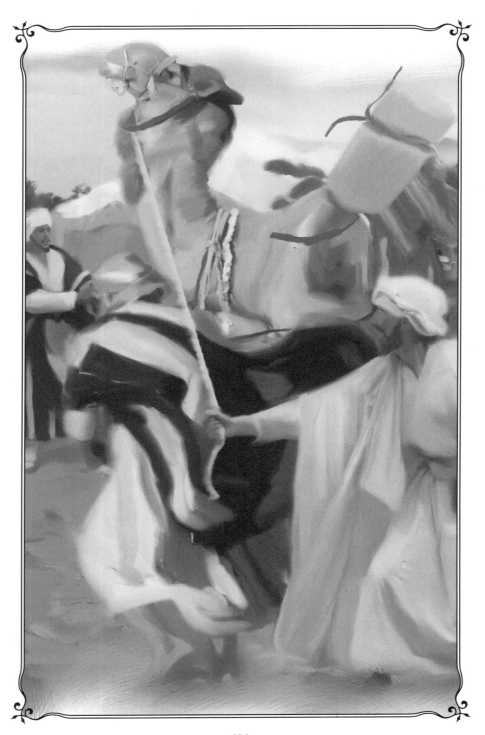

"When she took the first step and felt the cinches move, particularly the one near her udder, she ignited and came up out of the trench like an arrow piercing the night. She started kicking and bucking as though her intention was to land that pack load in the next wadi. Rijab, one of the caravaners, came running up to try to help Fedaht, who was barely able to stay ahead of her while running in a circle.

"It all happened so fast, and all Nuka was doing was trying to get that horrible thing off of her back that was attacking her. By now everyone was laughing and enjoying the action until they heard a scream and a crackling sound like a large, dry branch breaking. They looked to see Rijab go limp as one of Nuka's hoofs caught him just below the knee, snapping the bone like a twig and forcing it sideways through the skin.

"Several of the men rushed over to see what had happened. Poor Rijab was lying on the ground in extreme pain. Two of the men carried him back to camp, while Great-grandfather Abdul had two other men put two pots of water on the fire. One was to boil the frankincense resin, and the other was to boil the myrrh resin. One of the men pulled Rijab's leg straight, while another pushed the bone back through the skin and into place, causing him to lose consciousness for several minutes.

"The story goes on to say that while they were taking care of Rijab, Fedaht was still hanging onto Nuka and calling out commands like he would to one of his mules. Finally, his arms became so tired that he couldn't hold her any longer, and she pulled free, running and bucking everywhere. The packs came loose and Nuka scattered frankincense and myrrh resin for 500 meters across the hills."

By then Kaleb was laughing uncontrollably, and we were laughing as much at Kaleb as we were laughing while trying to imagine how it must have looked seeing all that resin go flying. In reality, it wouldn't have been fun, as none of us would want to be running around in the desert trying to find pieces of resin in the sand, but it sure sounded funny.

I waited for everyone, especially Kaleb, to get control of himself so that I could finish the story. "Fedaht and several of the other caravaners ran after her, trying to gather up the frankincense on their way. When they caught up to her, she was standing and shaking but starting to calm down as she realized there was nothing on her back that was going to hurt her. When Fedaht slowly approached her and softly commanded, 'huet, huet,' she unexpectedly knelt down and allowed the men to come near and reassemble the pack without any fuss.

"They led her back to camp and then hurried over to see what she had done to Rijab. Great-grandfather Abdul had the men scurrying to get the myrrh and frankincense ready for him. When the brown liquid from the myrrh cooled, Great-grandfather poured it into the open wound to kill any infection and start the tissue repair.

"Next, he made a poultice from the oily, white paste of the frankincense and packed it into the wound, covering a large area of the skin. They put a stick on each side of his leg and then wrapped it tightly so that the bone couldn't move. When Rijab regained consciousness, he had very little pain. His biggest concern would have been the possibility of infection, which could cause the loss of his leg.

"The legend says that because Rijab was hurt, the caravan had to stay camped until he was able to travel again, so Great-grandfather Abdul decided to have his men start training the other 20 milking camels to be led with packs on, like Nuka. What he thought would be lost time turned out to be a good opportunity to start preparing his little camel train.

"Great-grandfather had a unique attitude for his time. He never looked at difficulties as problems but as blessings cloaked in adversity. He believed that the greatest gifts come from self-discovery out of that adversity. Very few people ever seemed to grasp Great-grandfather's ideas, and yet those who did had success in their lives.

"Each day fresh myrrh and frankincense were boiled, and the dressing on Rijab's leg was changed morning and night. Great-grandfather said that frankincense was a gift from God and would heal both flesh and bone, while myrrh would cleanse the blood and prevent any 'evil deities' from entering the wound. In two weeks, Rijab was up and walking.

"The men remade the mule packs for the camels and had them ready to load. The camels responded without a problem, and even Nuka was ready to go. When the small caravan moved out, the packs that were on 20 mules and 45 donkeys were now on 10 camels.

"Everyone was greatly impressed with how easily the camels carried their heavy loads and how much faster they could travel, arriving in Marib several days ahead of their expected time. The donkeys and mules were able to keep up, since they were carrying very little, and after the last leg of the journey, Great-grandfather could see clearly that he now had little need for them.

"That must have been a great moment when they arrived in Marib. You can imagine the shock on people's faces. I'm sure they looked at the caravan in disbelief, and although some laughed, most were enthusiastically celebrating Great-grandfather Abdul's amazing accomplishment, one that most people never thought possible.

"He sold his donkeys and mules for a handsome profit and was able to buy 100 camels, most of which were young bulls with only a few cows. He had 16 of his men start to train them as the other men rested, traded goods, and took on more freight bound for Najran and Makka. He hired women in the city to make pack blankets and pack bags for the camels as well as halters and cinches made from hemp and coconut fibers and hired several men to pack the bags and blankets made from camel wool.

"I think the first camel caravan that rolled out of Marib must have been an unforgettable sight with all those camels carrying newly made blankets of different colors, breast collars, halters, and packs. It was said that it was the largest train to ever cross the mountains to Najran. People from all around the countryside must have come to see that new sight—the first camel caravan in history.

"Wouldn't all of you have liked to have been there and seen it?"

"I would have been the first," Jona quipped, "but let's hear the rest."

"When Great-grandfather Abdul first arrived in Marib, he had a simple pack train with 45 donkeys and 20 mules, which was a good achievement then.

"Great-grandfather Abdul became the owner of a pack supply station and a camel ranch, specializing in breeding, raising, and training camels for packing.

"Fedaht moved his wife and children from Shigum and stayed in Marib to oversee the camel training so that he could still work with Great-grandfather but not have to travel anymore with the caravan. I know some of his descendants who live in Marib who are still training camels. Sometimes when I am there, we visit and talk about the old stories.

"But let me finish this one. The word spread fast throughout the land, and everywhere Great-grandfather traveled, the people lined the streets and celebrated his arrival with food and festivities. It seemed that he became famous overnight, and his caravan grew from 120 camels on the first train to 250 camels on his return trip from Makka. A few years later he commanded three pack trains of over 300 camels each.

"It must have been exciting to think that the first caravan from Najran to Makka had taken 140 days, but with the camels, he had made the same trip in 72 days. With fewer animals, gear, and man-hours, the cost was greatly reduced, and with the camels able to carry bigger loads, the profit was greatly increased. Now, I would say, 'That's a good way to do business.'

"The villagers told how the owners of the mule and donkey trains laughed and said that it was too far to travel and that they knew it would never work. Some people said that Great-grandfather Abdul had been in the desert too long and that his mind had been burned up by the sun. Camels were not pack animals. They were for milk and meat.

"There was quite a big difference in price between the animals. At that time a camel cost 50 denarii, a donkey 125 denarii, and a mule 200 denarii. So when Great-grandfather sold all of his donkeys and mules, he made a great profit and was able to buy more camels, saddles, and packs.

"I can imagine how he must have felt with his new camel caravan, just knowing how I feel every time we come home with all the people waving and cheering. Men, just think about how you feel when the villagers celebrate our return. It's such an exhilarating time. Great-grandfather Abdul must have felt 2 meters tall when his caravan returned home 84 days later with 250 camels heavily laden with goods for market. What a great sight that must have been—a sight that changed the course of caravanning forever, and that's how the camel claimed its noble place in our world."

My men were still laughing about the camel story as they retold it in their own words. They would have been thrilled to be a part of that experience and have all the fun. It was late as they headed for their beds, but the chatter continued for a while as the campfire slowly burned down to ashes.

As we walked back to our tent, Kaleb kept asking questions, wanting to hear more, and Jona just shook his head and chuckled. As we closed our eyes, Kaleb still had the urge to laugh but contained himself, as we all needed to get some sleep.

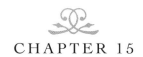

CHAPTER 15

Grandfather Azaad's Awakening

After resting for four days, it was time for the caravan to head for Yathrib. Many suggested that we take the old trail along the east side of the mountains. We would have less chance for any encounters with pirates, although it would take four to six days longer, and we would have to double back. The coastal route would be much easier for the wagons and chariots as well. It was 320 kilometers to Yathrib, and it would be faster and save a lot of time if we could avoid crossing the lava fields. The lava always caused so much damage to the animals' feet and would mean that we would have to make leather boots from camel brisket skins for them.

The second day out I repositioned the wagons of Queen Balkis to the rear of the caravan to reduce her exposure. However, she and her entourage had to deal with more dust. I had her men pull off all of the fancy embroidered work, ropes, and gold chains from the camels that she had insisted on putting on them. I didn't want anything to catch the sun and make a reflection. Her opulence and display of wealth never impressed anyone and just created disgust and resentment.

The first three days we stayed west of the lava fields and east of the shoreline, hoping that we would not be as visible to the sea pirates who would raid inland as far as a day's walk. By the fourth day I held the caravan until late afternoon before moving out and then traveled until the moon began to fade into morning light. This gave us only three hours of sun exposure where our dust could be seen. Once we crossed back into the mountains south of Yathrib, we could travel during the day again, which delighted everyone, especially the Queen.

The farther north we traveled, the less fanfare she would put on with her multiple tents for dining, bathing, lounging, and even socializing. That night as we camped in the mountains, the Queen's priest came over to inform me that he had an entire family down with dysentery, which included the grandfather, 7 sons, and 23 grandsons, who were all getting sicker by the hour. They had brought their caravan out of Taiz loaded with myrrh and joined us north of Marib. The priest was afraid it would spread to other camps, and the risk of death was high. I called to Kaleb, "Go find Enos and have him come."

The priest had four men, by order of the Queen, building an idol to make a sacrifice and worship in hopes of warding off this "evil deity." I said to the priest, "You need the real God to intervene, not your sun god."

He bristled in response, "What do you and your God know?"

"What I know is that the God I worship is my best friend and not some evil thing to fear and believe that He cursed you with a disease because you did something wrong. My God is the God of Abraham, Moses, and Solomon."

"I'll hear none of that foolishness," he snorted and turned to leave.

"Maybe not today," I challenged him, "but mark my words, before this caravan reaches its destination, you will see the miracles of my God!"

When Kaleb returned with Enos, I said, "Take three men and ride into the mountains. There you will find some springs, and along the edge of the water, gather the menthe and achillea, fill two sacks each, and bring them back. If you find any ruta, bring a sack of it as well. Remember, we bought some in the market in Najran." I mounted Sultan and rode over to see the Sabaean family from Taiz as they were setting up camp.

When I stepped inside the grandfather's tent, I found him lying on goatskin and sheep fleece, shaking with tremors from the fever and chills. I could see that his life force was slipping away and that the angels were close. I called him by name, "Azaad, can you hear me?" When he nodded his head, I continued. "Do you believe in the God of Abraham and Moses?" He shook his head *no*.

Three of Azaad's sons and four grandsons were there in the tent, also with fever and chills, although not as weak. They were listening and wondering, since it was an insult for one of a younger generation to have a different belief. "Azaad, do you believe that your sun god will save you?"

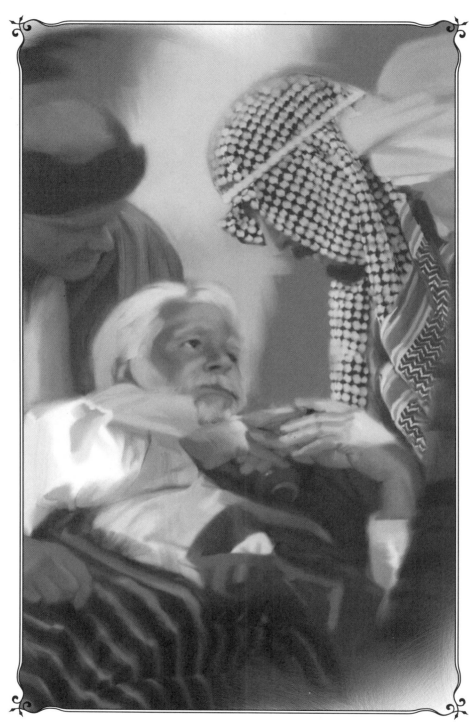

He responded with the same shake of the head as before.

"Azaad, I watched the God of Abraham and Moses, my God, heal my father's broken back after he fell down a muddy ravine and his camel rolled down, landing on top of him. I watched that same God direct me in saving my entire caravan in the Rub al Khali sandstorm. Azaad, you don't have to die. You have nothing to lose except your life, and that is soon to go. Azaad, look into my eyes."

The old man slowly turned his head to the sound of my voice, barely opening his eyes with all the strength he seemed to have. "Azaad, if you are willing, I will anoint your head with this luban that I believe my God provided for the healing of His children. If my God is not real, you will die and your children's children will know that the God of Abraham is not real. But if my God is real, you will be healed and will stand and walk and from this day be a witness that the God of Abraham lives."

He nodded his head in acceptance, so I took the vessel that hung around my neck that was filled with luban oil and poured a few drops on his head. At the same time, I asked the God of Heaven to heal Azaad and make him whole that he might become a mighty voice to teach his children about the One True God. As I ended my prayer, Azaad's fever broke, his stomach stopped heaving, the inflammation in his bowels quieted, and he rose to his feet. He raised his hand to the sky and cried, "Oh, mighty God of Abraham, Thou art real!"

"Now, Azaad, bless your children and heal them that they may stand with you," and I placed my oil vessel in his hand.

The priest was in the next tent chanting to the sun god Ra over Izeed, a second son. The guard was told by the priest not to let anyone in until he came out. Azaad walked towards his son's tent, but the guards would not let him pass. The priest was next in power to the Queen, and no one dared interrupt him.

The fires flickered in the early light of the moon, and as it climbed higher into the black sky, the priest came out of the tent and announced that the god Ra had taken Azaad's son. But as he stood there, he realized that Azaad and his other sons and grandsons were well, which brought a look of disbelief on his face, which quickly turned into one of amazement. Kaleb and Enos returned with the plants, which they steeped with the luban resin, and gave drink to all those in camp. The priest stayed out of my sight for the rest of the night. While the story of Azaad's conversion and healing spread quickly throughout the camp, many speculated that there would be a confrontation with the high priest.

When Kaleb, Jona, and I finally retired, Jona reached over to me and said, "Shutran, my friend, you certainly know how to stir up people."

"Jona," I said, "You know that until people feel pain or heavy sorrow for a deep cause, they don't know they are alive. Many just go through life as an uneventful experience and die with no conviction or commitment. They leave nothing of value behind that will improve or change another person's life for the better. They take no chance to do something different or investigate a different belief and discover something new. They are afraid of criticism and afraid of not being accepted simply because they have no identity and are only comfortable with another group or community or with someone they feel has the authority to tell them how they should think and feel.

"Jona, how can you know if you are alive unless you have tasted death on your lips? How can you know success when you have never experienced failure? How can you know loneliness when you have never been alone? How can you know who you are until you face adversity, destruction, loss, pain, ridicule, change, sickness, or separation? These experiences create the character, integrity, creativity, passion, and desire for adventure. These are all aspects of God, and only when you find them will you start finding God in yourself."

"Shutran, are you saying that God is within each of us?"

"Yes, His Spirit is within us, around us, and always with us. Ask those who know Him and they will tell you. Jona, ask!"

"Shutran, what I have seen this day with the Sabaean family I will never forget."

"I hope you don't, Jona, because that was God in action. Now, let's all get some sleep."

"You're right," Jona whispered as he lay his head down.

"Papa," Kaleb asked, "how do you know God is there? I mean, around us?"

"Kaleb, did you ever have a conversation with a friend without that friend being present?"

"No, Papa,"

"Well, God is the same. If you talk to Him, He will be present for the conversation."

"Thanks, Papa."

"Good night, Son."

Yathrib was a welcome stop for food and supplies. So far, things had been relatively peaceful. Tamrin was making an effort to win back his position by attempting to be respectful, even though it was an irritation to him. After resting for two days, making repairs, and acquiring new supplies, our next stop for food would be in Al-Ula, 275 kilometers and approximately 14 to 15 days from now.

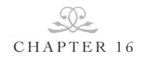

CHAPTER 16

A Reason to Live

At home, Mirah took Joshua and Armin and walked along the wadi leading down to the ocean. The three held hands as they walked, feeling the warm sand on their bare feet. Joshua looked up as he spoke, "Mama, you really miss Papa, don't you?"

Mirah choked back the tears that started to well up in her eyes. "Yes, Joshua, I surely do, and you?"

"Yes, I miss Papa playing with us, with Kaleb and me. I miss the wrestling and chasing and most of all Papa just holding me and telling me stories."

"Me, too," piped up Armin. "Do you think Papa is thinking about us? I mean, he's so busy."

"Armin, Papa thinks about us every day and every night," Mirah said, reassuring them.

"Do you think Kaleb misses us and thinks about us?" Joshua asked.

"I'm sure he does. Now, you need to know that when Kaleb returns, he will be all grown up. He will think and talk differently, and his voice will be a man's voice."

"Why, Mama?" Armin asked. "Why won't he come back the same?"

"It's because he will be almost two years older and will have the responsibilities of a man. He will not be the boy he was when he left. When he comes home, that might be difficult for you, both of you, because you are still children. Kaleb will see things that will change him. He will probably see and hear people lie, cheat, steal, kill, be killed, get sick, die, and may even help dig their graves. All of those things change a boy into a man really fast."

"Mama," Armin asked, "Will you know Kaleb when he returns?"

"Yes, of course, and I will feel his spirit. Your brother Kaleb is a wonderful boy with total love in his heart."

Then Joshua spoke up, "Kaleb loves me even when I beat up on him, doesn't he, Mama?"

"Yes, Joshua, even when he gets tired of you. Now, enough, you two are going to make me cry. I miss them so much at night that my heart hurts. Come, let's sit down in the sand and hold hands, and with our eyes closed, let's ask God to show us Papa and Kaleb so that we can know where they are and that all is well."

Within a few minutes Joshua said, "Mama, I can see them sitting by a fire talking."

Then Armin chimed in excitedly, "Mama, Mama, it's working! I saw them and then they went away."

Joshua interrupted, "Armin, they went away because you are making too much noise. Mama, tell her to be quiet."

"Joshua! Armin! Just listen very quietly and see if you can hear them talking." No one made a sound and only the big waves crashing on the beach broke the silence. Finally, Mirah stood up and took each child by the hand and started walking back towards the house.

On their way back, they met Samira walking by herself. Mirah asked her how Ahsein was doing. Samira said that he had been very sick and that he couldn't stop thinking about Nahor's death. With deep sadness in her eyes, she continued, "Nahor was everything to Ahsein. He tries with the other children, but his heart is not there. He really tried after Shutran talked with him, but it helped only for a short while; gradually, his pain has intensified. I am afraid that one day when I return home from market, he will be gone."

"Have you been burning luban at home?" Mirah asked.

"No, Mirah, I haven't—probably not for two months."

"Samira, you must start again. It will take the evil deities from his mind. If you need me to come and help, let me know. Perhaps I could go to the market for you."

"Mirah, thank you. You are so kind. How long has it been now since they left?"

With a faraway sound in her voice, Mirah responded, "Exactly four months and two days."

"Have you seen Salmah lately?" Samira questioned.

"Yes, I have. She is with child and when Jona returns, he will have a new baby. It will be such a surprise."

Samira's countenance brightened, "I'm going to go see if she needs any help."

Mirah suggested, "Why don't you take Ahsein with you? Perhaps it will lift his thoughts if he is able to be of help." The two women embraced before parting and bid each other a good night.

Mirah returned to the house, feeling exhausted and ready for bed. Joshua asked if he could make some tea. "Yes, that would be nice. Please make it for all of us," Mirah replied.

Armin look quizzically at Mirah, "Did you see Papa?"

"Yes, Armin, I saw him sitting by the fire talking about the day. Then he stood and went into the tent and laid down, putting his hands under his head as if looking into heaven. I heard his words in my mind as he said how much he and Kaleb miss us and that they are more than halfway to Jerusalem." After they drank their tea, Mirah took Joshua and Armin to her bed that night to sleep and held them tightly. "Just hold onto these precious moments," she said as they drifted off to sleep.

The next morning Joshua came running in all excited, "Mama, Kala is having trouble!"

"What's wrong?"

"She's trying to have her baby, and it won't come out. She's Papa's best breeding camel, and it will be terrible if something happens to her."

"Joshua, go get Mr. Ahsein and ask him to come and help. Hurry, run!" Mirah ran out to the stable where Kala was thrashing with pain. The baby camel was apparently breech and large. Mirah felt a little panic, since she couldn't hold Kala and help her at the same time.

Then Shutran's words came into her head. "Remember, when you need me, close your eyes and plead with God to bring me to you."

Mirah closed her eyes and cried, "God, please bring Shutran to me now; I need him and I need his help. Oh, God, please give Kala peace so she will lie still." No sooner had she spoken those words than Kala stopped kicking. Mirah tried to push the baby back in hopes of turning it, but the contractions were too strong and close together.

"Armin, run into the house and put one of the big bags of myrrh on to boil, one that's about 4 kilos. Hurry!" Mirah started to sing to Kala, which seemed to calm her down, slowing the contractions and making them less intense. She tried again to push the baby but with no success.

Closing her eyes she silently pleaded, "Shutran, what shall I do?" Then she heard his voice, "Mirah, all will be well. God will touch Ahsein's heart," who at that very moment was telling Joshua he couldn't do anything. Joshua watched him as his countenance changed, and even though he was shaking his head *no*, he stood up, grabbed some linen, and called to Samira to come with him as Mirah needed his help.

It was truly God's answer when Ahsein arrived as he was able to push the baby camel back and reach in to retrieve the other hind leg that was in a forward position preventing the delivery. He then helped Kala bring her baby into the world alive. Joshua ran to help Armin carry in the pot of myrrh water so that Mirah could coat the umbilical cord before the placenta was expelled, while Kala was licking and bonding with her new baby.

Mirah wrapped her arms around Ahsein with a big hug, thanking him over and over. "Ahsein had you not come, we would have lost both Kala and her baby, and you know Kala is Shutran's pride and joy."

Ahsein started to cry as he barely uttered, "Thank you, Mirah. God has changed my heart."

Now everyone was hugging and crying, not only because the new baby camel was out of danger and doing well but because Ahsein had come out of the black cloud he had been in for months. He stayed with Kala until she was strong enough to stand and then helped the baby get his first meal. Ahsein fell asleep in the stable with his arm stretched out over the baby, while Kala was sleeping all tangled up in legs.

As the night faded into the dawning of a new morning, Ahsein awoke with a new heart and again cried silently, thanking God for his deliverance from the shackles of the dark world. Samira came to the stable with hot tea and bread, which he enjoyed after helping little Ahsein feed, the name they had all decided to give the newborn, since they thought it was only right that he should bear the name of the man who saved his life.

Ahsein, now for the first time since Nahor's death, felt a zest for life rekindle in his heart, knowing that he had saved not just one life but two. By midmorning Ahsein had little Ahsein up on his wobbly legs and sucking lunch by himself. Ahsein felt such a bond and duty that he never left the stable until the next day after he felt assured that the new little one was doing well and could make it on his own and that Kala was eating and doing well herself.

When he walked into his home, he grabbed his children and cried again, realizing how much he needed them and was needed. From that day forth, Ahsein, at the end of his daily labors as a brick maker, would go visit all his neighbors to see who needed help or who was ill, desiring to assist them in any way possible.

The news traveled throughout the community about how Ahsein facilitated a breech birth, and before long he was asked to help deliver another baby camel, then a goat, and then a colt; soon it seemed that Ahsein had found a new path in life. He grew to love the animals like his own children, and many baby goats and sheep followed him around just like they did their mother. His own children were with him wherever he went, and his home became a happy place again.

Many weeks later Mirah asked Samira what happened. "What changed him? He said, 'No,' when Joshua went to ask him if he would come and help."

Samira said that when she finally felt safe to ask him, he said that he saw Nahor standing in front of him, who said, "Papa, go. You are needed. The baby will die if you don't help."

"Mirah, I don't know if he was imagining it, but that is what he believes. I really don't know if he did or did not see Nahor, but he certainly had a change of heart."

Mirah spoke softly, "Samira, I believe that he did see Nahor and that God used the birth of the baby camel to help Ahsein, because saving the lives of these two animals was powerful enough to take Ahsein's pain away, and I could not have saved them by myself. God always wants to do what's best for us. We will never know exactly what happened, but thankfully you have him back, and Shutran has a beautiful male camel and will be so happy with both."

Later Mirah, Salmah, their children, and some of the others from the village went to the mountains to harvest some luban. Salmah, speaking to Mirah, asked, "Is it because I am carrying Jona's new baby that I miss him so much, or is it just different this time?"

"Salmah, it is different for me, too."

"Do you feel sometimes Shutran isn't coming home?"

"Yes, Salmah. I continually have to push those thoughts out of my mind, because in my heart, I know that he will come home. But you are right. There is something different this time. Perhaps it is because they are going to be gone longer."

"Yes, I suppose that could be it," Salmah responded. "You know, it is a feeling like something is going to happen. But where? With us, our men, or the caravan? We can only trust that God will protect them and bring them home to us."

Mirah was quiet for a moment just looking at the ground and stirring up a little dirt with her right foot as she pondered what had been said. Then she looked into Salmah's face and with much concern spoke, "Salmah, you have to put your mind to other thoughts, or the baby will feel there is something wrong and may not want to come into this world."

"Mirah, how can that be?"

"A wise man once said that whatever we think, will happen. If our thoughts can be so strong, maybe the baby will feel it also, and it might have a bad effect.

"Salmah, remember when they were caught in the sandstorm that took Nahor's life? Remember how Samira was so sure something was going to happen, even before they left? Well, I remember one of the prophets saying that the very thing you fear will come upon you. Salmah, please think only the best thoughts. We have to do our part to help protect them. I am sure it is hard for Jona and Shutran to be gone, and I am sure they have their own demons to deal with besides all the caravan problems."

"Mirah, at least they have something to occupy their minds."

"Then, Salmah, you must get something to occupy your mind like Ahsein did. You used to make the most beautiful goat-hair rugs. Why don't you do that now?"

"Oh, I have just become too busy with the children and am too tired."

"Well, then, let's do it together."

"Yes, of course, but where shall we do it?"

"Salmah, I will come to your house. Then you can be there for your children. My children are older and I can come over more easily."

Mirah was a godsend for Salmah like Ahsein was to Kala. The weeks passed into months, and Mirah and Salmah made several rugs with goat and camel hair and sold them in the market. But Salmah could not quit talking about something bad that was going to happen, no matter how much Mirah tried to help her change her thoughts and stay positive. She kept going back to that same bad feeling.

That night Mirah and the children were holding hands again as they sat on the beach running the warm sand through their toes. The gentle breeze was refreshing as it caressed their faces. Their thoughts were with Shutran and Kaleb, and they pondered their separation in the quietness under the stars that twinkled brightly. They could feel their father's presence, which was comforting but yet intensified their longing. They prayed for Papa and Kaleb and were certain that they would feel their message of love and know that they were in their thoughts so far away at home.

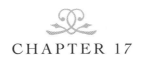

CHAPTER 17

The Black
Scorpion Strikes

I was sitting near the campfire and could feel Mirah's presence so strongly that I moved away from the fire to be alone. I went into my tent and laid down on the sheepskin bed, putting my hands behind my head while staring upward. The presence of Mirah and the children was so strong that I could smell the cistus and jasmine water that Mirah used to rinse her and the children's hair with before going to bed. I looked over at Kaleb, who had long since fallen asleep.

My promise to bring Kaleb home safely weighed heavily on my heart. The feeling overtook me as I reached over and put my hand on Kaleb's shoulder. Again, the picture of my family at home came into my mind, and the tears welled up in my eyes as I watched them in my mind walking on the beach until I drifted off into an exhausted sleep.

When the caravan rolled out of Al-Ula, it swung west away from the large lava fields. The village people said that the north trail was bad because the water from the monsoon rains had made it impossible to get the wagons through the pass. They said it would be best to stay on the west side of the mountains. As I sat on Sultan watching the caravan pass by, I made mental notes of how things appeared. I felt a change in the air that I didn't like and was trying to determine the reason.

The supply wagons, chariots, and loaded camels moved with ease and showed no signs of fatigue. The caravaners were walking well, and the sentries were riding ahead and watching for the best location to cross the wadi and the dunes and for any possible problems. All appeared peaceful, but that gnawing feeling in my stomach told me something was coming.

We had traveled for three days, and everything was fine. Still no problems and those who had been bedridden with dysentery were recovering and regaining their energy. Why did I have that sick feeling inside that kept nagging at me? That night I doubled the guard duty and pulled Kaleb off. He wasn't happy with me, so I told him I wasn't feeling well and might need his help during the night, which made it all right.

Shortly after the cook fires burned down and everyone had retired, we were startled by a woman's bloodcurdling scream that pierced the night like a flaming arrow. It seemed to come from a tent near some rocks that was shared by four of the Queen's servants. The ladies could not have known that as the night air grew cooler, the predators that lived under the rocks went visiting in search of a warmer place to sleep. The four heat-producing bodies were very inviting to these night visitors that crawled into the fleece blankets to snuggle closer to the heat source, not expecting their new bed partners to turn and lay on them.

The black Arabian Fattail scorpion did not like being disturbed in his sleep and protested violently with a deadly injection from his stinger into his victim. When the first lady screamed, the other ladies startled awake, wondering what happened. As they scrambled to get out of bed, the rest of the scorpion family quickly came awake, striking out to give the same punishment to the other three ladies, who had disturbed them in their newly found warmth.

Khadija, the Queen's masseuse, was stung three times on the left side of her back near her armpit. Tamahrah, the hairdresser, was stung on her foot. Laahruht, the second hairdresser, was stung on the ankle, and Kharehn, the Queen's wardrobe mistress, was stung on her hip.

When I arrived at the tent, many people had gathered around, and Kharehn, Tamahrah, and Laahruht were lying outside on their robes shaking and crying. Kharehn was having mild convulsions. Four of the Queen's soldiers were holding torches to help. Ayaar, the Queen's latest in command, came running up and asked what all the screaming was about. The Queen was upset that she had been awakened and wanted everyone to stop the noise immediately and be quiet.

I turned to Ayaar and forcefully said, "There is only one person who needs to be quiet, and that's you. We have three women in severe pain and who appear to have been stung by black scorpions."

One of the guards spoke up, "Captain Shutran, four women slept in that tent," pointing to the tent on his left. The tent was open so he went in and

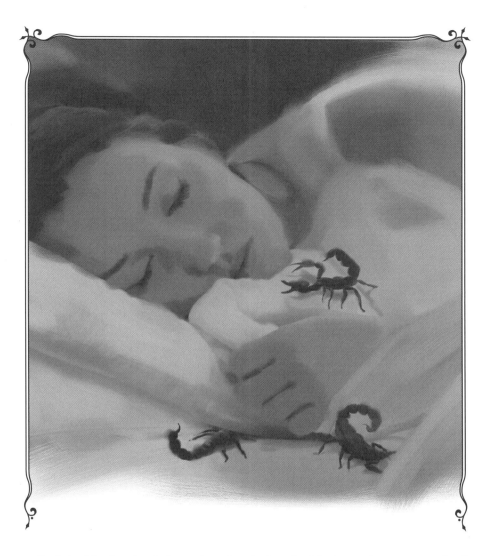

pulled the blanket back from the other lady. The black predator scurried off of Khadija's paralyzed body and disappeared into the rugs. When I went in to look, as soon as I saw her, I knew she was already dead.

Kaleb and Enos came with pots of hot myrrh, cassia, and spikenard and began applying the oils to the injection sites. The women were already running fevers. Enos was helping them to drink the water with the oils that had been made earlier to stop the dysentery. This would help increase their body fluids to dilute the venom. Kaleb rubbed frankincense on their feet, and Nadab brought more blankets. Ayaar stood outside listening until he knew enough of what was happening and left, most likely to give Queen Balkis a report. I handed the guard the torch as I stepped out of the tent. "The black death," I said, as many eyes were questioning.

Everyone knew that a single sting from a black scorpion in the right place was usually fatal. Many Bedouins died every year from their sting. Khadija had been stung three times, once very near to her heart.

The Queen finally showed up with Ayaar and Tamrin. She wasn't concerned about Khadija. Her only question was what we were going to do now.

I looked straight at her and raised my voice so that everyone could hear me, "Tomorrow the caravan will not move until Khadija is buried and every person has gone through blankets and clothing to make sure we do not leave here with more of our deadly friends. Separate your bedding with sticks and check before you lie back down tonight. It appears that the tent was visited by a whole family of scorpions.

"Ayaar, have your servants get a couple of sheepskins for the ladies to lie on over in the Queen's tent that she uses to receive her visitors." Turning to the Queen, I said, "Queen Balkis, I am sure you won't mind, will you?" She never answered but just glared at me and then turned and went back to her tent.

We didn't move the ladies until they were a little more stable and had calmed down and stopped crying. They were frightened and shocked. Khadija was a dear friend, and the ladies had all become very close over the weeks on the trail.

The mixture of myrrh, spikenard, and cassia had stopped the action of the venom, preventing any paralysis. The swelling was receding and the women were now out of pain. They seemed to feel all right to be walked over to their temporary tent. Kaleb and Enos stayed with them through the night, keeping them hydrated and giving reassurance that they were safe and that all was well. Many of the people did not return to their beds out of fear of what they had just seen.

Seven scorpions were found in Khadija's tent the next morning as it was being removed after her burial had been completed. When all the tents and bedding had been checked, 17 scorpions had been found and killed. After four and a half months on the trail and only three deaths, I still felt we had been blessed.

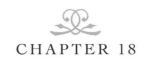

CHAPTER 18

Hagban—
A Fight to the Death

I wondered if the feeling that I had had for the past three days would leave now. I asked Kaleb and Enos to send word to all my captains, including those from the Sabaean caravan, to come to my camp. Everyone had gathered and finally Queen Balkis arrived with Ayaar and Tamrin, demanding to know what the summons was all about. "Queen Balkis, this is all about your safety. Any more questions?" She was silent.

"Comrades, I have carried a feeling of warning with me for three days. I have doubled the guard duty at night, as you know. After Khadija's death I thought that the feeling would leave, but it hasn't. Tomorrow I will take four scouts with me to look for a wadi to take us back through the mountains to the desert. I feel we are increasing our risk if we stay by the sea."

Ayaar spoke up, "Captain, the terrain here is much easier, and we are making better time. It is also easier for the Queen's wagons and her personal chariot."

"Yes, I agree. But I have been thinking about how some of the people in the village encouraged us to go this way and were almost too happy when we changed our direction and followed their suggestion. Do you remember?"

Grandfather Azaad stepped forward, "Yes, Captain, I remember. They seemed eager to help and overly friendly."

The priest spoke up, "That's ridiculous. I found them to be very hospitable people, who were just trying to help."

Tamrin added, "I think they were concerned for our Queen and wanted her to have an easier journey."

Mahmoud, another caravan captain who had joined us in Marib, spoke up, "If we turn back through the mountains, we will have to cross the lava fields. It will be hard on our animals as well as on those walking. The sharp lava could cripple some of our animals."

"Yes," I said. "That is a strong possibility."

Queen Balkis sarcastically asked, "Captain Shutran, what are you afraid of? Don't you believe your God will protect you?"

"Yes, but only if I listen. We are near the place where the sea narrows and divides the water to the west and to the east. On the west side, near the narrow water, Necho II opened a waterway for reed vessels to enter the Nile perhaps 300 to 400 years ago. I have heard stories of the water around the canal being filled with pirates who raid inland as well as on the seas."

"Captain Shutran, are you going to make us walk through sharp lava because of some campfire tale?" the Queen jeered with a cynical smile.

Kaleb was standing beside Seth, taking it all in, no doubt remembering what I had said about standing strong when you know you are right, regardless of what everyone is saying at the time. I couldn't help but smile inside and wonder, "God, are you trying to make a point here for Kaleb?"

All of the caravan captains started debating with each other. No one wanted to leave the comfort of the easy, flat sand of the coastal plain that stretched farther than the eye could see. While everyone was engaged in conversation, I disconnected myself from their noise and went into the feeling I had. I knew God put that feeling there, and I needed to decide how I was going to act upon it. If I listened to Him, I would be blessed and protected. If I didn't, I would be on my own for the experience of what lay ahead.

I realized that I would deal with ridicule, regardless of my decision. The question was which ridicule would last the longest, and then the next time when I needed God's counsel, would He be there if I ignored Him now? I remembered my father saying years ago, "Son, sometimes the easiest decision is not the best." Of course, the easiest would be to stay on the coast.

Finally, Ayaar said, "Captain, what do you fear?"

"Ayaar, for me, nothing! But for the caravan and those traveling with it, it is different. If a group of desert brigands and sea pirates join together, we could lose the caravan and many lives."

"Do you think that could happen?"

"Yes, I do."

"But, Captain, there are nearly 1,700 of us."

"You are right, Captain Ayaar. But how many are trained in combat and are master archers and swordsmen—10 to 20 at best? We have women and young men. Three to four hundred raiders could take this caravan easily. Captain Ayaar, do you know what a sea pirate would do to a woman like the Queen or much worse to a servant?"

Balkis was now listening quite intensely. "Captain Shutran, if they know we are coming and are waiting for us and we don't show up, don't you think they will follow us?"

"Yes, I am sure of that, but then it would be on our terms, not theirs."

Jona stepped forward and spoke, "I think we need to hear what the Captain has to say before we make a decision." Silence spread over the camp, acknowledging the request.

"Tomorrow I will send three of the scouts to ride two days ahead of the caravan to look for signs of trouble, while we look for a wadi where we can cross over before reaching Shaghb. If we don't find a wadi, we will turn the caravan east and travel towards the lava fields until we do find one where we can pass through to the other side. Then we can travel east of the dunes until we reach Tabuk. This will add only three to four more days to our journey."

Mahmoud spoke up again, "Captain, if your son were not with us, would you be more willing to stay on the plain?"

"No," I answered without any explanation.

A captain from another caravan came forward wanting to be recognized and said, "My name is Hagban and I think we should take a vote. I think Captain Shutran is getting old and prays too much to his imaginary God of Abraham. Wasn't Abraham the one who sacrificed his own son? Come now, people, are we going to listen to any more of this and waste our time?"

Jona moved to shut him up, but I grabbed him while shaking my head. "No," I said, "let's hear him out." Jona shook his head in disgust and stepped back.

Hagban went on, "I think we should stay on the coastal plain. We'll be in the red rock city of Selah in about 20 days. If we go east into the lava fields, we could add another week or more." Hagban had everyone's attention and they were nodding in agreement. "Come on," he hollered, "let's vote."

I spoke again, "Hagban, is another week a terrible price to pay for the lives of all these people? You can vote, but the real question should be, can you fight?" You could hear a pin drop as the air became still.

"Hagban is pushing to vote and many of you want to stay the easy course. I looked sternly at him and called, "Hagban, come over here. Jona, take this camel blanket out 100 meters and hang it on that nard bush. Kaleb, hand me that bow and quiver," which I passed over to Hagban. "Put your arrow through the hole that's in the blanket."

"I can hardly see it," he said.

"Yes, and you might not see the enemy, either." Hagban was nervous. He was not an archer and he missed the blanket. He handed me the bow. I easily placed the arrow in the hole, and turning to Ayaar, I said, "Now you place your arrow." He also missed and handed the bow to Mahmoud, who missed as well. He didn't even come near the hole.

I stepped forward with my arm stretched towards those listening and called, "Now is the time to see who will defend the caravan."

Hagban said, "I am not an archer, but a swordsman." I drew my sword and spun while at the same time cutting the leather string that held his jambiyya and opened his thobe to his chin without drawing blood, and he hadn't even touched his sword.

Looking him in the eye, I roared, "Hagban, you are dead."

I turned to the crowd and yelled, "Now you can all choose to follow Hagban, who can't defend you, or an old man like me, who can and who also has an 'imaginary' God who can protect you." As I sheathed my sword with my eyes still on Hagban, I raised my voice and gave the command, "We move out at first light," and then walked away, with Jona, Kaleb, Enos, Seth, and Alimud right behind me.

Jona spoke, "Well, Captain, you certainly know how to make enemies. Now I have to add Hagban to the list of those to watch."

A few minutes later Balkis rode up in her chariot to where we were about to begin repairs on some pack saddles. "Very impressive, Shutran. But I have a question. Do you think you could take Hagban in hand-to-hand combat? We might see something different."

"You might," I responded. "You may think he could best me, and I haven't seen his hand skills."

"Don't you think you should?"

"Queen Balkis, think about it. By the time the enemy came close enough for hand-to-hand battle, Hagban would likely be dead."

"Yes," she said, "but different people have different strengths."

"You're right," I replied.

She continued, "Just because he is not a good archer or swordsman, you don't think he could lead the caravan, even though his strength might be in his hands."

"Do you think that alone would qualify him to lead the caravan?"

"No," she retorted, "but I think it qualifies him to question your decision."

"Pardon me, oh Queen, but you are like a myrrh thorn in a pack saddle blanket." As we bantered back and forth, Ayaar came riding up with Hagban, followed by many others from camp.

Jona looked up and shook his head, "Here we go again."

Kaleb was lacing a pack pad and stood up to see what was happening. "Papa, what is going on?"

"Well, Son, I guess we haven't had enough entertainment yet today, and our good Queen wants to make sure that everyone has sufficient."

Queen Balkis was in her element pitting people against each other. She spoke up, "Now, Shutran, if Hagban bests you, would you say he is strong enough to lead the caravan?"

"No, Queen Balkis. It takes a lot more than being a street bully."

"But would you listen to his opinion?"

"I always listen when something of value is spoken. So far, I haven't heard anything of value except the desire to create contention and separation. But if you are looking for a fight, and if that will please you, then let's get on with it as I have work to do."

Jona leaned over to me and whispered, "What are you thinking? Hagban is 25 years younger than you and 25 or 30 kilos heavier. I've heard around the camp that he is a brawler and has never been beaten."

"Well, Jona, I guess it's time for him to have a new experience."

"Shutran, you're not even listening. If this man gets his arms around you, he'll crush you to death."

"Jona, you sound like you have little faith in this old man!" I looked at Jona sideways and winked and nodded towards Kaleb, who was listening.

Jona understood immediately and changed his tune. "Ah, Captain, I just had to give you a bad time. In reality, I really feel sorry for that big boy. He doesn't know who he's dealing with this time."

I saw the expression on Kaleb's face change as the tension went out, and he relaxed as Jona spoke. The men and a few of the Queen's servants were trying to get into a good position to watch. I thought, "How sad that people get more excited over a fight, death, pain, and war than they get by knowing God." I realized that what Jona said was true and knew this was not a fight of strength. For me, there was no question about his strength. He could easily best me. This was going to be a fight of wit and skill for me. Hagban was counting only on his strength.

I knew I had to position myself for the first blow and the change that would come after the first hit. Moving over by the cook fire to get a drink and take off my jambiyya, I looked on the ground for an equalizer, like a right-sized stone that could bring balance to this unfair fight. Hagban dropped his jambiyya and moved in closer to engage. I looked up at him, a head taller than me. He made me look small. His eyes were glistening with easy anticipation of a quick conquest. I said, "Hagban, do you wish to settle this discussion a different way?"

"No," he retorted. "You made a fool out of me with your bow and sword. Now I will make ground meat out of you."

As we circled to where I wanted him, I said, "Hagban, I have another question. Are you ready to be made a fool of again?"

"No!" he yelled.

"Well, then, you should go back to your camp before it happens."

Rage visibly overtook him. "This is good," I said to myself. "He who angers you, conquers you. One more jabbing statement and I'll be ready," I thought as I moved into my final position. "Hagban, is it true what they say about you?"

"What?"

"That you've never been able to make it with a woman?" As I said it, I clipped him lightly with a left hook on the cheek. With blood in his eyes, he charged forward, expecting to get his crushing arms around me.

I dropped fast to one knee as he lunged, tripping him flat out into the cooking fire and driving his head into the terra cotta cooking pot, smashing it and dumping the goat stew all over him. His thobe caught on fire as he lay stunned for a moment. Then shaking, he came up out of the fire like a raging bull, slapping at the flames until they were out. Then standing in front of me with both fists clenched, he yelled, "Come on! Come on!"

The people were laughing and cheering him on. I said, "Hagban, I think you have made a big enough fool of yourself." I had grabbed a stone that was on the ground when I was down on my knee, an elongated, smooth stone that fit perfectly in the palm of my left hand to use as my "equalizer." Wrapping my fingers around it, I knew it would keep me from getting any of my fingers broken. "Come on, Hagban; let's end this foolishness."

"No!" he yelled again. "Come on!" I reached my right hand out to shake his hand, which infuriated him even more. As he swung to knock my hand out of the way, I threw a left hook with all my weight behind me, smashing my fist that clenched the stone across his right eye and parting the skin on his eyebrow like a meat cleaver. Even though the blood gushed out, blinding him, he came at me swinging and grappling like a crazy man. I came up with a right hook to his gut, stopping his forward movement, but with no other effect. It was like hitting the side of a camel.

As I spun away and kept moving to his right, I landed another right hook to his nose. The blood squirted but that never slowed him down. He kept coming with his huge arms like giant clubs that never stopped swinging. As I ducked, waiting for an opening to his left eye, he clipped the side of my head, knocking me to the ground. Dazed, I started immediately crawling to find a space to get back on my feet. I knew I had to get up fast, but then I felt his kick bounce off my hip into my side, throwing me into the crowd.

I grabbed someone's thobe and pulled myself up and around behind him just as Hagban hit the man, knocking him unconscious. It bought me enough time to get away from him and move back around into the camp circle while catching my breath. I knew I couldn't make another mistake. This wasn't a fight any more. This was a death duel for Hagban. He had one plan and that was to kill me.

This was the first time Hagban had tasted his own blood, which made him act crazy as if he had lost his mind. He came through the crowd after me as I moved into the open. Kaleb grabbed Jona. "Jona, please stop it. He'll kill Papa; please, Jona."

"Kaleb, what did your father teach you? Believe in your God and believe in your father."

"But, Jona. . . ."

"If I stop the fight, it would disgrace your father. He would rather die."

I punched Hagban in the nose and in the eye again to keep the blood running. His right eye was swollen completely closed. I continued to hit and move fast. I knew my game, knowing I had to strike his left eye. I took a chance to get closer but took another blow to the side of the head that put me on the ground again. I rolled and rolled to gain distance so that I could get up.

Hagban was almost leaning over me as I rose up from my knees. I knew it was now or never, and I swung with all that was left in me, hitting my mark. The blood squirted from his left eye, blinding him as it ran down his face, disorienting him for a moment and giving me the chance to move away and breathe again. My head was pounding and it felt like I had been kicked by a mule.

Hagban came swinging blindly, but I sidestepped him and hit his left eye again. Just then I felt someone grab me from behind and yell, "Hagban, here."

As I tried to push away the two men who were standing behind me, I heard Jona yell, "No!" as they shoved me into Hagban.

As he grappled his arms around me, picking me up and shaking me like a rag, I heard my ribs break. I knew he would squeeze me until I couldn't breathe. As my ribs were breaking, I cried out, "Oh, God, deliver me!" I raised both of my hands while cupping them and then came down as hard as I could over both of Hagban's ears. He shrieked in pain and dropped me as both eardrums exploded.

I tried to move away, feeling that I was going to lose consciousness. I saw Mirah's face and then Armin's and Joshua's and then heard Kaleb screaming, "Papa." I was still backing up, trying to stay conscious and put more distance between me and Hagban, who was yelling, screaming, and floundering, looking for me.

The spectators wanted death and were chanting my position so that Hagban could find me. He kept moving as the crowd directed him to the right or the left. But I kept moving in circles, trying to find an opening in the crowd. Kaleb yelled, "Papa, over here," as some of my men were trying to break the crowd open. Hagban could still see enough from the left eye and kept coming after me.

I was weakening and knew it. I cried, "God, I didn't ask for this. Give me the strength to end it." I suddenly felt my head clear, and the power of renewed strength flowed over me. I stopped for a second and then went straight at Hagban, which took him by surprise, and I ducked his swing as he tried to hit me. He recoiled and then started to lunge toward me again.

I came up with a half-open fist, driving my knuckles into his throat and shattering his Adam's apple. As he dropped his head, I cross-chopped the bridge of his nose and then planted a left uppercut with the palm of my hand squarely on the front of his nose, driving the bone into his brain. His knees shook and he stopped in his tracks, falling backwards to the ground. The laughing and cheering stopped immediately, and the crowd went silent while staring in wonder at what they had just seen.

Kaleb's voice was all I could hear as he ran over to me in a panic. "Papa, Papa, you're hurt." I sensed that Jona, Seth, Ibram, and Enos had also reached me.

As we started to walk away, with one of my men under each arm holding me up, I caught the staring eye of the Queen. I looked over to the crowd where I had been pushed and said, "You might break my ribs, but not as fast as my God can heal me."

Turning back to the Queen and Ayaar, I said, "The caravan moves out at first light. Do you have any questions?"

With a flustered look of defeat on her face, she stammered, "No, Captain," as I turned and walked away.

As the crowd parted, letting me pass, there stood Grandfather Azaad. "Captain Shutran, God heard you, as I did, and He delivered you."

"Yes, Azaad, He did!" I barely made it to my tent with the help of Jona and Seth, as Kaleb parted the way through the spectators. Several of my men had gathered at the tent to help.

Jona spoke, "Shutran, you can't ride tomorrow."

"Yes, I can and I will. Kaleb, fetch the frankincense, myrrh, balsam, and spikenard and help rub it on me. Tomorrow will be a long day."

When Jona and I rode out of camp with the scouts early the next morning, I gave Kaleb the charge to lead the caravan out one hour later. At first light Tamrin rode up to Kaleb, not knowing where I was but wanting to inform the Queen and asked, "Where is the Captain? Is he staying behind until he heals?"

Kaleb turned in the saddle and asked, "Healed from what? The Captain left over an hour ago with the scouts." Tamrin's face became sober as he turned and rode back to the Queen's wagon. Kaleb swung his arm over his head and with a great motion of triumph signaled the caravan to move out.

At the end of the day as the sun had just about disappeared into the sandy, desert floor, I returned with Jona and the scouts as the camp was being prepared for the evening. I called my captains together to inquire about our scouts who went northwest. Only two of the three had returned. Musilum spoke up, "We found an old wadi that runs through a narrow strip of the lava bed that would cut off the distance of maybe 15 kilometers and get us away quicker from the coastal plains."

Two of my scouts, Musilum and Hussin, described what they had found of a caravan that had been raided maybe six months ago. Apparently, not many men had been killed, since the scouts found the remains of only a few men and camels. The rest must have been taken as slaves. All the tracks headed toward the coast, not inland.

"Where is Zenith?"

"We separated to cover more ground, but he never met up with us as planned. We waited until morning and then felt we should get back with the report. One thing is for sure, a caravan this size doesn't move without everybody talking about it, especially being the Queen's caravan with all of the wealth and merchandise."

Seth spoke up, "Captain, remember when Sabah rode off in the middle of the night to give our location to the brigands?"

"Yes, I was just thinking about that, and maybe Zenith is walking that same, dark path. It wouldn't be the first time someone on the caravan turned traitor." Turning to the scouts, I asked, "Can you tell me how many you think were in the raiding party?"

"Well, the caravan was small, with maybe 300 camels, and they were apparently easily overtaken. Not much sign of them is left. I would say there were probably around 200 raiders—maybe a few more."

Ayaar spoke up, "That small of a raiding party would not attack our caravan."

"Not unless we were strung out in a narrow wadi for several kilometers. Men, go back to your camps and start packing. We will move out in two hours. If Zenith joined with them, then he has to feel pretty safe, knowing our numbers and position."

Ayaar protested, "Captain Shutran, the Queen is not going to like this."

"You're right," I answered. "Many are not going to like it! However, I wonder if they would rather be dead or be slaves. First of all, we need to get over the lava terrain, as the raiders will not be expecting that. That's number one. Second, we will travel by night. They definitely won't expect that either, so let's get started."

Ayaar, realizing that we were in a vulnerable position, responded, "Captain Shutran, you are right. I'll do my best."

"Ayaar, tell the Queen and then get everyone else ready. She won't have any choice but to go."

The wadi was narrow and precarious as we took the wagons and the chariot through. We had about 600 men spread out and around with small torches to move and roll the rocks out of our way. Some big rocks had to be pulled out of the away with mules to make way for the wagons. By dawn we were across and headed toward Tabuk, a small village where we could rest the caravan for two hours without unloading and then move on.

When we finally stopped for the night, everyone was exhausted and excited to think that we had not encountered any pirates and obviously had outsmarted them. The next night we stopped in the village of Al Bad, where we were able to trade for more food supplies and let everyone rest and bathe, for which we were all grateful, even though we had had the frankincense smoke in the tents at night to mask the stale, musky stench of men and animal sweat.

After leaving the old village of Al Bad in the Midian Valley, we stopped in Elim, where there were 12 springs and large groves of trees. This was a refreshing oasis, a place where we could rest the caravan for three or four days and let our hunters gather some meat from the mountains to make jerky for the next few weeks. Here everyone could enjoy bathing in the fresh, spring water, and the animals had, for the first time since we left Marib, lush grass to replenish their fat energy supply.

At night around the cook fires was the time to bring out the instruments, and as soon as the music started, people began coming from all over the camp. It was more enjoyable for the men, since this time there were many young women from the Queen's camp who joined them. Soon they were all singing, clapping hands, and moving around as if trying to dance.

It was amusing to watch but in a short time there was a lot of excitement growing, and the stress and worries of the day disappeared into the loud volume and distinct rhythm of the music. The sound echoed through the hills long into the night.

I enjoyed this peaceful moment sitting around the fire and talking. I told them that this is the valley where Moses brought the Israelites when they first came out of bondage. There is still evidence of the encampment where 400 years ago they built stone altars and carved images of their sacred cows in the rocks. We could see the blackened mountain top from where the Israelite legends say that the voice of God thundered from the mountain when He gave Moses the law.

From here we would follow the King's Highway through the ancient land of Midian, now known as the Edomite Kingdom, a three-day journey from Selah that was being built because of the self-indulgence of Nebaioth, the firstborn son of Ishmael. The original inhabitants built the first stone city called Beitha. These people were the cave dwellers who started the first stone construction some 600 years ago. Seth remarked, "This history is very interesting."

"Yes, Seth, it is a strange feeling to know that I am in the land of my ancestors. It is sad that so much history has been lost that we will really never know."

"Shutran, tell us more."

"Well, a lot of it comes from the fragments of age-old legends and different people's opinions. But supposedly Nebaioth, Ishmael's first son, as I mentioned, and his people conquered the land of Moab. Gilead and his descendants were the Nebaioth people, who some of the Hebrew prophets talked about. They were gifted scribes and wrote some of their own history that we have today.

"They were also great craftsmen and I believe that one day a great stone city will be built in Selah and that these people will create trade between many countries. They will be successful because they understand the value of resins, which they began trading when the small village fort of Aila, the White City, was built at the mouth of the great water."

"Why do they call it the White City?" Kaleb asked.

"Quite simply because it is built of white limestone.

"This past year the Nebaioths put in a taxation port at Aila for all merchandise coming off the ships. Because the winds are so strong, only the Nebaioths' boats, with their specially designed lateen sails, are able to track the wind. They are the only ones who can bring the merchandise in and out of the village, which gives them control over the port."

Jona asked, "What is a lateen sail?"

"It is a sail that has a triangular shape and can turn to catch the wind coming from different directions. Most sails you see on the dhows are square and very big and can't turn with the wind, so if the wind is not moving in a direction to push the sail, they simply can't move or the wind can even push them in the wrong direction."

Jona then asked, "How is it that you know so much about so many things?"

"Reading!" I said.

"Come on, Shutran, you can't read."

"No, but Mirah can. When I'm home, she reads to me while I'm working, and then I often go down to the water and study the boats."

"Why?" Jona asked again.

"Well, men, I am thinking of going into the shipping business when we get back."

Seth spoke up with excitement, "Captain, are you serious?"

Ibram, Mohamed, Abdul, Micah, and Kaleb became very excited as well, and all seemed to ask at the same time, "Captain, will you take us?"

I smiled and asked them, "Who's going to help Jona?"

Ibram blurted out, "Jona can hire Tamrin and Ayaar." They all roared with laughter.

Jona mused, "Captain, are you trading your legs for fins?"

"No, Jona. I want to stay home and run the business from there and just make short trips like I used to when I first started my caravan.

"Whenever we stop near a port city, I ride down to the water to look at the Nebaioth boats. They are new, very different, and so fast that they sail right past the Egyptian boats that are using the same amount of wind."

"Why do you want to start a new business?" Enos asked.

"Well, I feel the time is coming when the caravan will become a thing of the past—not for a long while—but it will happen.

"Remember the stories we heard our grandfathers tell about Queen Hatshepsut coming in boats from Egypt 600 years ago, and every year someone built a better boat? So much is changing and our lives will never be the same."

Jona responded, "Well, I'm staying with my camel." We all laughed again.

"I'm sure we will see more and more demand for frankincense now that trade with other countries has started and they have discovered the great value of incense. Look what our forefathers said would happen when Egypt learned of the great gift of frankincense, and how many tons are we taking to Solomon on this very caravan?

"The caravans will just become bigger and bigger. They will be busy just getting the luban from the mountains to the ships. That would really make a great business. If all of you are interested when we return, we'll make plans for you to get started."

Micah blurted out, "Captain, tell us more. Keep talking!"

"Well, I believe the ships will take over one day. They are limited in numbers now, but when the demand starts to grow, there will also be a need for the caravans to pick up at Aila and transport to Gaza, Jerusalem,

Damascus, Nineveh, and even Alexandria.

"Caravans will always be needed to cross the Empty Quarter to Gerrha from the mountains to the seaports. We could set up a caravan company to transport all through Arabia, if some of you are willing to move to different locations such as Aila, Najran, or Marib. That would be easy for those of you who don't yet have your own families. We could establish a main company station and create relays so that no one would have to be gone for more than two to four months instead of six months to one-and-a-half years. Would this interest any of you?"

Micah spoke first, "Captain, it sure would. I would really like to work out of Aila, because it's close to my home in Gilead."

Enos spoke up next, "Captain, I would like to work out of Marib or the port of Qana."

Hussin asked, "But you'll still need scouts, won't you?"

"Yes, of course, we will. As long as there are political differences, borders to determine, new trails to open, and, unfortunately, thieves in the land, scouts will always be needed.

"We will have a lot of time on the return journey home to plan, if you would like, but for tonight until we talk again, give some thought to what you would like to be a part of in this new business."

"Sounds good, Captain," Seth said.

"We had better turn in. We are already in the Edomite Kingdom and are one day from Aila. We could still meet with some problems."

As the fires burned down and the excitement waned, everyone gradually wandered back to their tents. Fragments of music were heard drifting off with the breeze until sleep had taken over the night and the camp was silent, except for an occasional sound from one of the animals.

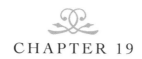

CHAPTER 19

The Abduction

As Kaleb, Jona, and I walked to our tent, the pain in my stomach became so strong that I wanted to vomit. My walk slowed as I grabbed my stomach. Kaleb, concerned, asked, "Papa, are you all right?" I barely heard his words as I felt Mirah's presence. I knew instantly that something was wrong at home. I heard Kaleb ask again, "Papa?"

As I became aware of his voice, I noticed that Jona was also looking at me. "Yes, Son, I'm fine; I was just thinking about home. Go ahead and get into bed. I'll be there shortly," and turned and walked over to the fire. I bent over to put on another piece of wood and then sat down on a rock.

Jona came over and sat down beside me and asked, "What's wrong, Shutran?"

I shook my head and with a pain in my voice said, "Jona, I don't know, but something is not right."

"Shutran, you look sick."

"Yes, I feel that way."

"Any idea what it is?"

"No, Jona, not yet. Even though I can feel Mirah's presence, I sense there is something else."

At that very moment Mirah awakened out of a deep sleep after having had a vivid dream of Shutran fighting to save Kaleb from bandits who had stolen him from the camp. She could see that they had taken him, thinking that Shutran's son would bring a high ransom from some other caravan commander and even a greater price if sold as a slave to the Pharaoh of

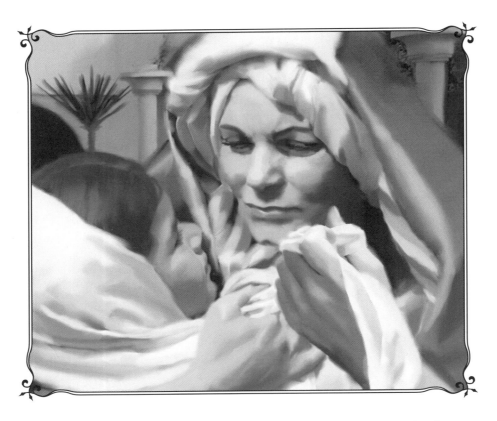

Egypt. She was sitting on her bed in a cold sweat trying to get the dream out of her mind when she heard Armin faintly whimper.

Mirah walked quickly into the children's room to check on her. As soon as she put her hand on Armin's little back, she could feel that she was burning up with fever. Mirah awakened Joshua and asked him to hurry and bring a bucket of water and some cloth. Then she started taking off Armin's nightwear so that she could wash Armin's body in the cool water. When Joshua returned, she had him put a pot of water on the fire to boil with some cassia, menthe, and frankincense. "Please hurry!" she called.

Armin was drifting in and out of a conscious state crying, "Mama, where is Papa? I need him. I'm so hot like the fire."

"Armin, Papa is far away."

"But, Mama, I need him. Tell him to please come home."

Mirah was fighting back the fear that was gripping her as Joshua lit the torch. In the pale light Mirah could see Armin's little, white, ashen face and gently asked, "Armin, when did you start feeling this way?"

"Yesterday I felt sleepy all day."

"Yes, I remember."

"And today I felt hot before I went to bed."

"Armin, why didn't you say something?"

"Mama, I didn't want to worry you any more; besides, you were worried about Papa."

"Yes, Armin, I was worried about Papa, but you are my precious little daughter, and I always want to know when you are not feeling well."

"Yes, Mama, but please tell Papa and Kaleb to come home. I want Papa to hold me and pray me better."

"I do, too. Mama will send Papa a message to come home. But you have to get better because it will take them many days to get here."

"Oh, Mama," Armin sobbed.

Joshua kept bringing cool water from the spring, and Mirah kept changing cold cloths every 15 minutes. "Joshua, is the tea almost ready?"

"Yes, Mama, I'm coming with it now."

Putting her arm around Armin, Mirah coaxed, "Here, sit up and drink this tea. It will help you feel better."

Armin tried to sit up but was too weak and fell back against Mirah and cried, "Mama, I just want to sleep."

"No, Armin, let Mama help you!"

"Mama, I just want to go and see Papa."

"Oh, my dearest," Mirah pleaded, "please don't go; Papa is too far away."

"No, he isn't, Mama; I can see him." Fear grabbed Mirah's heart as she fought back the tears, wanting to cry aloud.

Her mind flashed back to just two years earlier when she had sat with her sister and little nephew, who was the same age as Armin. Mirah had her arm around her sister as her sister held her little boy, who, after being kicked in the head by a camel, developed a high fever. Armin was saying the same things that he had said as he slowly slipped from this life into the next. As tears ran down Mirah's face, she remembered something Shutran's father had said, "When life is the very blackest, you must pray to God for direction. You must trust and know that He will be with you and will give you strength and comfort."

Mirah cried inside pleading, "Oh, God, please don't take my little girl now! Please let me have her until Shutran and Kaleb come home! I don't know how I could make it if you take her away while they are gone! Please, oh, God. She wants to see her papa and brother. Please, grant us her wish!"

But as those words came out of her mouth, she knew that it was not what she wanted God to hear. She begged God for forgiveness for doubting and thanked him for Armin's healing. Mirah held Armin tightly in her arms, rocked her as she tried to see Shutran in her mind, and thanked God for the great faith and wisdom of this man. She prayed for his safety as well as for the safety of her firstborn son, Kaleb, and thanked God again for His great blessings.

The caravan was quiet, as most of the men and animals were already sleeping. The crackling of the sparks from the fire made an eerie sound in the dark night. Mirah's voice still seemed to echo in my head. I turned to Jona and asked him to check to see if Kaleb was asleep. As Jona turned toward the tent, I stood up, still feeling very nauseous. I walked between the tents and into the stillness of the night to a small bluff with an outcropping of rocks. I found a place to kneel down and asked God to let me see Mirah and the children.

As the picture came into my mind, Mirah was holding Armin and rocking her. I could see that she was wrapped with cloth, which told me she was sick. I pleaded, "Oh, God, heal my little Armin. If you must take her, for which reason I know not, I beg, give us a little more time with her. Please let us have her until I can return home."

The nausea subsided and I thanked God for granting my request. I knew her fever was decreasing, even though I could feel her slipping in and out of consciousness. I could see Mirah putting a few drops of the frankincense tea on her lips so that it could run into her mouth until the flask that was next to her was empty. Gradually, the vision faded from my mind, and my thoughts returned to Kaleb.

As I stood up, the pain was suddenly more intense, and I felt that my anguish would overtake me. I looked up into the sky and then closing my eyes silently asked, "Father, what is it?" A frightening scene loomed in my mind as a chill went up my spine, the chill of death. At first I thought God had not granted my request, but then I could feel that this was different. I ran towards the camp, realizing how foolish I had been to leave my sword and whip in the tent when I went for my walk.

I broke out into a cold sweat, and the nausea increased as I felt that something terrible loomed before me. The flow of adrenaline surged as I ran around the rocks, gaining speed. My anxiety continued to mount as the feeling of death grew stronger. I couldn't imagine what was happening, but I knew this feeling very well.

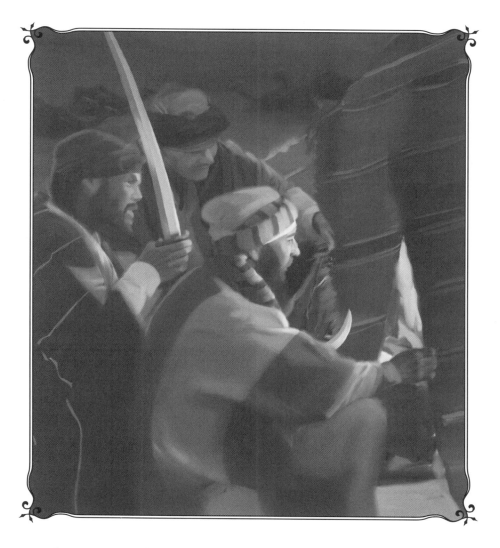

As I came in sight of my tent, on the other side of the cook fire, I could sense something was very wrong. Just then the tent flap parted, and Jona stumbled out backwards, tripping over the tent rope and clutching his side as he fell down. A burly looking pirate followed him out with his sword raised, ready to make his kill. He didn't see me in the dark, as he was totally focused on Jona.

Without a moment of hesitation, I headed straight towards him, not 8 meters away. Pulling my jambiyya from my belt, I threw it overhanded as hard as I could. The pirate's arms were extended to strike the death blow when my jambiyya buried itself deep inside his throat, splitting the jugular vein and spewing blood in every direction. He gasped and choked with a gurgling sound, as there was more blood than air. His hand went limp and his sword fell as he staggered sideways and crashed to the ground, dead.

I ran to Jona and knelt beside him to examine his wound in the faint light coming from the burning embers of the cook fire. Blood was running from a large incision in his right side just below the rib cage. When I touched him, he realized who it was and spoke with what little strength he had left, "Shutran, they've taken Kaleb. You've got to catch them before they get to the water."

In shock I felt myself sinking into a dark abyss, only to be stopped by the rage that came boiling up, giving me a ferocious desire to fight. I tore a piece of cloth from my clothing and plugged it into the hole in Jona's side while at the same time yelling for Seth, Ibram, and Micah to come fast. I could feel the life leaving Jona as he slipped into an unconscious state. I knew that without help from God, he would surely die. I looked to the heavens and in great anguish cried, "Oh, God Almighty, heal Jona, like you healed my father. Make him whole so that he can finish this journey by my side. Thank you, Father, for his healing."

Ibram was the first to reach me. "Shutran, Seth has been killed. He went to relieve himself and didn't come back. We just thought he went to put wood on the fire and find something more to eat. I fell asleep until I heard you yell and then tripped over Seth as I ran to you."

Micah came running as did Ahmad, Mohamed, and Enos. "What happened, Captain?"

"Raiders hit our camp and took Kaleb while Jona and I were away from the tent. The pirate who remained was looking for things to steal after Kaleb was carried off. Jona was attacked when he walked into the tent. Micah, you and Enos take care of Jona. Ahmad, come with me. Mohamed, get to the other captains and see if anyone else is missing and find out how they got inside our camp." A thought flashed through my mind. "Zenith!" I said under my breath.

As we rode out, Tamrin and Ayaar were waiting for us. "Captain Shutran, I heard that the pirates have taken Kaleb."

"Yes," I answered.

"They have also taken four of the Queen's servants, and we have lost two more guards. The caravan from Taiz is missing four camels, and one of their guards is dead," Tamrin reported. "Apparently, the pirates knew where to strike. Is there anything else?"

"Yes," I answered, they killed Seth and wounded Jona badly."

Ayaar spoke up, "What do you want us to do?"

"Ayaar, as soon as it is daylight, do a complete assessment to see what the damages are, reassign new guards, and double them."

Just then one of Ayaar's chiefs came running into camp and reported, "Captain Ayaar, 11 of our horses are missing, and both guards who were in charge of the horses are severely wounded and could die."

"Keep the caravan here until I return," I ordered. "If I am not back in three days, take the caravan on to Selah. If I don't meet up with you within two days after you arrive, follow the King's Highway north to Wadi Dana and down to the old copper mine. Then cross at the south end of the Salt Sea and go to Ein Gedi. Camp there and send scouts into Jerusalem to notify Solomon. He will send his military to escort you. I will find you in Jerusalem, but I will not be back until I have Kaleb and the others."

Haashrun, one of Azaad's grandsons, also came running up, out of breath, and exclaimed, "Four of my brothers have been taken."

"Ahmad, ride back and get Ibram and Mohamed."

I turned to Ayaar, "Can you give Ibram eight of your best archers and horsemen?" Speaking to Haashrun, I asked, "Can your father spare six or eight men? I mean fighting men. These pirates are after slaves to sell to the Pharaoh in Egypt. They will split and take the camels and some of the horses and likely go southeast as a decoy. The rest of the pirates will take the slaves and a few horses and head to Aila, the White City, to put them on a boat to go up the Red Sea, taking the canal over to the Nile and sailing up to Luxor. Ahmad, have Salah gather some torches and come with me. We cannot lose another minute."

"What happened to Kaleb?" Ahmad asked as the other men listened intensely.

"Apparently, the pirates lifted the back of the tent, crawled in, probably hit him on the head to knock him out, bound his hands and feet, and carried him out. They could easily have thrown him over the shoulder of one of the robbers and run between the tents until they reached their horses."

By the time everyone was assembled, the captains reported that 10 young men, 6 young women, 6 camels, and 25 horses had been taken. These desert pirates knew what they were doing and had exact information about our camp formation and the location of the young men and women. I would suspect that it was Zenith who sold them the information, which is probably why he didn't return from his scouting trip with the other two.

As Salah and Ahmad returned, I was circling the camp looking for tracks. On the south side of the camp, maybe 200 meters, I found where they had all joined and then split up. I now had Ahmad, Ibram, Mohamed, Salah, eight of Ayaar's archers, and six men from Azaad's caravan, who were all seasoned fighters with bow and sword.

"Ibram, this is where they split into two groups. You take Ali, who is one of the best with sword and bow, another archer, and two other men. You and Ali are good trackers and will easily be able to follow this group. They are traveling with all of the camels and 18 horses of their own but only ten men. The other raiders, who we will track, have all of the stolen horses and the captives and have headed into the desert towards the mountains.

"They hope that their clever diversion will get us to follow the wrong group with horses and camels to the south. When they are far enough away, they will turn to the west and go in a different direction, thinking we will then lose the trail completely. Then they will double back to meet up in Aila.

"The raiding party is small, with only 45 men and horses. They slipped in quietly and moved quickly, knowing exactly where they were going. They took their victims, slipped out, and killed anyone who got in their way. They will be easy to follow once you pick up the trail, but stay out of sight and be aware that they will have a rear scout watching for you. You must kill him first but wait until they are in the open desert, and then let the archers take out all of them.

"You each have two horses, so as soon as it is light and the trail is visible, ride hard and then change horses and keep riding. Do not stop until you have found them. At best, they probably have only one hour on you. They will gain distance while it's dark, and it won't be light for another seven hours. You won't be able to move as fast because of having to watch for the trail. By daylight they could be ahead of you by 25 to 35 kilometers. Knowing that, they will feel secure, thinking they can stay ahead of you. When it's daylight, they will probably relax as they head into the mountains, confident that they have lost you.

"They won't think that you'll be taking a second horse to ride. As soon as you have light, by riding and switching horses at a steady gallop, you can gain perhaps a couple of kilometers or more per hour. You should catch them by noon if you don't lose the trail. By mid-morning when the sun casts your horses' shadows no more than ½ meter from your horses standing sideways to the sun, start watching for their scout. He will be watching for your dust, so spread out. Bring their ears back and spare no life.

The caravan will wait here for three days and then will move out for Selah. Men, this is a no-defeat battle. When we are finished, any future raiders will think twice before they attack another caravan or kidnap anyone. Let's ride!"

I rode to the outskirts of the camp to look for any signs of the pirates. When I stopped and dismounted, Salah handed me a torch to better examine the tracks. One of Ayaar's men rode beside me and stepped down off his horse to look at them. "Captain, how can you be sure we are following the pirates who took your son and the others?"

"Look here; I'll show you. See this horse track? This horse is being led by this one, and these two are tailed-up."

"What do you mean?"

"The second horse is tied to the tail of the first horse and so on. It is very easy to see the hoof prints in this sandy soil. That is why they are headed towards the mountains, so they can hide their tracks. Approximately 35 men are in this group and no camels. You can see in the depth of the mark from the inner part of the horse's hoof where it makes contact with the ground first and also in the mark of the hoof ring that this horse has no rider. When you know what to look for, hoof prints give much information. If you look at the tracks over here, you can see that this one has a rider, but a smaller rider like my son, who weighs maybe 46 to 48 kilos."

"I can't see any difference," he said.

"You can if you know what to look for. Look closely at the depth in the dirt and how the hoof comes up out of the dirt. This horse looks like it is dragging its foot a little. See how the toe rounds the front, top rim as he comes up and moves forward? The depth is another half a centimeter deeper," I explained.

He replied, "But, Captain, maybe this horse is just a bigger horse."

"No, and for two reasons. First, the hoof is just a little smaller than those of the other three horses. Second, look at the area of the inside of the hoof. If the horse were bigger, it would have a wider hoof imprint and would be larger. Now if it were daylight and we could follow every track, in about two hours you would see that one of our boys is riding this horse."

Enos spoke up, "Captain, how can you tell?"

"That's easy. The boys will get down to pee right beside their horses. Because they are nervous and scared, they will have to pee in about two hours. The women, even though they are also scared and nervous, will hold it until it starts to break light. Now, let's mount up and ride. Every

15 minutes I will check the tracks to make sure we are still on the trail. After we have traveled for about two hours, I will start watching the trail more closely. Enos, look. This horse is being ridden double, which would slow them down a little. One of the women can't ride by herself."

I walked with the torch, following the tracks, and could see that the pirates were having problems. The pirates who were leading the riderless horses were ahead, while the pirates who were with the captives were riding a bit slower, trying to keep them moving. They had probably tied some of the captives onto their horses and were leading them. We came to where they had stopped and readjusted the riders and could tell that now three horses were each carrying two riders.

The night air had cooled the dirt and sand, and the early morning chill had set in. Once I found what I was looking for, I would feel better. Ayaar's men were pushing for me to move faster, as they were anxious to make the capture. "Captain Shutran, if we hurry and ride, we can catch them before they get to the mountains."

"You're right, but I need to know all that I can before we overtake them. When I feel ready, you had better be ready to ride." Shortly after that I found what I was looking for—to know for sure that the horse I was watching was the one Kaleb was riding.

I could see that their horses had stopped again; this time one of the horses had turned completely around, and I could see in the sand where Kaleb had written his name in the dirt as he peed. Several of the boys and pirates had stopped to relieve themselves along the way. The sand was still wet, which told me they were not too far ahead. I started to feel Kaleb's sense of peace, knowing at that moment that everything was all right.

I had the information that I needed, and so I swung up into the saddle and was now ready to ride, and ride hard. I thanked God for healing Armin and for delivering the pirates into my hands. I held that image in my mind and saw nothing else. Daylight was breaking and the pirates' horses would be tiring. Kaleb and the other young men would delay as much as they could when the pirates stopped to change horses. I hoped that one of the boys would be able to let his mount break free, which would delay them by 20 to 30 minutes because of having to catch and bring the horse back. Every minute was precious.

In the meantime the pirates led their captives towards the mountains as quickly as they could, although they couldn't move as fast as they wanted; but they were still certain they would lose us in the night.

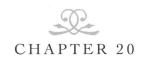

CHAPTER 20

Kaleb's Trial of Faith

My head was spinning as I tried to figure out what had happened to me. I felt the pinch of the leather around my wrists and realized that I was tied to my horse. All I could hear was the sound of the horses. I wondered why I didn't hear any voices. Then I looked around and saw the others from camp, and like me they had scarves binding their mouths that were tied around their heads to keep them from talking. I recognized several of the young men, including Azaad's four grandsons, who I had come to know on the caravan. They were also tied to their horses, and when I nodded to them, they nodded back, acknowledging me.

The pirate in charge, who called himself Alwadi, came around to the captives and said to us very sternly, "If you want to live, do what you're told and keep quiet. If you make any sound, the man who is closest to you will kill you," as if he thought his hostages could talk with their mouths tied shut. Then he called out to me, "Kaleb?" and I just nodded my head in acceptance. The others followed my lead, nodding their heads as well.

I knew I had to keep the thoughts of fear from building in order to mentally communicate with Papa. Any other thought would interfere with the signal. If I practiced what Papa taught me about absolute *knowing*, God would protect me, and so I kept that vision in my mind, allowing no doubt to enter. That would be the only message God would get, regardless of how things looked at the moment.

I remember a conversation with Papa when he said, "When you're in a bad situation and in great danger, just ask yourself, 'What is the worst thing that could happen?' Use your imagination to see how you would handle it, even if you might be killed, but how bad would that be?

"Of course, it would be terrible for those who love you and are left behind, but for you, you would be with God in His glorious kingdom, although He might give you an assignment to come back. So you never need to fear death. Once you have seen your fear and have gone through all of the pain determining how you would survive, then you don't have to think about it again.

"But *the first step* is to believe and to see it as you want the outcome to be and then take the next step. This is how you begin your journey to come *to know* God." I kept thinking about this conversation with Papa while trying to combat my fear.

After the pirates were certain that they had gained enough distance from the camp, they stopped to let us get off our horses to stretch and relieve ourselves. They untied our hands and took the scarves off our mouths. It was a relief to feel that freedom, but the pirates put a lot of fear into their captives, threatening us should anyone think of yelling or trying to escape. I peed my name into the sand, knowing Papa would see it. He could track anything, so I wanted to leave him signs that the pirates wouldn't notice. We only had a few minutes before they ordered us to get back onto our horses. They were determined to get to the mountains before morning.

As we started moving again, I went back to thinking about my family. In my mind I could see Mama in the kitchen. She was listening to that conversation and making a comment now and then while she prepared our evening meal. I thought about how much I missed her and wished I were eating that evening meal right now. Mama loved to listen to Papa teach about God. She said it helped her when Papa was gone for such a long time.

Joshua went outside to gather more wood for the fire, and Armin wanted to go with him, so for the moment, we were able to talk about more serious things. I continued asking, "Papa, what comes after believing?"

"Most people never get this far."

"Why?" I asked.

"What you talk about is what you get. You have to form the thoughts in your mind to convince yourself, but there may be no real foundation for your belief, and you may still change your mind.

"*The second step* is faith, which is just a stronger conviction of your belief. It's a little like magic. Children see magic as real, and the more they see it, the greater is their belief until it becomes their truth. But does that make it real? Then, when the children become older and gain more knowledge, what happens to the belief and faith?

"Son, this is where most people are in the world, and this is why their lives don't work or why people who are sick don't get well. Look at your friends who believe in many gods. They have faith and even go through various rituals and prayer ceremonies to pray up their faith. However, it doesn't change the fact that the sun is not a god." I wondered what the other captives were thinking. I doubted they had very much Godly conviction to help them through this frightening time.

The third step, Papa explained, was coming to really *know* God and how He works. "Knowledge is information learned through actual experience, stored in the mind and not questioned." I could have chuckled to myself thinking about this very real experience that I was having that would change my life forever. But I wasn't amused, even though I knew that through all of this, I would see God's power in my life if I stayed strong in my *knowing*.

Thinking about the things Papa had taught me was very reassuring. His words came clearly into my mind, "Son, many people will try to convince you that what they think is true. But when you develop your own relationship with God, your knowledge of truth will come directly from Him, and you can have the outcome you seek. Life is a continuous experience of problems and challenges, but these are the things that help you develop that relationship. You don't need someone else telling you what you are supposed to believe. Besides, their truth could easily be false and just another form of magic."

I love to hear Papa talk about God; he has so much wisdom. I always listen to every word. I want to have that same *knowing*. I love the caravan and being with Papa all day. Although he is my father, he is also a great Commander, a side of Papa I hadn't seen before. He told many fascinating stories of things that happened on the caravans. I listened in awe and wondered if I could ever be like him. I was learning so much and seeing life in a different way, a man's way.

But if there was a time to call upon God, it was now. As small children, we were taught by Papa and Mama to pray to God and trust in Him. When Papa was home, we would sit at night on the warm sand near the seashore and talk about God and His world. Papa always said that it was very important for us to know God so that we could call on Him when we needed Him, especially when Papa was gone with the caravan for such a long time.

One night, when just the two of us were sitting around the campfire talking, I asked him if he would teach me more. "Of course," he replied. As I rocked back and forth in the saddle, watching the pirates and the other captives, I wished they could hear Papa's words.

"*The fourth step* is to act with certainty, *knowing* that God has granted your request." Papa said, "It's like the story about your grandfather when he fell with the seven camels down to the bottom of the ravine and ended up underneath them, lying on the rocks with a broken back and paralyzed legs. Only God could have saved your grandfather. He didn't ask for my help or send me to get help. He didn't pray, 'If it be God's will.' He prayed with a powerful *knowing* and simply asked God to heal him. Then he thanked God, stood up, and walked."

What an amazing experience that must have been for Papa. I wish I could have been there. But now I was having my own experience—and not one I wanted but which I was certain would be a story I would tell to my children. Then I thought about Joshua and Armin. They would be excited to hear about my capture, but Mama would be anxiously waiting to hear about my rescue.

I often wondered what Papa meant when he said, "God is not a *will* God; He is a *knowing* God." That was difficult for me to understand as a boy. Papa explained that to say "Thy will" released a person from any responsibility. But now I understand that if a person offers a prayer and yet does little or nothing to help the situation, then God will usually allow nature to take its course. Then it becomes easy for that person to say that it was God's will and take no responsibility for the outcome.

Papa explained that there were times when God doesn't fulfill our requests because there is a higher purpose for what is happening at that moment, and we just don't have enough understanding. Sometimes God will intervene when it would be better for our well-being. We just have to have enough faith and know and trust in Him. Now I was beginning to understand what Papa meant.

"But how does it work? How do you do it?" I had asked.

"Simply by acting. People ask God for many things, but they doubt in their hearts and deny the possibility of having their prayers answered. You have to act as though your prayer has been answered, not the opposite."

It seemed like we had been riding for a long time, when the pirates decided to stop again. We were anxious to get off the horses and move

172

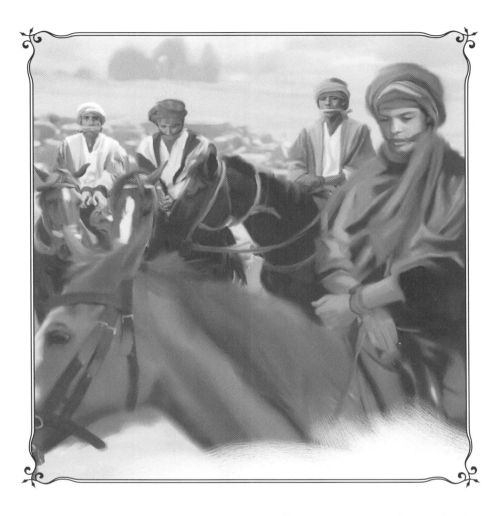

around. This time Mahrus, one of Azaad's grandsons, tried to make it look like he was having trouble with his horse and let it escape. Alwadi sent his men running to catch it. He was furious and came over to Mahrus and struck him so hard that he fell to the ground. Alwadi put his hand on his jambiyya as though he were going to kill Mahrus, and in a very harsh voice, he growled, "If you ever let go of that horse again, I will kill you," and kicked him as he went to check on the others.

It took the pirates several minutes to catch the horse and bring it back. They were very angry as they handed the rope to Alwadi, who was still fuming because of the time they had lost. He just looked at Mahrus, whose face was bleeding a little from his mouth and nose, and snarled,

"Now get on your horse and don't try anything else."

I was sorry Mahrus had been struck, but I knew that the time he caused the pirates to lose would help Papa. We were moving quicker as the pirates pushed to recover the lost minutes, but with the difficulty of moving the captives and all of the extra horses, they didn't gain much.

I went back to my conversations with Papa. We had talked a lot about the night Azaad's son, Izeed, died, but Grandfather Azaad was the sickest. Papa simply thanked God for healing Azaad and then went on with what he had to do, as though his request had already been answered. At the same time in the next tent, the Queen's priest and physician was chanting and carrying on all night over Azaad's son, who died anyway.

All these things gave me strength to block my fear from the thought of what Papa told me pirates did to slaves in order to get a higher price. I watched the other captives bouncing as they rode and thought how terrible it must be for the ladies to have to ride on a horse with one of the pirates and hang onto him. It was a relief when they stopped to rest the horses, and we were allowed to get down and stretch our legs for a short time.

If only I could share with them the things that Papa had taught me about God, then they, too, could have the *knowing* that we would soon be rescued. A time like this is when we find out how important it is to have a belief in God. They probably didn't have anything to hang onto, which must have filled them with a panic and a horrible fear. Whenever I had the chance, I would nod to them as a way of giving them reassurance.

I wished I had some frankincense resin in my pocket. We always burned it at home so that we could breathe the incense while praying. Papa said it was a physical way that would help us connect to God, and the smell could open our minds to greater things. Papa would chuckle and say, "If you can't burn it, chew it, because it will still bring about a peaceful feeling and block the evil thoughts from coming into your mind." I was certain Papa would be chewing luban right now.

The thought even crossed my mind that maybe I should thank God for allowing me to be captured, since this was helping me to develop my relationship with Him. But I didn't keep that thought very long. I determined I didn't need to be a captive in order to learn about God. Just then I felt a sense of peace come over me and sent Papa a mental message to let him know that we were safe for the moment. I could feel his presence and kept thanking God, knowing that Papa would come soon.

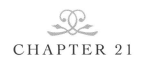

CHAPTER 21

The Rescue

y men and I stayed steady on the trail but couldn't move as fast as we would like and were anxious for the morning light. One of the men rode up, interrupting my concentration. "How close do you think we are?" he asked.

"I will be able to tell better when morning comes and I can clearly see the trail." As I focused ahead, I reached for some luban resin. I loved the feel of it in my hand and for a couple of seconds just let my fingers feel the surface. Then I popped it in my mouth and started chewing. It seemed to ease my thoughts and take away the heavy feelings.

My thoughts went to Mirah, knowing that she must be worried. I was concerned about her and started sending messages to let her know that Kaleb was safe and that he would soon be with me again. I also sent Kaleb a message to let him know that it wouldn't be long before I was there and to be alert so that he would be ready when the signal came.

I kept thinking about the plan that I had made and how it was going to work when we caught up with the raiders. I closed my eyes for a moment and let Sultan follow the trail. He was a smart, aggressive stallion, who sensed my feelings and seemed to know what he was to do. The pirates had taken some mares, and Sultan could smell them. He periodically would drop his head to check the scent. I always knew when we were on the right trail because he would increase his speed.

I relaxed the reins and let Sultan take the lead, so I could focus in on Kaleb. Within a couple of minutes, I could see him tied to his red gelding.

He seemed peaceful and confident, which was reassuring to the others. He was looking for landmarks that he could mentally send to me. Then I heard his voice in my head, "Oh, Papa, you're there." Daylight would come soon, which would make it easy for me to actually see the landmarks that Kaleb was seeing and sending to my mind.

Ali, one of my scouts, lost the trail twice as we crossed the rocks and hard ground. When that happened, all I had to do was drop the reins and pat Sultan's neck and say, "Take the trail and find Kaleb." He would make a circle and in less than two minutes, he would find it again. We knew we could travel faster in the daylight and would probably sight them by mid-morning. We stopped for only a moment to water the horses and change mounts.

At first light and with fresh horses, we doubled our speed. By the time the coolness was gone from the ground and the temperature rose, we stopped, switched saddles, and then kept going at a full gallop. As I received more mental images from Kaleb, I watched the sun and shadows to figure out our distance from the pirates, which I had determined was about one hour, more or less.

Now we had to be careful, because if the pirates felt the least threatened, they would kill one captive at a time until we gave up. As of yet, they were not aware that we were behind them, but they would be if we were not careful when we got closer. I didn't want them to see us until I was ready to put my plan into action, which was to allow their scout to see us riding away in the opposite direction. The pirates had gone into the mountains to cover their tracks and were traveling northwest towards Aila.

I called out to Mohamed, "We will split up here. You take Azaad's four men and two archers. Stay on the trail and stay back far enough so that they won't know you're behind them. Spread out and watch for their rear scout. We are getting close to Aila, so they are pushing hard now, but their horses will start fatiguing by mid-afternoon, and they should run out of water before then.

"They will probably camp in the mountains and then pass through the city while it is still dark before the morning light to board their captives without being noticed. You are outnumbered seven to one, so do not make contact. Our captives, including the ladies, might be killed before you could surrender. I'll take my men and ride south by southwest away from their trail until I get to the western mountains. Then I'll turn north and try to get in front of them and reach Aila first.

As we dropped down out of the foothills and onto the valley floor, Ali rode up, "Captain, the pirates will see us."

"Yes, that is my plan. As we ride away, I want them to think that we have lost their trail and are going in the wrong direction. As soon as they see that, they will think that they have succeeded in losing us and will slow their pace. They will pull their rear scout in closer, which will reduce Mohamed's risk." I could feel Kaleb's concern as he felt me leave. I sent my thoughts to him of our plan to try to get more space between us and the captives, so he would know I wanted him to delay them as much as possible.

While the pirates were resting their horses, Mohamed and Ahmad were crouching down behind the rocks on the hillside a half a kilometer away, watching their activity to determine how many men they had and if all the captives were still with them.

Shortly after the high noon sun, their rear scout rode up all excited. Kaleb pretended to not pay any attention but overheard the scout telling Alwadi that Shutran had lost their trail and was headed south with his men. Alwadi was very pleased and said, "You know, it isn't hard to outsmart these dumb caravaners. They are just a bunch of camel herders, not fighting men. We have nothing to worry about. Tomorrow, by early morning, we will be on the boat headed for Egypt, while they are still wandering around in the desert."

I took Micah, Enos, and the other men with me and rode toward Aila. I gave Sultan my heel, sending him into a full gallop for an hour, going west. Then we stopped, changed horses, and rode at a hard gallop for another hour. We switched our horses again and turned north. By changing, riding, and changing again, we arrived close to Aila by mid-morning.

When we stopped to rest, I turned to Enos and said, "I want you to find the highest point for observation. The pirates are staying in the foothills west of the Wadi Rum, making it difficult to track them. My feeling is that they'll stay east of the King's Highway, the old Israelite trail, and make camp for the night.

Before the morning light they will come down into Aila but will wait to enter until they are sure we are not there. Then they will pass through the city in the dark to board their ship. Micah, I want you to scout around the city and check for any pirates. I'm going down to the shore to see what ships are there. I hope to be back before dark. We will meet here."

As I rode in, I kept going over all the possibilities of the worst thing that could happen. The warmth of the morning sun was bringing the little port village to life, and from where I stopped, I could see three Nebaioth ships built with triangular sails. One of them or maybe all three of them had to be the ships waiting to carry away the captives. I secured Sultan to a tree behind some rocks on a hill above the city and found my way down to the water's edge where the ships were tied.

I kept asking myself, "What if the pirates got by us and made it to their ships?" That would make it very difficult or almost impossible for us to get Kaleb and the others back. I had to make sure they didn't sail. I eased into the water, swimming below the surface so as not to catch attention. I came up under the rear of the first boat by the rudder and carefully climbed up. It was a dhow with a semi-open hull. My blood turned cold and I shuttered as I saw chains and leg shackles in the hull awaiting the captives.

Only one guard was on this ship, and he was sound asleep, enjoying the morning peacefulness in the warmth of the sun. My jambiyya made a quick slice as I sent him into a deeper sleep as he departed into the next world. I hurriedly climbed out of the ship and back into the water to swim to the third one, where I had seen another guard.

There wasn't a sign of anyone on the second ship, so I decided to check that one last. Either the pirates felt confident that two guards were sufficient, or the third guard was in the town marketplace. Nevertheless, these three ships were slave-trader ships. I couldn't be sure if they all belonged to the pirates and were the ones meant to carry Kaleb and the others away, but no matter, I was going to make sure that they would never carry slaves again.

The second guard was sleeping just like the first one, so it was easy to send him to meet his comrade. The ships were loaded with supplies and contained food, olive oil, dried fish, salt, and some cotton bales that obviously had been taken from previous victims. The sails were up, which told me that they were expecting to leave at any time.

With both guards deep in the sleep of the dead, I went to work rigging the ships. Using the oil, I soaked the bales of cotton and then made a rope, which I wrapped around the mast, part way up towards the sails. Then striking my flint, I started a fire in the hull, where it would burn slowly until the heat became so hot that the deck would burst into flames and travel up the mast to the sails. I had to move fast to get the other two ships prepared and ignited before the first one became a raging fire on the water.

As soon as I had the last ship burning, I climbed down into the cool water to cut the ropes that anchored them to the shore. By the time I made it back to Sultan, the three ships had drifted out into deep water and were in full blaze. The villagers stood on shore wondering what had happened, while I quietly rode out unnoticed.

Night had settled in by the time I reached camp, and the men were gathered around a small fire in the rocks. I quickly ate some boiled jerky and lentils that were still hot, while everyone reported what they had discovered. "We'll get as close as possible to the camp with the horses, but the archers must be in position when the pirates start to move," I instructed.

I thought we had possibly five hours before the pirates would know about the ships if their scout returned. "We need to move now," I said. "Remember, these pirates live by the sword, which is how they get their money. They are not going to take any chances that anyone might try to run. Most likely they will have all the captives staked to the ground with leather straps. The pirates will be sleeping close by, so we must make sure we take out everyone positioned for night duty. After two nights of not being pursued, they will be a little less edgy.

Our plan was for Mohamed and his men to attack from the east. I was sure they were hiding in the rocks watching the pirate's camp and waiting for Salah's jaguar scream, which was the signal to move. The attack had to be fast, taking them by surprise before the pirates had time to kill any captives. Mohamed's archers were ready, knowing that when the flaming arrows lit up the sky, they would have only enough light to get a single arrow in the air, and they couldn't miss.

I started sending messages to Kaleb, telling him to wake up and go relieve himself so that we could see his position. Within ten minutes Kaleb was up, moved as far away as his tethered rope allowed, and peed slowly, taking his time while looking around. Only a sliver of the moon gave a glimpse of light, while in the rocks it was dark, but I could see him.

I whispered to Salah, "Take Enos and move to the picket line; cut all their horses loose and then make your jaguar scream. Remember, no standing when the fighting breaks out, unless you're engaged in hand-to-hand battle; otherwise, stay down or be on one knee so that we know who you are. Remove your gutrah, as we will not kill anyone whose head is bare."

We all knew what to do and started to crawl into camp. The archers were ready to set the flame to their arrows, so Mohamed's archers on the other side of the camp would be able to see the guards to take them out, and we would be able to see the captives. We were ready when Salah's blood-curdling scream pierced the night, causing the horses to go crazy.

The flaming arrows shot swiftly upward, lighting the sky so that the archers from the other side could find their targets. Alwadi and his men jumped to their feet in a panic and started running toward the horses. The sky was bright from the burning camel fat and frankincense resin wrapped in wool strips around the shafts of the arrows. I heard one man holler, "Get the horses," as he came running in my direction.

Another man yelled, "Alwadi, the captives. . . ." But he was struck down with a flaming arrow that set his thobe on fire.

Alwadi, who was running towards me, yelled, "Kill them."

I sprang up on my feet squarely in front of him and buried my jambiyya deep in his stomach. He had a shocked look on his face as he tried to catch his breath. "Who, who are you?" he moaned, as he lost the grip on his sword that fell to the ground. His punctured gut made a gurgling sound as the blood mixed with the air. His knees started to weaken but I grabbed his thobe with my right hand to steady him so that he could have a final look at who killed him.

"I am Shutran, the Commander of the caravan. You robbed the caravan and killed one of my best captains, wounded my best friend, and kidnapped my son. Now you can go to the dark abyss of your endless torment." Then I jerked him upward, which opened his abdomen more as I pulled back while withdrawing my jambiyya, and dropped him on the ground.

Within a few seconds I reach Kaleb, and while cutting him free, I handed him my jambiyya and pulled out my sword. "Papa!" he yelled. I rolled over just as a sword came slicing down. But before I could thrust my sword, an arrow found its mark, and the pirate pitched forward, landing face down beside me. With weapons in hand, Kaleb and I ran to cut the others free. Mohamed was cutting the bindings on the women as the hand-to-hand fighting started with the pirates who had escaped the archers' arrows.

I was cutting one of Azaad's grandsons from the stake when he hollered, "Watch out!"

I turned abruptly just as one of the pirates was about to attack Kaleb. I yelled as the man came at him with his jambiyya raised for the blow of death. Kaleb turned and dropped to the ground as I lashed with my whip, catching the pirate's face. Kaleb jabbed hard, sticking his jambiyya in one of the pirate's legs, who then stumbled and yelled as the blood sprayed out of a severed artery.

The pirate's hatred kept him going after Kaleb, who stabbed him again. With blood running down his leg, the pirate half crawled and half ran in a circle as he tried to stab Kaleb but missed as my whip caught his arm this time and jerked him around. With my sword drawn, I lunged towards him as Kaleb came up onto his feet, driving his jambiyya into the man's side.

He stopped in his tracks and gasped for air as a foul-smelling liquid from his punctured bowel drained out with the blood. Not wanting to be defeated by a boy, in his last dying moment, he grabbed Kaleb's clothing and wrestled him to the ground in one last attempt to kill him. I chopped a sideways blow to his head, and he collapsed dead on top of Kaleb.

"Papa, get him off me," Kaleb moaned. As I rolled him away, I saw that Kaleb was covered with blood but was not hurt. I turned as other attackers were approaching. In the dark I could see three more marauders coming towards us, and two of the young men still hadn't been cut free.

"Kaleb, get to those boys and cut their ropes while I deal with these three."

"Oh, Papa, I've never been so scared in my life!"

"Go, Son. Get the boys and take them to the horses."

Kaleb was half crying as he yelled, "But, Papa, you need me!"

"Kaleb, go now! There is no time to lose."

The three pirates charged me while swinging their swords. This was going to be a challenge. These men lived by the sword and would certainly die by the sword. They were not like Tamrin's men, who thought sword fighting was a chance to test their skill with the sword, or like Bedouin bush thieves, who got into a fight once or twice in their lives. These men probably fought more for pleasure than others did for survival. I could hear swords clashing around the camp, which told me the battle wasn't over yet. I knew that I probably couldn't expect any help. It was dark and even though my night vision was good, it was almost impossible to see their swords or determine their stance.

The coals from the small fires helped somewhat, even though they were burning low. I knew I couldn't survive in a hand-to-hand fight with three skilled swordsmen of their caliber. I would need more wit and cunning than just skill. After several quick swings and blocks, they became so confident that they would finish me quickly that one of them stepped back to watch his comrades carve me a little at a time. He would be the one to come forward for the finish. They were going to have fun

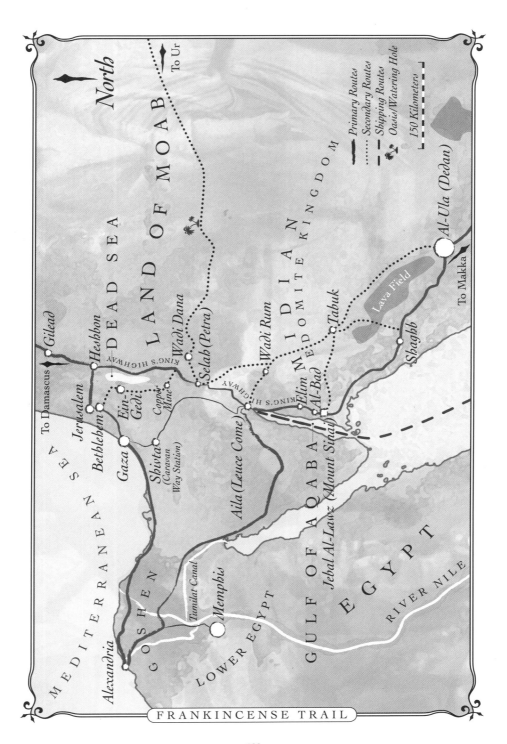

North

MEDITERRANEAN SEA

DEAD SEA

LAND OF MOAB

To Ur

MIDIAN

EDOMITE KINGDOM

Lava Field

Al-Ula (Dedan)

To Makka

Gilead

To Damascus

Heshbon

KING'S HIGHWAY

Wadi Dana

Selah (Petra)

Wadi Rum

Tabuk

Shaghb

Jerusalem

Bethlehem

Ein-Gedi

Copper Mine

KING'S HIGHWAY

Elim

Al-Bad

Gaza

Shivta
(Caravan
Way Station)

Aila (Leuce Come)

Jebal Al-Lawz (Mount Sinai)

GULF OF AQABA

GOSHEN

Tumilat Canal

Memphis

LOWER EGYPT

EGYPT

RIVER NILE

Alexandria

Primary Routes
Secondary Routes
Shipping Routes
Oasis/Watering Hole

150 Kilometers

FRANKINCENSE TRAIL

182

and enjoy this, like three pumas playing with one rabbit. I retreated slowly as they advanced with the gleam of the kill in their eyes.

Back home, in Al-Balid, Mirah was still nursing Armin back to health and had had little sleep for the last three nights. Now, finally, for the first time, as Armin was sleeping well, Mirah laid down and fell asleep, exhausted. She had barely closed her eyes when she started having a nightmare of me engaged in a sword fight with pirates. As the fight intensified, she could sense that my fate was about to be determined by the end of a sword.

She wanted to scream but felt herself shaking and heard the faint sound of a voice calling, "Mama, Mama, wake up. Papa needs us."

Mirah slowly realized that it was Armin's voice she heard. "Armin," Mirah questioned as she awakened a bit in a daze, "Are you all right?"

"Yes, Mama, but Papa needs us now. Something awful is happening." As Mirah's head cleared, she connected her nightmare to what Armin was saying.

"Yes, Armin, Papa needs us. Come now; we must ask God to help Papa. Let's wake up Joshua to come and pray with us."

I could see the faces of Mirah, Joshua, and Armin, as it looked like my end was coming near. I thought to myself, "I wonder if Kaleb reached the horses and if any of my men survived. If Kaleb wasn't safe, I couldn't die. It couldn't end here." At that moment a burst of energy surged through my veins, even as the blood ran down from a slice on my cheek and on my upper right arm. A small cut across my abdomen was bleeding as well. The pirates were not going to do this quickly. They were going to enjoy every minute of the kill.

I was retreating again, trying to time every move, knowing that I didn't have many left. I sent a message of love to Mirah and the children to let them know how I missed them and longed to put my arms around them. Within a moment's time my mind cleared, and I again focused on the advancing pirates as they closed the distance to finish off their prey.

Without hesitating, in one motion I dropped down on my right shoulder with my arm and sword to my side and rolled quickly to my left. Then coming up partway on my right, I swung up and across with my sword, opening the abdomen of both men, causing their innards to fall out. In the same swing with a backwards overhand twist of the wrist, I came up on both feet and opened the first man's chest and the throat of the second. They were both dead before they hit the ground.

I turned in the dark, preparing for the third one, when I felt an impact as though I had been kicked by a mule as the jambiyya of the third pirate sunk deep into my right shoulder. I stumbled sideways, avoiding him as he charged for the kill. I could feel the strength drain from my body as the blood gushed down my arm and off my fingertips. Breathing heavily, I tried to keep my head clear and be ready for battle. I blocked three strikes and drew blood from his right side.

He was now enraged and careless as he came at me again, swinging wildly, hitting my sword with such force that I was knocked backwards. I was losing a lot of blood with every movement as the jambiyya stuck in my shoulder cut deeper. He knew that if he kept me moving, the jambiyya would bleed me out, and he could finish me off.

I asked God to give me the strength to stay on my feet. I struck his face, exposing all of the teeth on his left side and severing half of his nose. Even that didn't slow him down as he came forward swinging. I stepped back enough that he missed, but I dropped my sword to my side and stumbled backwards as if I were letting go of life.

He paused for a moment and then raised his sword slowly just as Kaleb screamed and came charging from behind. Seeing his new opponent and thinking I was finished, he turned and raised his sword to fight Kaleb. I swung up, pivoting on my left foot, and with my knees bent, I lunged forward with everything I had left. My sword pierced his rib cage, opening him up from the back to the front, as Kaleb cut him across the left arm and chest in seconds. The pirate hardly knew what hit him as he collapsed to the ground.

I glanced up to see Kaleb rushing towards me. I tried to reach out to him but couldn't move. My head was spinning as I felt myself fading into complete darkness.

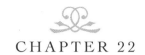

CHAPTER 22

A Son's Love

When I opened my eyes, I first saw Kaleb staring anxiously at me and holding a cup of luban and cistus tea in his hand. Moving my eyes, I realized that I was lying down. Kaleb whispered, "Papa," with the sound of relief, "you're awake."

"Yes, my son." Kaleb could see that I was struggling to remember what happened and how I came to be lying down in this unfamiliar place. As recall slowly came to me, I asked, "What happened? Is everyone safe?"

Just then Queen Balkis walked in and inquired, "How is he doing today, Master Kaleb?"

"He is awake, Queen Balkis."

"Well, then, I am sure the Captain will want to move out at first light. So you men stop standing around like puppies waiting for mother to wake you for feeding time. I'm sure you have things to attend to in camp."

With great amusement I heard, "Yes, my Queen," and then I saw Jona kneeling, with his hands on my feet.

"Captain, if you ever scare us like that again, I personally will. . . .," and then he went silent, dropping his head. I could feel this big man silently sobbing as he squeezed my feet. When he regained his composure, he said, "Captain, I am so relieved I won't have to face Mirah with different news. She would have killed me," he chuckled.

Barely lifting my hand towards Jona, I said to him, "You are alive, my friend! God has blessed us."

Ibram stepped up and touching my shoulder said, "You have a great swordsman there in your son. He saved your life, and, Captain, we did what you said. There was no defeat for us, and for them, no survivors, and it was the same with Ali and his men. We recovered everything that was taken, plus another 45 horses."

"Where are we?" I asked. "Papa, you have been sleeping for seven days. Ibram rode back and brought the caravan to us, and they have been here for five days," Kaleb informed me.

Queen Balkis spoke up, "Captain Shutran, you can be very proud of your son. He stayed at your side constantly as he didn't want anyone else to touch you. He and Jona hardly closed their eyes for seven days or nights, changing the dressings on your wounds and putting the drops of frankincense and cistus in camel milk and honey on your lips. Kaleb had half the men in camp boiling myrrh, balsam, galbanum, frankincense, and cistus and mixing the paste with honey and mustard for the wraps to be put on your wounds and kept changing them every hour, without fail.

"You lost so much blood that even the priest said there was no hope that you would live. But, Captain, I told everyone that we wouldn't be so lucky. You were too stubborn to die," she said with a slight smile on her face and then winked at Kaleb as she turned and walked out.

When I started to move, I could feel where the attacker had hit his mark. My shoulder still hurt quite a bit, but I was anxious to be up and moving and wanted to talk with my men who had been with me and made the rescue.

After a couple more days of rest, I decided to make the three-day journey with the others to Selah to buy supplies and food and to do a little trading. Because I was still healing, my men didn't think I was ready to ride and wanted me to stay in camp, but I was never one to stay behind. Kaleb tried to hide his concern and suggested, "Captain, I could stay in camp with you, and then we could go over some of the things from my record book."

"Kaleb, I know what you're trying to do, but I have not been doing my job for the last few days," I said chuckling. "Why don't you ride with me to Selah, and then you can keep an eye on me."

Realizing that there was no chance that I would stay in camp and trying to keep from laughing, Kaleb just blurted out, "You're the Commander. Let's go."

Jona interrupted, "Shutran, do you feel ready to ride?"

"Yes, I think I do. I want Kaleb to see the red rocks of Selah, and he won't go if I stay back."

The rock houses carved out of multicolored sandstone were an amazing sight. I remarked to my men how smart and industrious these people are and that I believed that in the future Selah would become a major trading center along the incense trail.

This would be a perfect location for them to build a great city with a treasury house large enough to hold the immense amount of merchandise that would be stored there. They would capture the trade from the southbound caravans coming from Nineveh going through Damascus and on to Gaza and from the westbound caravans coming from Babylon on the Silk Road to Gilead.

News of the pirate raid had already reached the talk around the campfires, and, of course, my men were more than happy to retell it in the most exciting way imaginable.

Towards evening after a day's activities, I felt a bit weak, so Kaleb and Jona helped me walk back to our tent as we left the men to their storytelling. "This has been a good day, but sleep will be welcome," I said. "We move out at first light."

Jona turned to look at me and in a serious tone of voice said, "Shutran, more and more I can see why you believe in the One God that you speak about. Your wounds were so severe that you should have died within hours. You shouldn't be alive."

"God is real, Jona, and you know what else? Abraham and the other ancient prophets talked about a new Messiah, who will come and teach more about this One God."

Jona was quiet and then responded, "That sounds very strange to me, but when I think about all that I have been through with you, a warm feeling comes over me."

"You know, Jona, there is so much we don't know or understand. We have trusted in 'the wise' to tell us what we should think and believe. But as I have experienced life, it has occurred to me that just because we can't read or write doesn't make them smarter.

"Jona, when I realized that we had given away our power too easily and had just become sheep and followed blindly, I decided I had to know for myself, and so I started asking questions. To my surprise, many of those so called 'learned people' never had a satisfactory answer for me. Their response was always something vague like, 'Well, you just have to believe because that is what the King or Queen or even the High Priest says.'

"But, Jona, you know this multiple god theory never made sense to me. The Egyptians believe in the sun god known as Ra; the god Horus, the falcon god; and many others. Queen Balkis believes in the sun god from her ancestry. So much of what we are taught is ancestral belief, and much of that is just blind superstition. To me, if you believe in those things, you lose your freedom."

"What do you mean, you lose your freedom?" Jona asked. "Shutran, how?"

"They teach you to believe one thing and control you in that belief out of fear. How can you be free when you fear what you believe? What kind of God is it that you have to fear?"

"Shutran, that's an interesting thought."

"It's only my feeling. I think we are just beginning to see the dawn of a whole new society that will try to control people as they start embracing the One God concept.

Well, it's late and morning comes early enough. We'll talk again. Good night, Jona."

"And to you, also, Shutran."

I laid there listening to the sounds of the night thinking about Mirah, the children at home, the caravan, and all the things that had happened while on the trail. Remarkably, we had suffered very little loss of life to this point.

I thought of my men and the commanders of the other caravans who had joined us and was so happy for them to think how they had led their own caravans, some with just two or three camels, men like Azaad, 25 years older than me, who almost died from dysentery, yet lived, only to bury one of his sons.

I wondered about that first morning when I was up and starting to walk around and Tamrin rode into our camp. He just couldn't wait to let everyone know in a very loud voice that surely the ultimate fight was soon to take place. That fueled my anger towards him and seemed to give me more strength, but I restrained myself and acted as though I couldn't be bothered with him. He took that as another insult and turned and rode off in a fury towards the Queen's camp, causing the dust to fly in every direction. I just knew that the outcome of his constant antagonism would not be good.

I thought about how Queen Balkis had come walking into my tent shortly after I had regained consciousness. She was always cold and distant, so her visit had surprised me, and even more so when she looked straight at me and loudly spoke as if to be giving an order that I, the Captain, would want to move out at first light. I wondered why she even came, since she had never shown any concern for me at all, except when she was trying to control me and get her way. She was a difficult woman to understand, and yet it was easy to see that she was very unhappy. I wondered who the real Queen was under that beautiful, dark skin.

Thinking about Tamrin, the Queen, and this immense caravan carried my thoughts back to my captains, Ibram, Mohamed, Ahmad, and Micah, and how grateful I was for their leadership and loyalty to me and the responsibility each one carried. Most of us had experienced several caravan treks together, while others were new and just beginning to build that trust and friendship. Together there was a powerful feeling of unity and protection for each other.

I was impressed with how much Enos had grown and how he took charge when there was a need and how he watched out for Kaleb and the great friendship they had developed. Enos had finally found his self-worth and his identity and had become a man on this caravan. Even Alimud, with the humiliation he faced every day, had made a big change.

At the same time a smile broke out on my face and my eyes watered when I thought of Jona. What a great friend and companion he had been over the years with his tough exterior and gentle heart. He displayed such genuine concern as I lay at death's door, relieving Kaleb and hardly sleeping until I was conscious again.

I felt a pain in my heart for Hagban's family as I reflected on how the outcome could have been different. His character was what it was, but he still had a family that loved him and would greatly suffer when they received the news.

But my greatest pain was the loss of Seth. Like Jona, he had become a great and trusted friend over the years. Seth had been the third in command for the last six caravans, a man who was not replaceable in commitment and loyalty. His dedication to his family and his responsibility was an example for everyone. Our homecoming would be bittersweet, as I had to take this dreadful news to his family. I said a quiet prayer for Seth's family and the others who would mourn the loss of their loved ones.

But then my thoughts turned to Kaleb, my firstborn son, and my heart seemed to overflow with adoration and pride. He gave such strength to the others during their captivity and boosted their belief in their rescue through his example of courageous and calculated action. I felt his fear when the pirate turned on him as he came to my rescue, but he was ready to do sword-to-sword battle without hesitation. I could hardly breathe as I thought about the raid and his captivity. I choked back the tears as I reflected on how he acted against my orders and turned back to fight.

Had he not, I would be dead. His courage was most remarkable.

I was impressed with how seriously he took his responsibilities; his daily journal entries and detailed records were a blessing to me. He had become very disciplined and was trustworthy in all of his duties. But most of all, I was happy to see how his relationship with God had grown. He had left home as a boy facing the unknown but had become a man to be reckoned with as life evolved each day on the caravan.

How could a father be more proud? I felt overwhelmed with gratitude as the knowing came to me that God does love me. Look at the witness He has given me. Then I thought about my family, Mirah, Kaleb, Joshua, and little Armin, and the tears started to run like a river down my cheeks until I couldn't wipe them away fast enough.

At that moment I felt Kaleb gently touch my arm, "Papa, are you all right?" he whispered, not wanting to wake Jona.

I turned and put my arms around my son and said, "Yes, Kaleb, I am. I just miss your mother, little Armin, and Joshua."

"I know, Papa; I do, too."

"Kaleb?"

"Yes, Papa?"

"I want you to never forget, no matter what happens, how much I love you. I am so proud of you and the wonderful young man you have become, and I thank you for saving my life."

"Oh, Papa," Kaleb cried as tears filled his eyes, "I love you, too."

The two of us lay there in silence, allowing the emotion of that moment to settle. Then Kaleb broke the silence, "Papa, I have a question."

"Yes, Kaleb."

"Would you be disappointed in me when I tell you that I was very scared when the pirates captured me? You have always told me to trust in God and not be afraid, but when the fighting started and that pirate stuck the jambiyya in your shoulder, I was really scared. I wanted to run, but yet I wanted to fight."

"Kaleb, we all feel fear at times, but how we deal with it is what matters. If you let the fear take control of you, then you are defeated. If you had run or done something different, the whole outcome for the other captives and your papa would have been different."

I leaned over and kissed him on the forehead and whispered, "You have done well, my son. Now, let's get some sleep."

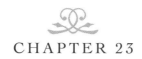

CHAPTER 23

The Treacherous
Crossing

orning seemed to come too early, but everyone wanted to get moving. There was a busyness of anxious commotion about camp as the smell of breakfast fires aroused the appetite. Some of the men were quickly eating, while others scurried to finish packing the camels. Kaleb came into the tent to check on me. "Captain, are you ready to ride?"

"Yes, Kaleb," I replied. "I'm just a little stiff this morning."

I asked Kaleb if he had seen the westbound caravan from Nineveh yet. "No," he answered, "why?"

"I was just curious to talk to them about the caravans coming out of the Indus Valley and over the Silk Road. I want to hear about the Emperor's interest in the luban and myrrh that we traded in Gerrha last year. A lot of the silk we have been carrying on our caravans has come from China the last three years.

"Queen Balkis has been planning this trip for a long time, ever since Solomon married one of the Pharaoh's daughters. Egyptians of royal blood are forbidden to marry outside of Egypt, so the Egyptians have been in an uproar against Solomon, and Solomon has used that to show his greater power, making the Egyptians even angrier. Kaleb, I just can't help but feel that Queen Balkis has a hidden reason for going to Jerusalem. I think the Pharaoh's daughter might be the Queen's sister."

Just as Kaleb and I stepped out of the tent, Tamrin, impressed with himself as usual, rode up and condescendingly greeted us, "Oh, Captain, I am glad to see you on your feet. We have a duel in Jerusalem, if you remember. I'm just checking to see if you'll be up to it."

"Tamrin, you need to worry about yourself. I am surprised that you are so anxious to die!"

"Captain Shutran, I have been insulted by you for the last time," he snarled as he rode off.

Tamrin's dust was still in the air when Jona rode up to let me know that all of the camels were packed and everything was ready. When daylight broke, the great caravan pulled out of Selah and headed north up the King's Highway. We had a three-day journey to Wadi Dana, and the climb out of the valley was slow. I had a foreboding feeling as I journeyed farther from my precious family and into the vast unknown of what might lie ahead.

The third night out of Selah, we camped at the top of the Wadi Dana Canyon. While eating, Enos asked, "Captain, why is this trail called the King's Highway?"

"One reason is because legends say that this is where Moses led about three million Israelites from the land of Midian back to Israel. Just north of here is a city called Heshbon, where Moses supposedly was attacked by the Amorites led by King Sihon, who Moses and his army defeated. Heshbon is a trade city for the caravans coming out of Babylon going to Jerusalem and out of Damascus going to Alexandria. This caravan trail has been a main travel route for probably 500 years from Aila, the White City, to Damascus."

"If the trade route crossroad is at Heshbon, why are we going to cross here?" Alimud asked. Silence fell on everyone as all eyes turned to look at him. This was the first time that he had interacted with the men since we left Marib four months ago.

"Alimud, that is a good question. Going down the wadi is more difficult, and staying on the King's Highway certainly makes more sense.

"However, I have a couple of stops I want to make. First, at the mouth of the canyon is a copper mine, where I want to leave a list of things to be picked up on our return from Jerusalem. Second, we must stop at Ein Gedi, which is on the west shore of the Salt Sea, to unload some balsam and frankincense trees as well as the resins. This will be our last stop before entering Jerusalem. As soon as we arrive in Ein Gedi, I will send a messenger to notify King Solomon, since I am sure he will want his army to ride out to meet us and escort us into their great city."

While we were talking, Tamrin rode up unannounced again and stopped his horse in front of us. "Captain, how are you feeling?" he queried. Without waiting for an answer, he continued. "In how many days do you figure we will be in Jerusalem?"

"In five days," I answered.

"I'll tell the Queen," he said and turned to ride away.

"Tamrin," I called as I stood up. He stopped his horse and turned back to face me.

"To answer your question, I am feeling better every day."

"That's good, Captain," he smugly retorted and turned and rode back to his camp.

As I squatted back down, Mohamed questioned, "What was that all about?"

"You know what that was about," Jona quipped.

"All right, men. Let's call it a night. It's been another good day."

Just before daylight Hussin came riding in to let me know that earlier rains had flooded the wadi, taking out the trail. Moving the wagons through it would be next to impossible without a lot of work. I sent Kaleb to tell Nadab to notify the Queen that we would be camped here for probably two days while we cleared the trail. I told Jona to send all of my captains out to notify everyone else that we would be camped here for about two days and that they were to bring their men, mules, and camels to move boulders and debris.

After we saw the condition of the trail, it was easy to determine that two days would not be enough time to open it to get the wagons through. I rode back up to camp with Jona and Mohamed to meet with the Queen to let her know my thoughts and discuss our possible solutions. After seeing how the trail had been gouged out and washed away, I knew that we would need at least two weeks to make it passable for the wagons.

"Captain," the Queen asked, "what do you feel we should do?"

"We have several choices. We can take two weeks to open the trail so that we can pass through with the wagons, or we can open it enough for the animals to get through and leave the wagons here until we return. We could also send the animals around the wadi, which would be a little easier but would take longer, and then we would still have to come back for the wagons. However, we can take the wagons apart, pack them across the slide, and reassemble them after we get through the canyon."

I had felt her anxiousness to get to Jerusalem ever since we arrived in Selah. "Well, Captain, what are you waiting for?" she questioned.

"After the trail is open, the caravan will take two to three days to get across the slide. I suggest that you stay here, and Tamrin can bring you across on your horse when we're ready. When the wagons are disassembled, he can bring the mules back to start packing them and your possessions. This will take another three days."

"Whatever you say, Captain. You know what's best."

Tamrin bristled, "Why can't you take the Queen around through Heshbon without the entire caravan? It would be much easier and we could make better time."

"Tamrin, it doesn't matter to me, but I do not believe the Queen wants to enter Jerusalem without her caravan."

"Captain Shutran is right. Now let's get every man working to open the trail."

I gave Tamrin an order, "Take as many men as you need and start dismantling the wagons and her chariot." Tamrin scowled at me but didn't say a word as he turned and rode away.

Five kilometers down the canyon, another flashflood had come in from a cross wadi and had saturated the ground so badly that much of the mountain, 300 meters wide, had slid down into the canyon below, completely taking out the trail. I called to Ibram, "Take 200 slaves with spades and have them start digging out a new trail across the mountain. Tell them to watch for underground water, and if they see any, pull back and go higher up the side of the mountain. If they dig where it's soft, the rest of the mountain could come down and bury all of them. I'll ride through the wadi and see if I can get down into the bottom and find a way through to check the other side. In the meantime, get the mule teams moving the big boulders off the trail."

In two days we had the trail open enough to get the camels across and down the wadi to the mouth of the canyon where we had set up a second camp. Then the men started bringing the camels across with limited packs of about 150 kilos. The mountainside was soft, but once past the slide area, the trail was solid. The camels were nervous and did not like the insecurity of the steep mountainside and soft ground. I told the men to walk no more than three camels across at a time.

Joktel, one of Tamrin's men, was the fifth to cross. Since the others had crossed without any problem, Tamrin told him to take five camels at a time so that they could get everything over the slide area before dark. When Grandfather Azaad saw what Joktel was doing, he hollered out, "Captain Shutran said not more than three camels at a time!"

Tamrin turned and yelled at Azaad, "Silence, old man. These are my camels and I am in charge; you're going across next, so get your camels ready, five at a time."

Joktel was only halfway across when the back foot of the fifth camel slid a little, which made him nervous and caused him to pull back, stepping off the trail. Joktel stopped and in a panic started yelling at the other four camels to hold steady, but they could feel the tension and were becoming unsettled.

The fifth camel started to slide a little more and couldn't recapture his footing, pulling the other camels backwards until the fourth one came off the trail, creating a chain reaction. Joktel was trying to pull the first one forward, but it was too late. The camels were out of control and trying to keep their footing, but there was no way to stop them.

Joktel didn't notice that he had stepped over the lead rope, and as the camels started to slide, it wrapped around his ankles. He was still yelling as he slid the first 20 meters down the mountain. When the camels began to cartwheel into the ravine 300 meters below, all that could be heard was the crashing of rocks, the snapping of branches, and the faint braying of camels. It was a terrifying sight, and those who saw it were in shock as they looked to the bottom of the canyon. The mountain quickly became quiet as the dust that filled the air silently settled to the ground.

Tamrin, with no concern for what just happened, turned to Azaad and hollered, "You're next. Get your camels across; we have to keep moving." Meanwhile, Nadab sent a couple of men down the ravine to see if any of the camels were alive, what damage there was, and if there was any sign of Joktel, who probably didn't survive the fall.

Jona had taken charge of getting everything into the new camp before dark and was on his way back to the slide area with some of the men and camels with empty packs to reload. The dust was still in the air when he noticed the two men climbing down the steep face.

Azaad had untied his camels and was about to start crossing with one of them when Tamrin came riding up and hit him with his whip, yelling, "I said you're taking five camels across!" Azaad refused so Tamrin hit him again. Jona had already started to cross from the other side with three camels and saw Azaad trying to protect himself from Tamrin's whip. When Tamrin saw Jona coming, he abruptly turned and rode up to the top of the trail to the Queen's camp and remained there.

Jona quickly reached Azaad, where the men were standing and holding loaded camels and mules ready to cross. After hearing what happened

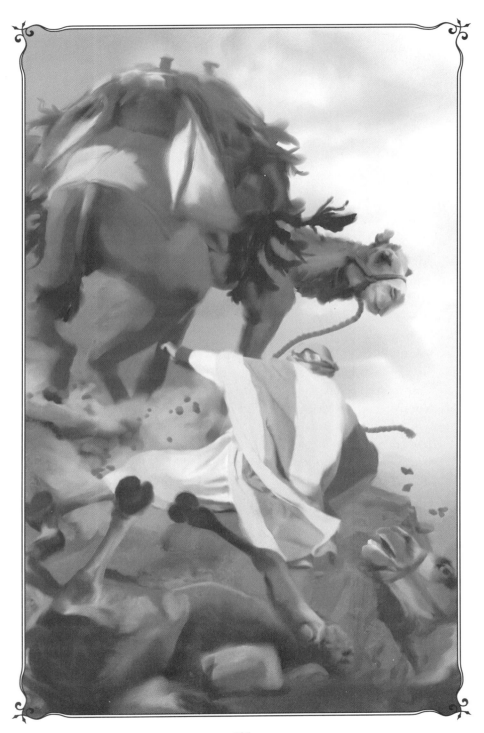

and assessing the situation, he said, "Men, only the mules are to cross until we can re-establish the trail and after that only one camel at a time."

When the two men reached the bottom, they found two camels dead and three alive, but there was no trace of Joktel. Jona yelled down to the men to repack the three camels, take off their lead ropes, and let them find their way out of the wadi. Then he turned back to the others and yelled, "Let's get some more men with spades on the trail. We have to get across before dark."

When I finished the trade agreement for the copper to be picked up on our return trip, I rode back to camp. When I arrived, there was a lot of commotion about the slide down the mountain. Jona had just arrived with the last of the loaded camels and said that two men and three camels were still in the bottom of the canyon.

I called to Ibram and Alimud, "Go with Azaad's two sons and take some food, water, and six mules to go and find the camels. The rocks in the bottom of the ravine are so big that the camels can't get through carrying full packs. But I feel that the mules could get through, and if the packs on the camels are reduced in size, they would most likely be able to follow the mules. If it gets dark before you get through, then stay there until morning to avoid the risk of breaking a leg in the rocks."

I then turned to Jona and asked, "What happened?"

"Tamrin, again! He told Joktel to take five camels across, and the last camel became nervous, started to pull back, and stepped off the trail, dragging the rest down with him, including Joktel."

"What happened to him?"

"They said that so much mud and dirt went down with them that he must have been buried. They didn't find him, and the packs of the two camels that died are still at the bottom and have to be brought out."

I could feel my blood boiling as I anticipated what I felt I had to do. The fight would not wait until Jerusalem.

I mounted Sultan and rode over to Kaleb and Enos, who were getting the mules ready to go with the men to help retrieve the camels and packs from the bottom of the ravine. "Kaleb, I'm going to ride up the trail to check on the Queen and make sure the wagons will be ready to cross in the morning."

"Be careful, Captain," Kaleb's voice resounded as I turned to start up the trail.

Jona came around one of the tents, moving quickly to intercept my departure, out of Kaleb's sight. "Captain, wait, I have to talk to you." I reined Sultan around in his direction to see what he wanted. "Shutran, where are you going?"

"You know where I am going."

"Yes, that's what I thought. It will take you six hours at best to cross the slide and reach the camp in the dark. Do you really think that's wise? You have been pushing hard all day, and you are still recovering. You do not need to engage in a fight in your condition. Shutran, as tired as you are, and with Tamrin having done nothing all day except give orders, you will be at a great disadvantage."

"Jona," I said with a slight grin, "you sound just like Mirah," and rode off into the dark of the night. Calling back to Jona, I yelled, "Make sure you get all the packs and the camels out of the wadi in the morning." Jona never responded. He had already gone looking for Mohamed and Micah.

When I arrived at the slide area three hours later, the moon was climbing overhead, illuminating the deep canyon. I gave Sultan the lead, because he could smell the trail, and started across slowly.

He was a high-spirited Arabian that always seemed to know what to do no matter what the situation. I raised him from a colt and had been riding him for 15 years. He had taken me across the treacherous desert, through the rugged, high mountains, and along the dangerous coastal plains of Arabia that were infested with pirates. His speed brought me safely through raging sandstorms, and he stayed close to me in battle as I outmaneuvered my opponent. I never had to question his loyalty. He was strong, powerful, bigger than most, and never seemed to tire. After 14 hours in the saddle, he was still as energetic as when we started.

I was always amazed at how he could follow a trail, like when we were following the pirates who captured Kaleb. I simply dropped the reins and let him go, even across the rocks. In reality, I spent more time with Sultan than I did with my wife. I never had to tie him to the picket line because he never left my tent except to water and feed. If I fell asleep in the saddle and he thought I should be awake, he would act as if he were stumbling to wake me up. Then he would wiggle his ears as if laughing at me.

Sultan could easily find his way through the dark. As soon as we were over the slide area, he moved swiftly on the trail. I thought about Queen Balkis and everything she was carrying with her. It would take all day to get the wagons and the Queen's camp across.

I kept rehearsing in my mind what I would do to Tamrin. I should have killed him months ago when I had my sword at his throat. My anger grew with intensity as I thought back over the months since I had come to know this disgusting individual. Under his command five men had lost their lives because of his arrogant, self-impressed attitude and complete lack of caring for another human being. The more I thought about him, the more enraged I became.

I reached the camp about two hours before daylight. The guards on duty were alert and acted as though they were expecting someone. I stepped down out of the saddle as one of them spoke, "Captain Shutran, you must have ridden all night to get here. Is everything all right with the rest of the caravan?"

"Yes, men. Everything is fine. Listen, I need you to watch the trail. I think I have possibly been followed by a couple of men on horses. Take them by surprise, tie them up, and hold them until daylight. I have a meeting with Captain Tamrin, and I do not want to be disturbed."

"But, Captain," Awad spoke up, "Captain Tamrin is asleep."

"Yes, but he knew I was coming. He won't mind being awakened early."

"Captain, he wanted me to let him know if you came."

"Awad, I would be more concerned about the two men following me if I were you. I can find Tamrin by myself."

Now with this information I knew Tamrin would have his tent guarded, and they would be on the alert for me. I loosened Sultan's cinch and secured him to the tree behind some rocks. Then I circled around the back of the camp to the picket line. The guard was leaning against a large rock, half asleep. I walked up to him from his blind side and stuck my sword tip against his throat. He came fully awake with such fear that he peed down both legs. As I whispered to him not to make a sound, I stepped around in front of him so that he could see me. Then slowly I lowered my sword. He gasped with a sigh of relief, almost losing his breath.

"Oh, Captain Shutran, I didn't know it was you."

I looked at him and sternly asked, "Do you know what the punishment is for sleeping on duty?" In the moonlight I could see the blood drain from his face.

"Yes, Captain, I do!" His voice was shaking as I told him to be quiet.

"If you promise to never fall asleep again and do exactly as I say, I'll keep this quiet. I am here for a meeting with Captain Tamrin, but no one must know until we are finished. Saddle his horse for him so he can leave when we're ready." Reaching down, I handed him Tamrin's saddle and saddle blanket in which I had just stuck four large thorns. "If anyone asks, just say that you are following Captain Tamrin's orders."

When the guard cinched down the saddle, Tamrin's horse kicked the horse beside him and then started to stomp sideways and back the other way, making a lot of commotion. When the other two guards outside of Tamrin's tent heard the noise, they went to see what was happening. At that moment I crawled to the back of the tent and cut a small hole with my jambiyya to see who was inside. Sure enough, Nadab and Ayaar were there with him.

I went back around to the front near the opening and whispered just loud enough so that they could hear me, "Captain Tamrin, Captain Tamrin, something is wrong with your horse." Tamrin turned over and nudged Nadab and Ayaar awake and told them to go see what was wrong with his horse. As soon as they left the tent, I crawled in from the back and then stood up and kicked Tamrin in the side and said softly, "Get up, now!" He startled half awake and stood up. He was mad and a little disoriented as he turned to see who had awakened him.

Before he was able to really see my face, I shoved my fist tightly gripped around my jambiyya right into the pit of his stomach, followed by another jab to the left side, breaking his ribs. I hit him again so fast in the stomach that he couldn't even take a breath and that caused him to stumble backwards, catching his feet in Ayaar's blankets.

Then with the butt of my jambiyya, I made a smashing blow to his face, making a cut from the left temple across the eyebrow between his eyes. With the blood running down his face, I drove my fist directly to the point of his nose, causing the blood to gush out as he went down on his knees. I followed with another blow across the right eyebrow, splitting it wide open. As he collapsed on the ground, I could hear the wheezing as he tried to breathe, wrenching with pain.

I wrapped his gutrah around his neck, dragged him out of the tent, and jerked him up to his knees. With the pent-up rage inside of me, I drove another crosscutting blow to the right of his chin. His jaw snapped and he went over sideways. He was barely conscious as I grabbed the gutrah and pulled him back up on his knees. I held onto him until he quit wrenching, while he tried to open his eyes.

"Tamrin, I am not going to kill you here. I am going to let you have the audience you want in King Solomon's court, but so help me, I will kill you." Then I drove another crashing jambiyya fist into his face, crushing his cheekbone, and said, "That was for Azaad and Joktel." As I let go of the gutrah, he went face down into the dirt.

I was standing over him when the two guards came walking back from the picket line. Daylight was breaking and they recognized who I was. They did not see Tamrin on the ground until after they spoke. "Captain Shutran?"

"Yes," I said, looking down at Tamrin. "One of you needs to go get the Queen's priest. Tamrin needs help. It looks like he tripped coming out of his tent when he heard the commotion."

Just then Nadab walked up and gasped when he saw Tamrin, who was barely moving and was moaning with pain. As he came up on his knees, blood-soaked dirt stuck to his face and the front of his thobe. His face was not recognizable as he tried to talk, and he whimpered with pain greater than he had ever imagined in his life. Nadab knelt down beside him and asked, "Captain, what happened?" In the same breath he turned and ordered one of the guards to go for the priest and two others to help get Tamrin into his tent.

Nadab looked up at me with a question on his face. With complete calmness as if to answer his unasked question, I said, "He killed Joktel," and I walked off. I tightened Sultan's cinch, swung up into the saddle, and rode out to where the guards were. There sat Jona and Mohamed, captive as I had ordered.

Jona was the first to speak, "I don't suppose you had any idea that they would think we were thieves, now, did you?"

"I wouldn't think that, Jona, unless you were sneaking around trying not to be seen, especially when no one would think you would come up the trail to visit anyway."

They could easily see that I was trying to hold back my laughter as I nodded to the guard to free them. "With all you had to do, what are you doing here?"

Jona turned to speak to Mohamed as though I weren't present, "Did we miss the trail into the canyon when we were looking for the last three camels?"

"I think so," Mohamed chuckled. "It was getting dark when we left."

As Jona stood up and faced me, I said, "Jona, thanks for your concern. I may be 25 years older than Tamrin, but he has no salt. He is just a pretty bully who thinks his position has given him the right to whip and beat slaves and peasants. Tonight he got to experience what a beating feels like. It will be several weeks before he forgets, and, I hope, never. You and Mohamed had better start back. I am going to stay to answer questions from the Queen and to get her camp moving early.

"With the Queen's four wagons and her chariot dismantled, it will take until noonday to pack the 45 camels and get them across the slide. Jona, by the time you get back to the caravan, it will be early afternoon. Have the men go over all the pack equipment and make sure we do not have to stop later for repairs. Have everyone ready to start loading early in the morning. Organize all the gifts for Solomon on the first 500 camels. Load the luban first and then the myrrh, balsam, gold, diamonds, ivory, and silk in that order. Have Kaleb and Enos make a full accounting of all the goods. This will be a good use of the time."

"Captain, now that we know you don't need any help and that you are all right, we'll ride fast and be ready when you arrive tonight."

When I rode back to the Queen's camp, it was full light and the sun was making its climb to the top of the mountains. I thought to myself, this is a good day. I felt so light and free to have released six months of locked-up anger towards Tamrin. It felt good to know that he wouldn't be interfering with the caravan for the rest of the journey or be beating anyone for a long time. Even though I knew I had to have a conversation with Queen Balkis, it was still a great day.

As I rode in, I could see servants scurrying in and out of Tamrin's tent. Queen Balkis was standing with the two guards who had carried him into the tent. Looking up as I came into her view, she immediately started speaking with a loud voice. "Captain Shutran, what is your explanation of Tamrin's condition? He is almost dead and may die before the day is over. The priest said Tamrin has lost a lot of blood and is in shock from the pain."

I stepped down out of the saddle in front of her and the guards while she was talking. I looked her in the eyes without flinching until she stopped to take a breath. I shot a glance at the two guards to see their response and was surprised to see non-responsive looks on their faces. As my eyes went back to Balkis, I hesitated to answer in a way that might provoke more anger, since she was steaming. Then she snapped, "I suppose you want this camp to move this morning?"

"Yes, Queen Balkis, we need to get the camp across the slide before noonday."

"What about Tamrin? The guards said they saw you standing over him. I demand an explanation." Her anger was growing. "I could have you. . . ."

I held up my hand and said, "Stop, Queen Balkis; let's be honest. You do not have one man in your military here who would dare approach me, and you know it. They have watched your Captain Tamrin for months beat your slaves, yell at your servants, insult and humiliate them, and even whip two of your guards. You are a long way from your home, and every man knows he does not have to return unless he wants to.

"Tamrin does not rule here, and neither do you, Queen Balkis, and not to be disrespectful, but do you want to know more?"

Her faced was hot with anger while she tried to show her power and superiority to all who were watching and listening. "Captain, you are a brutal and cruel man."

"For what, Queen Balkis? For beating a man half my age and 20 kilos heavier; who boasts to be a great swordsman; who boasts no man can beat him in hand-to-hand fighting; who whips men, children, defenseless slaves, and peasants; who kills with no feeling or regard for life? A man who will put your entire caravan at risk, and you still demand an answer?

"I question your reasoning and why it is that you want men to fear you and women to hate you. You hired me to lead your caravan, and you agreed to my conditions. I might remind you that over and over again I have had no help from Tamrin. He has caused nothing but problems with his arrogant and antagonistic attitude. Every time I turned my back, he has defied my orders and given counter orders, like yesterday. I gave the order for only three camels to cross the slide at a time.

"The moment I rode out to take care of other matters, he ordered Joktel to take five camels across the slide. They all went down the mountain, killing Joktel and two camels and destroying many of the packs and goods they were carrying. Immediately after they fell, he ordered Azaad to take five of his camels across, with no concern for what had happened. When Azaad refused to follow his order, he struck him. If Jona hadn't arrived, Tamrin probably would have killed Azaad. Men are in the canyon right now trying to find Joktel's body to give him a rightful burial and trying to retrieve all the packs and goods spread out in the bottom of the canyon.

"Queen Balkis, how many camels did you lose as a result of Tamrin's interference with my orders? How much time have we lost? And you want an explanation?" Several of her servants and six more guards had gathered around and were listening intensely. When the Queen noticed that others were listening to this conversation, she realized that she was not in a favorable position and had to immediately redeem herself and save her dignity.

She stepped forward, placing her hand on my arm very cautiously, and said, "Captain Shutran, I had no knowledge of yesterday's misfortune. You're right; Captain Tamrin will be stripped of his rank, and when he recovers, he will be given the place of a guard."

"What you do with him is of no concern to me as long as he never gives another order while on this caravan."

"Captain, I had no idea of all these charges against him. In spite of all of the problems, you have brought this caravan this far, and no man has accomplished such a feat. Captain, I just have one question." She just wouldn't leave it alone. "Do you know who beat Tamrin?" I looked her right in the eye, and before I spoke, she gently squeezed my arm and with a slight smile said, "Tell me."

"There was only one man, and it was a fight eye-to-eye, and when Tamrin can speak, he can tell you who it was. I am quite sure that there was no question in his mind."

She again squeezed my arm, "Captain, was it you? It was, wasn't it?"

I responded with only a slight smile on my face and then changed the subject. Nadab was standing nearby, so I called him over. "You take charge of the camp and get it packed and moving."

"Captain Shutran, could you tell us how to pack the wagons on the camels?"

"Yes, gather the men and camels and let me know when they are all here."

Nadab hurriedly called his chiefs to come and bring a few of their camels. When they were ready, I walked over to the group and began to explain what needed to be done.

"First, you have to take the wagon box apart and use the boards to make a flat platform for the bolsters. Second, place the reach on one side of the platform and the tongue on the other side. Third, roll a tent around each axle and place one along each side of the camel.

"Next, tie one rear wheel flat against the axle and then tie the second wheel to the other side. The front wheels are smaller, so you can tie two of them on each side of the camel. Take a rope and run it over the pack saddle, tying the top of the two wheels together in a sling. Each wheel weighs about 120 kilos, so it is extremely important that the camel is balanced. When the wheels are securely tied, you can hang the packs with the cooking gear on last, but make sure the camel stays balanced.

"As the camels are loaded and secured, take them across the slide one at a time and on into camp to unload. It will take seven camels to pack the four wagons across.

"Because the Queen's chariot is inlaid with so much gold and silver, you'll have to load two camels to carry it across. You'll also need two camels to carry the four heavy wheels for the merchant wagon. When the camels arrive at the camp, the men can begin to reassemble the wagons and chariot.

The rest of the Queen's camp was packed and lined up at the slide, waiting their turn. Queen Balkis came riding up to me on the black stallion that was to be a gift to Solomon. Looking at her, I shook my head and she immediately questioned, "What's wrong?"

"Queen Balkis, why do you give so much to one man who is already five times richer than you?"

"He doesn't know how rich I am," she responded.

"Queen Balkis, he knows all about his adversaries, and you can be sure your entire fortune is no secret to him."

"Shutran, why do you care?"

"I just never knew a woman to give a man such gifts except that she had a hidden reason."

"Perhaps I just want to gain his wisdom." Changing the subject she remarked, "You have not inquired about Tamrin."

"You're right and I won't."

"Well, for your information, Nadab took him up the trail to the Bedouin village so that they can care for him. Nadab left Tamrin's horse there so that when he is able, he can catch up with us."

"It would be better if he didn't."

"Tamrin wants to see King Solomon's temple, and he says he has a meeting with you in the King's court."

"We'll see."

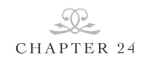

CHAPTER 24

Sheba's Change of Heart

Queen Balkis was sitting on her horse while looking at the trail going across the slide. It was obvious to everyone watching that she was anxious. I motioned to her to start across as I nudged Sultan with my heels. Not hearing any movement, I turned back to look at her and saw that she was still sitting on her horse, motionless. I called to her to follow, but she just looked at me and reluctantly asked, "Captain Shutran, will you lead my horse across the slide?"

"Queen Balkis, do I detect a note of fear in your voice? How unlike you, a woman who is as hard as the brass on the axle of your wagon," I said with a tone of amusement. She obviously was not amused and did not answer back, which caught my attention. I turned my focus away from the slide area to move closer to her, wondering what was happening. As our eyes met, I could see that her fear was real and that she was not going to go any farther. Not wanting to cause her further embarrassment, I said, "Of course, Queen Balkis; let's go."

I took the reins of her horse and headed towards the slide area. All of her camels were over, and just a few military guards were still waiting to cross. The big stallion was nervous and started prancing when we started. Queen Balkis was already breathing hard, which made the horse more nervous. He pranced sideways, switching back and forth, until we reached the slide. As the horse sensed the Queen's fear mounting, his prancing increased. His nostrils flared and he snorted harder; I could see that he was not going to calm down.

The Queen was almost in tears, and when I stopped and dismounted, she swung quickly out of her saddle and came running and wrapped her arms around me. "Shutran, I am so scared. I can't let my men see me this way. I'm afraid of heights and when I look down the slide to the bottom, I feel like I'm going to faint. I've never been so scared in my life."

Thinking to calm her down, I said, "Here, you get on Sultan and I'll bring the black."

"No, I can't do it. Please, Captain, don't let go of me, please," she begged and started to cry.

"Queen Balkis, get a hold of yourself. Your men are watching." But as the fear gripped her, she went limp into my arms.

I thought about my situation and wondered, "What next?" Here I was, ready to start across this treacherous slide with a prancing, snorting stallion about to jump off the trail; the Queen, struck with such fear that she passes out in my arms; and Sultan is looking sideways with his ears twitching back and forth, wondering what he did wrong. I would have laughed if the situation hadn't been so critical. I called to a guard to come and take the black. When I handed him the lead rope, the horse calmed down immediately. I shook my head and told him not to breathe a word of this to a single person and to pass that on to the rest of the men.

Looking at the Queen, the guard asked, "Captain, what's wrong?"

"She was so frightened that she fainted."

"The Queen, who is as tough as the brisket hide on a camel?"

"Yes," I said as he laughed. "You just better keep it quiet, because if this tough, brisket-hide Queen finds out you talked, she might end your life," I said chuckling. We retreated 20 meters to a small, flat ridge, where I could sit her down and lean her against a large rock. I poured a little water over her face and head until she started to cough.

While she regained composure and came to her senses, I sent all but one of the guards with the black stallion across the slide. I sent the remaining guard back up the trail to wait out of sight until he saw me cross and then to follow behind me.

The Queen, now fully aware of what happened, was sitting quietly, feeling a bit embarrassed. She didn't say a word but was just watching me to see what I was going to do. I mounted Sultan and leaving the left stirrup open, I motioned for her to take my hand and climb up behind me. As I came to the slide, she started breathing uncontrollably. I stopped Sultan and said, "Queen Balkis, you have a choice. You have to get control of your fear or stay behind with Tamrin."

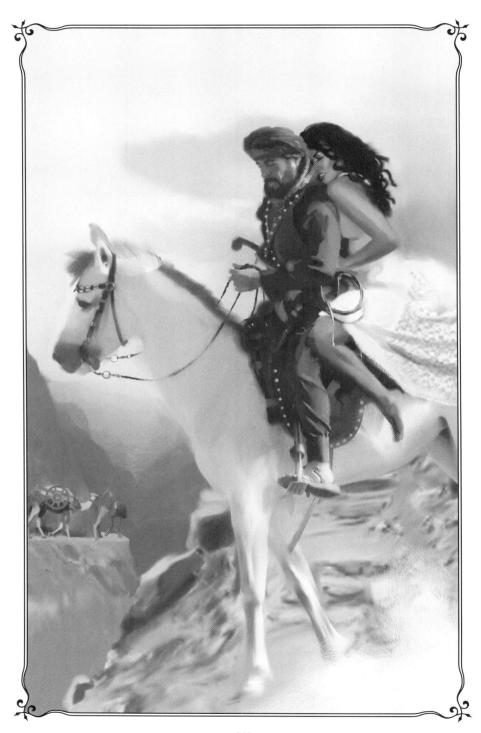

"Please, Shutran, don't leave me!"

I shook my head and thought, "How interesting." I could feel her trembling and so with a big sigh, I said, "Now, don't look down! Just think about when you were so mad at me that you wanted blood. Hang on and don't move because the ground is soft and still moving." With her face buried in my back and squeezing me until I almost couldn't breathe, we started across.

Sultan was very surefooted and steadily moved forward at his own pace, feeling the ground underneath him. It felt like at any moment the whole side of the mountain could slide again. It seemed like it took a long time, but we were to the other side in just a few minutes. Once we were safely across, the last guard followed without a problem.

I tapped the Queen's hand so that she would know it was safe and that we had crossed over the slide. I told her that we were on the trail that went past the copper mine to our camp. She relaxed a bit but never let go the entire three hours of our journey.

I didn't say another word while she tried to put herself back together and figure out how she was going to maintain her position and keep up her reputation. She was certain that the guards had told everyone about her fear and having to ride with Shutran across the slide. I could feel her squirming, looking for a way to start a conversation, but I remained silent, thinking it would be good to let her feel foolish and uneasy a little longer.

After some time had passed and the darkness of the night had settled upon us, she finally broke the silence. "Captain, the people will laugh at me, and I will lose the control and power I had over them."

"Well, are you afraid that they might see you as human? Everyone has a fear of something."

"Captain, do you have a fear?"

"Of course, I do—many."

"Like what?"

"Well, if I told you, then you would have an advantage, and I couldn't allow that, now, could I?"

"Come on, Captain, tell me one so that I can feel better."

"All right; I have a fear that I may not live up to God's expectations of me."

"That's not a fear," she said.

"It is for me. Sometimes I get caught up in negative thoughts and fears about my family when I'm away."

"No, Captain, I mean a real fear of something like my fear of heights. Surely you fear something that is more real."

"For me, Queen Balkis, those fears are real." I wasn't going to tell her that my one worst fear was that of the deadly viper snake of the desert, whose strike meant almost instant death.

"What do you do with fear when you feel it?" she asked.

"I simply look at it and ask myself, 'What is the worst thing that could happen?' For me, losing my family is the very worst, so I trust in God when I am not there."

"Captain, I hear you believe in the One God, the same as King Solomon."

"Yes, that's true."

"Why?" she asked.

"Why not?" I replied. "It makes more sense. Think about it."

Wanting to know more about the Queen, I changed the subject and asked, "Queen Balkis, you're not from the Hadhramaut originally, are you?"

"No," she said quite sternly. "When my grandfather, the Pharaoh of Egypt, was in Ethiopia visiting in the court of the Ethiopian King, he was taken by the beauty of my grandmother, a princess, who in time became pregnant with his child. Afraid that the child would be an embarrassment to Egypt, he left her and returned to his country.

"When my mother became a young woman, she traveled to Egypt to meet her father, the Pharaoh, who smiled on her and allowed her to stay in his court. She was a beautiful woman and fell in love with the young prince, Siamun, the son of the Pharaoh. When the Pharaoh found out that she was with child, my mother was sent back to Ethiopia, since it wasn't proper to marry outside our culture. Sometime after my twin sister, Makshara, and I were born, my father, Siamun, became the Pharaoh of Egypt, but he never saw my mother again nor knew anything about our birth.

"As I grew into womanhood, I wanted to meet our father, so I encouraged my twin sister and our mother's brother, our uncle, to journey with us to Egypt. When we arrived, our father would receive us only as visitors to his court and did not want to acknowledge us as his daughters. But when he saw us, he favored Makshara because she was fair skinned like him. I was dark skinned like my Ethiopian mother, who he did not want to acknowledge.

"I was much bolder than my sister and told him that I wanted my rightful place as a princess. I think he wanted to keep Makshara near him, but only Makshara, so he granted my wish and gave me the kingdom of

Saba, with the condition that I could rule and possess great wealth as long as I did not marry nor return to Egypt. However, at the time I agreed, I didn't realize the implication of his conditions and certainly had no idea of the location of this desert kingdom he gave me.

"I was so angry with my grandfather for abandoning my mother and then with my father for preferring my sister and rejecting me that I swore to never trust a man again. I would just use them like they used my mother and grandmother."

"Where is your father now?"

"He is the great Pharaoh of Egypt. After my mother was sent back to Ethiopia, he married an Egyptian princess. She bore him a son, who is my half brother, Shishak, who is the prince who will inherit the throne from my father.

My mother, who should have been the Queen of Egypt, has lived a very lonely and sad life. When the Pharaoh sent her back to Ethiopia, she was rejected by her own people and was left to take care of herself. While my father had great wealth, he never bestowed any of that on my mother. He could have taken care of her so that she could have lived as she deserved with a proper home in which to raise her twin daughters.

"My father lied to me saying that the Hadhramaut was a rich and luxurious paradise with great wealth. But then when I saw that the desert was a wasteland, I became even angrier and vowed that he would live to regret the day he gave me this miserable land. I set out to do that and have made it a rich kingdom. Later I learned that my father, Siamun, knew about the riches of the Hadhramaut from the stories passed down about our ancestor, Queen Hatshepsut, who was the first to discover the Land of Frankincense.

"By putting me there to rule as the Queen of Saba, or Sheba, as I like to be called, he thought he could take my Hadhramaut Kingdom under Egyptian rule. What he didn't expect was that I would become strong and fight against him, and now we profit greatly from his merchants who buy the resins of frankincense and myrrh as well as the rose water for his courts and temples."

Queen Balkis was probably for the first time dumping the pain from her heart as she told me how she had been betrayed by the most important people in her life. She had been rejected as a child and displaced as a young woman by her father and grandfather when all she wanted was for them to love her. She was sent to a place in a vast wilderness with all the odds against her, yet out of hate and determination, she fought and succeeded in building a mighty kingdom that her father thought she would just hand over to him or that he could easily take from her.

"My feelings became hard when I came to Saba," she continued, "and the people laughed at me because I was a foreigner and a woman. Because of my beauty, men tried to use me, until I realized that I could use my beauty and riches to control them. I would let them think I would be their mistress until I got what I wanted.

"Shutran, you are the first man to reject my affection, and I hated you for it. I couldn't control you and yet I desperately wanted to. You are a strong man and you know what you want. I think if I had a man like you by my side, we could conquer the world. Think about it, Shutran—what you and I could do, the lands we could conquer, and the riches we could have with your vision and ability to lead my military. Shutran, you need a woman like me. You are the first man I know who I can trust and believe in, and you are also the first man I have felt a feeling for that is real. Shutran, I think I am falling in love with you."

"Queen Balkis. . . ."

"Stop," she said. "Please call me Sheba. My mother gave me that name when I came to the Hadhramaut."

"Yes, Sheba, but please call me Captain. I think the scare you just had awoke another side of you, which could be really threatening."

"What do you mean by that?"

"Let me see; how can I say this? Perhaps you realized that you have a desire for friendship and love, which made you feel somewhat insecure and probably very strange. You only let people see your rough, hard exterior, which attracts men like Tamrin. Sheba, the life you live can be great, but you have to see the greatness in everything around you."

"Captain, I have watched how you treat your men and how they respect you, like Jona, Ibram, and Enos. They love you but when I see that, it makes me angry. How do you do it? How can you treat them as though they are your family so that eventually they become that? Haven't you ever been betrayed by trusting and believing in someone?"

"Yes, of course. People have choices and if their spirit is not pure, they will betray you for personal gain. But they are the ones who lose, because once that happens, eventually someone will betray them. What goes out eventually comes back. It's just that sometimes it seems like it doesn't come around fast enough. You can't quit trusting people. You just have to be more selective and careful."

"Captain, right now you seem so soft, but I watched what you did to Hagban. You killed him and I know you beat Tamrin nearly to death. I do not understand how you can be so caring in one moment and in the next moment be so violent."

"Sheba, perhaps that is my character flaw. I would much rather be a peaceful, loving person than a fighter, but I cannot tolerate evil and injustice. I think God gave me the temperament to defend when necessary. There are not enough fighters for what is right in our world. That is why evil seems to always be one step ahead."

"That's why I said if we were together, we could conquer the world."

"Queen Balkis, the world is fine. It does not need to be conquered. People need to learn to respect our world and each other. Sheba, what is it that you want out of life?"

She was silent for a moment and then said, "I wish this moment would last forever."

"Now, Sheba, don't go soft on me," I chuckled. "What do you really want?"

"I want to conquer more land and have more power and more wealth. That is why I am seeking the wisdom of Solomon so that I can be a *female* Solomon, the most powerful Queen to ever rule."

"Well, if that is your desire, you will never know love or have a loving family. To have more power, you must create war and bloodshed. No one wants to have his land taken away. Look at Ramses 400 years ago. He enslaved and killed thousands of Israelites, and they just wanted to be at peace and work their land. He lost most of his army pursuing Moses and never won, and in the end three million Israelites left Egypt and became free. Think about it.

"How many great warriors, kings, and pharaohs died with great wealth, but died lonely? Look at Shutruk-Nakhunte, who was a great king of Mesopotamia. He conquered more kingdoms than any other king."

"Shutruk who?" Sheba asked.

"You see, you don't even know who he was, and he has only been dead perhaps 200 years. He was one of the greatest kings to ever rule. Yet Moses, who fled Egypt and became a simple shepherd who served God, is still talked about 400 years later. Why?"

"Captain, that is a good question, and I am sure you will give me the answer."

"King Shutruk took everything from the people, including their freedom.

Moses gave the people their freedom and gave them value, even though many betrayed him. You will only be remembered when you give back to the land and the people."

"Captain, what do you want?"

"I want to be remembered as someone who gave more than he took, to be an example, to help make a better tomorrow for our children, and most of all I want my family to love me and say good things about me when I am gone."

"Oh, Captain, you're too idealistic!"

"Idealistic? You will have to explain yourself."

"You want to be perfect!" she said.

"What's wrong with wanting to do better every day?"

"Come on, Captain. You've been around enough to know better than that."

"Well, Sheba, I don't believe everything I hear."

"Captain, I can see we do think differently, but I must say, I certainly feel safe in your arms."

I laughed, "It seems that I am the one in your arms."

"You know what I mean."

"Yes, and thank you."

"Captain, could we be friends? As we have been talking, I have realized that I do not have a true friend, and you are right, it is lonely."

"Sheba, you really could be a powerful Queen if you just let this side of you come out of the cage. And, yes, I will be a friend as long as the friendship is based on honesty."

"Captain, I could bed any man I wanted until you came along. I've never met anyone like you. I would really like to have you as my first friend."

"Sheba, you have to give of yourself and put time into a relationship in order for a friendship to grow. So only time will determine if we can be friends."

As we came in sight of the campfires, I knew the guards would be near, so I swung out of the saddle and gave Sheba the reins. "Ride into camp alone and have one of your guards take Sultan to Kaleb. They will have your tent ready for you."

"But, Captain, what about you?"

"Just tell Kaleb I am coming in with the guards. Now, go ahead."

Early in the morning, Jona had everyone up packing camels and getting the caravan ready. You could feel the excitement growing as the men were anticipating our arrival in Jerusalem.

Joktel was given a proper burial at daylight, since they found his body and brought it out with everything else they recovered in the canyon. I was going over some of the final details with Jona and Kaleb when Issa came running up out of breath, "Captain Shutran, Queen Balkis would like you to stop by her wagon when you have time. Captain, I think the Queen is sick. She has not been herself ever since she returned last night."

I looked at the ground and kicked some dirt with my foot and smiled. Jona, overhearing the remark, piped up, "Did you say she is sick, Issa?"

"No, not exactly. She just acts differently."

"Like what?" Jona probed.

"Well, she didn't yell and curse at anyone last night or this morning, and she actually asked if I could draw her some water. She was even carrying some of her personal things out to her wagon."

Jona grinned, "Sounds like a woman in love."

"Issa, tell the Queen I will stop by."

When Issa left, Jona looked up at me and had a smile on his face, "Well, well, Captain Shutran, amazing how a late-night horseback ride can change a woman," giving me a backhanded slap on the shoulder as he walked away, chuckling.

Trying to keep a straight face, I turned to Kaleb, "Check with Nadab and make sure they greased the hubs before mounting the wheels. If they haven't, then pull the wheels off and do it."

"Yes, Captain."

I rode across the camp to the Queen's tents, which were being taken down. To my surprise, Balkis was carrying out some of her things, just like Issa said.

Seeing me, she walked away from the wagon and came to greet me. "Captain Shutran, thank you for yesterday. I thought all night about the things you said, and I, too, want to be a better person."

"Then, Queen Balkis, you shall be. I am very happy for you. Just remember, it is not easy to change. Just keep going in your new direction and see how you feel about yourself and how others respond to you."

"Captain, could I ride beside you today?"

"Of course, there is less dust up front, and Kaleb would enjoy that. From here the journey to Ein Gedi will be easy, and we should be there in four days. We will unload all the balsam and frankincense trees and the cistus plants we are carrying. I'll send a runner to Solomon's court to let him know where we are. From there it will probably take only a day or two to arrive in Jerusalem."

"Captain, you told the men two weeks."

"I know! It could be just that, because I don't know if Solomon will respond in one day or ten days."

I enjoyed the early morning smell from the breakfast fires with boiling rice, lentils, wheat, and the frying meat of the ibex. But even more, I enjoyed the aroma coming from the pots of steaming frankincense and menthe, which most of my men drank to keep their bowels clear of parasites and their stomachs settled and feeling light after a heavy meal. After six months on the trail, it was interesting to see that my men who drank the frankincense tea never got sick. They slept better, woke up earlier, and didn't get lazy at midday. I was always pleased to see the results of what my father had taught me.

The men actually had a pleasant smell in the early morning after their clothing had been saturated with the frankincense smoke all night. Too bad it didn't last all day, because by midday they didn't smell the same.

Riding through the caravan, I saw Nadab's men replacing wheels on one wagon, which pleased me to see that Kaleb had carried out his job.

Jona, Ibram, Enos, Mohamed, and Micah came riding up together. "Captain, there is a different feeling in the air. This morning everyone is happy," Micah said. Enos naively suggested that maybe it was because Captain Tamrin wasn't whipping someone and the Queen wasn't yelling at her servants.

Ibram asked, "What happened last night during the journey from the slide, Captain?"

"Have you ever been really scared?" I asked.

"Yes," came several replies.

"The Queen was very frightened and when you're frightened like she was, everyone can see it and there is no place to hide. She needed a diversion and started talking about her father and grandfather.

"She has had a painful life and has taken her anger out on everyone around her, making her the hard person that everyone fears. But I believe there is a different person behind that hard exterior. She is demonstrating a desire to change, so this is our opportunity to help her. Men, pass the word to the others to compliment her on her behavior when it is deserved. We will see a different Queen by the time we reach Ein Gedi."

Ayaar came riding up, "We're ready, Captain."

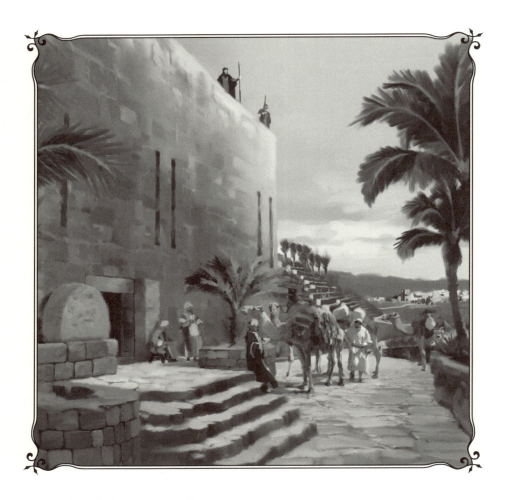

"Then let's move out!"

By late morning of the fourth day, we rounded a bluff and came in sight of the Ein Gedi Palace and Treasury House. The rustling of the breeze through the branches of the palm trees along the wadi almost sounded like music. The vineyards and the vegetable gardens were very beautiful. It was such a welcome sight and seemed so peaceful.

The Treasury House stood five stories high. The base was 1½ meters thick, and about midway up, the thickness of the walls was 1 meter. We were amazed to see the huge, round stone at the entrance way, which would be rolled in place if there was a threat of robbers. The side hills were a lush green and spotted with a wide variety of brightly colored flowers. The huge rose gardens that spread farther than the eye could see were breathtaking.

They were similar to the palace grounds of Queen Balkis.

The men immediately started unloading the camels and getting the trees and cistus plants to the gardeners. Azaad and his sons unloaded two camels, one each with myrrh and luban. Kaleb wrote the announcement of our arrival to King Solomon. If Hussin rode now, he would reach Jerusalem at dusk and be able to deliver our message before the day ended.

I sent Kaleb to tell the men to put up only the captains' tents and the minimum necessary for the Queen. I was sure we would be ready to leave for Jerusalem by morning. Now it was time to get out the decorated breast collars with the ropes and fine halters for the camels. We wanted to look our best.

I had Kaleb bring all my captains and chiefs to my tent for a meeting. "Men, tomorrow is the time to wear your best thobes, galabeyas, and gutrahs. After the camels are loaded and everything is ready, then you can change. Be sure to smoke your clean clothing for tomorrow with luban tonight. Go to bed early as it will take more time to prepare for the fanfare to meet Solomon. We want to leave with the first light of the morning sun."

Ayaar spoke up, "Well, what's so different about that?" and everyone laughed. "Does Captain Shutran know any other time to get up? Men, pass the word and make sure that every man has heard the Captain's orders." He then offered me his hand to shake with a grand gesture of respect. I shook his hand with gratitude for the changes that I had seen come to him and those of Sheba's command. "Captain Shutran, these last four days, without question, have been our very best. I believe Captain Tamrin really poisoned a lot of us, but never again. The change I see in the Queen is most astounding."

"Ayaar, what do you think Tamrin will do?"

"Captain, I think he will ride into Jerusalem and claim his fight with you. As his pain decreases, so will his memory of what caused it, and his desire for revenge will grow every day."

"Has Queen Balkis given you a new commission?" I asked.

"No, not yet."

I asked again, "Captain Ayaar, do you feel you could take a new commission and not let it go to your head?"

Ayaar responded, "In the beginning of our journey, I would have answered, 'No,' but today I can say, 'Yes.' Captain Shutran, you have been a powerful example!"

"Ayaar, thank you. I just work at doing my best every day. Do you have your horses, the Queen's wagons, and her chariot ready for tomorrow?"

"The men are working on it, but I best go check. Thanks again, Commander. See you in the morning."

Cook fires were burning bright, and everyone was excited about tomorrow. The men were singing with great vigor as some of the women from Sheba's camp had wandered over. Music was in the air as they played their flutes and picked at the strings on their wooden instruments. The more music they played, the louder they sang and the faster they danced.

Everyone was enjoying the grape wine that was already being passed around when Jona got word. He quickly stopped it and was a bit harsh with his words. "Tell me," he said to the men, "do you really want to look like fools tomorrow and embarrass the Captain and the Queen? If I see one of you drunk in the morning, I will cut your tongue out. Is that clear?"

Azaad spoke up, "Jona is right. Let's make our Commander proud. Now, let's get some rest."

As I laid in bed, my thoughts drifted to home. I could feel Mirah's presence and a feeling of concern made it hard for me to sleep. I kept hearing Armin asking for me to come home. Kaleb must have felt my concern and broke the silence, "Papa, are you all right?"

"Yes, Son, but Armin is not doing well. Something is wrong."

"Papa, let's pray for Armin before we sleep."

"Yes, let's pray." I was so proud of Kaleb for his growing faith. I hugged him as he finished his prayer and said, "Now you need to get some sleep. Tomorrow will be an exciting day, one that you will remember forever." The moon was climbing high among the twinkling stars when I finally fell asleep.

I startled awake when I heard a horse come in and the guards allowed the rider to pass. It had to be Hussin. I stepped out of my tent as he rode up.

"Captain, King Solomon is anxiously awaiting our arrival tomorrow."

"Good job, Hussin! You'd better get some sleep."

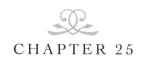

CHAPTER 25

Sheba and Solomon —
Hidden Agendas

The caravan was ready to move out by the time daylight had barely started to replace the night. Very few had taken time to eat breakfast because of their anxiousness to get moving. It was a sight watching them scurry about in their fine galabeyas and thobes with brightly colored gutrahs on their heads. From the Queen's wagons we could see the billowing smoke of frankincense wafting through the morning air. It was that same intoxicating aroma that I welcomed every morning from the campfire. Queen Balkis had her servants dressed in the best silk from China, with strings of pearls and sapphires adorning their necks.

The wagons that were inlaid with silver were decorated with silk embroidery work. The Queen's chariot was always beautiful with her four white stallions; however, beautiful could not begin to describe what we saw this day. The harnesses of the four stallions were gold studded with silk ribbons hanging from their bridles. Gold chains connected the horse tugs to the chariot, and gold ribbon was wrapped around the doubletrees. Silk tassels and ribbons with strings of gold were woven into the manes and tails, a sight that would have stopped a rich man.

When I thought I had seen it all and could hardly get my breath, the Queen came out of her tent. The chatter of every man there seemed to stop instantly. You could have heard a scarab beetle sneeze. She was, without question, the most beautiful woman any man here had ever seen. As she walked, it seemed as though even the animals were watching her.

Her gown was white silk trimmed with something pink that I later learned was called lace. Her long, black hair, that I hadn't seen let down since we left Marib, was braided with white silk and gold strings with diamonds. Her neck was covered with sapphires from India, rubies from Persia, turquoise from Mesopotamia, and diamonds from Africa. She wore gold bracelets and hanging earrings studded with diamonds.

Her full, flowing gown that accented her body fluttered in the slight breeze. The fragrance of her exotic rose water perfume, with jasmine, cassia, and sweet myrrh, permeated the air. I stood almost frozen as she walked up to me, stopping a horse length away. With an alluring look in her eyes, she said, "Captain, how do I look?"

"The horses look fine." Then realizing what I had said, I laughed, "Queen Balkis, you are a sight for tired, sand-filled eyes that would make a man forget to rub them." She chuckled with me. For the first time, Sheba responded like a woman caring about what someone else thought. I do not believe that one man saw her as the same Queen who left Marib. A transformation was taking place that warmed many hearts.

"My Queen, your six years of waiting are over. Today is your final journey to the Palace of Solomon. Sheba, are you ready?"

She took a deep breath and straightened her shoulders. As her eyes pierced my very being, with a sense of gratitude, she said majestically, "Yes, Commander, I am ready."

The caravan was a magnificent sight when it crested the hills above Ein Gedi west of the Salt Sea. Sheba took the lead in her chariot, flanked by Ayaar on her right, who held the reins, and Nadab on her left. I followed directly behind her with Kaleb, Jona, and Ibram. We could hear the trumpets sounding long before we came within sight of Jerusalem. But as they heralded the arrival of the Queen, we could see the flags of many nations blowing in the breeze as the sound pierced the air.

On top of the hill that looked down on the gates of Jerusalem, in a military, double-line formation, King Solomon's army, with 3,000 stunningly decorated horses pulling magnificent chariots, accompanied the King as he came toward us. We had heard that Solomon's personal chariot had been brought from Egypt at a cost of 600 shekels of silver. It was made from the finest aromatic, red sandalwood with superb craftsmanship of intricately inlaid silver and gold that accented the framework. The beauty was only increased by the bronze rims and polished brass hubs of the chariot that was pulled by four white Arabian stallions that were adorned with gold thread braided in their manes and bridles studded with jewels. Surely the finest in Judea. Certainly there was none more exquisite that had come out of Egypt.

I stopped the caravan and then rode up beside Sheba as Ayaar brought the chariot to a gentle stop. Once King Solomon saw that she was ready to receive him, he slowly approached until they could see each other face to face. With a wide gesture of his arm and with all the magnificence and power he commanded, he asked the question, "Who is this that cometh out of the wilderness like pillars of smoke perfumed with myrrh and frankincense, with all powders of the merchant?"

We all just looked in wonder as he spoke, as his voice demanded total attention and respect. It was my place to respond first, so when his arm relaxed, I came out of the saddle and stepped forward to introduce myself. "I am Shutran Abdulla Ismelacor, Commander of the great caravan of Queen Balkis, the Queen of Saba." I pivoted halfway back towards Sheba, and in a gesture of greeting, I said, "If I may, oh King, present to you Queen Balkis, the most beautiful Queen in all the land."

Ayaar pulled the Queen's chariot up beside Solomon's chariot so that they could exchange small gifts and the King could welcome her to his kingdom. Sheba handled herself with seductive majesty that mystified Solomon, yet with gentle warmth that I had not seen before. He invited her to join him in his chariot to ride into the city. Every man watching was struck with Solomon's grandeur and lavishness. The horses, the chariots, the 1,000 mounted soldiers, the entire entourage—all decorated with the splendor of Solomon's court—were a sight beyond description.

Between gasps of breath, Kaleb kept repeating, "Oh, Papa; oh, Papa." In his bewilderment, he couldn't find words to express himself. He just rode excitedly next to me, taking in everything with great wonder.

Jona looked over at me and very quietly uttered, "Never did I imagine anything so magnificent." Then Jona went silent. I hadn't seen him so speechless since Samira kissed him the first time. I turned in the saddle and looked back over the caravan, letting the splendor of it envelope my very being. I, too, felt speechless.

I turned my attention back to King Solomon and watched as Queen Balkis was being assisted into his chariot by Captain Ayaar. The King was stately and seemed to be a gentleman. However, he had a lust for beauty like the mighty Pharaoh for the riches of the world. He was infatuated with the Queen, who would perhaps be his greatest conquest.

As I looked at him, I could feel Sheba's disappointment that Solomon didn't have the masculine physique that she had created in her mind, like Tamrin's. The King obviously had the best chefs in the land, and it showed around his waistline. He was my height, just slightly shorter than 2 meters, but outweighed me by 20 kilos. His face was round and jovial, and his head didn't appear to have much hair left on it. In spite of his appearance, he had an air of superior authority.

I couldn't help notice his hands when he greeted the Queen. They were not hands that had seen much work. They were soft, without broken nails, cracked skin, cuts, or scars. I looked at my hands and wondered that Mirah would even hold these hands of hard labor, calloused from cutting myrrh and luban since childhood and scarred with cuts and rope burns from training camels and horses and from putting ropes on packs and pulling them off. I even had one scar across the back of my hand and forearm from a sword fight. I wondered if I was doing all of this so that my sons wouldn't have to grow up and have hands like mine.

Solomon tried to contain his excitement in her presence. It was easy to see that he was smitten by her beauty, since he could not take his eyes off of her as she introduced Ayaar, captain of her military; Nadab, her second-in-command; and then Jona, Kaleb, Ibram, and Mohamed.

Solomon acknowledged them graciously and invited us to follow him into the royal court of Jerusalem next to the great temple he was just completing. All of our men with their heavily laden camels just wanted to off-load, take the camels to pasture, and find their place of rest to bathe and sleep. They wanted to be free to move about and see the great city. Solomon seemed to understand how everyone felt and dispatched his servants immediately to take care of our every need.

First, we pulled the Queen's four wagons near the temple, and then Solomon assigned servants to escort her and her entourage to his palace. King Solomon's court was immense, with countless corridors and rooms. Queen Balkis, Captain Ayaar, her chiefs, and her ladies-in-waiting were given rooms where servants prepared tubs of hot water scented with jasmine and eucalyptus to soothe away their aches and pains from the long journey and served food and drink of immense variety.

Since I was the Commander, Jona, Kaleb and I were given private quarters. Servants were there to draw our baths and attend to our every need. Jona winked at me as we watched the expression on Kaleb's face. It was a look of amazement as though he were in some make-believe world. After the first hot bath in months that washed away the dust of the trail, a massage with the essences of jasmine and rose in olive oil was

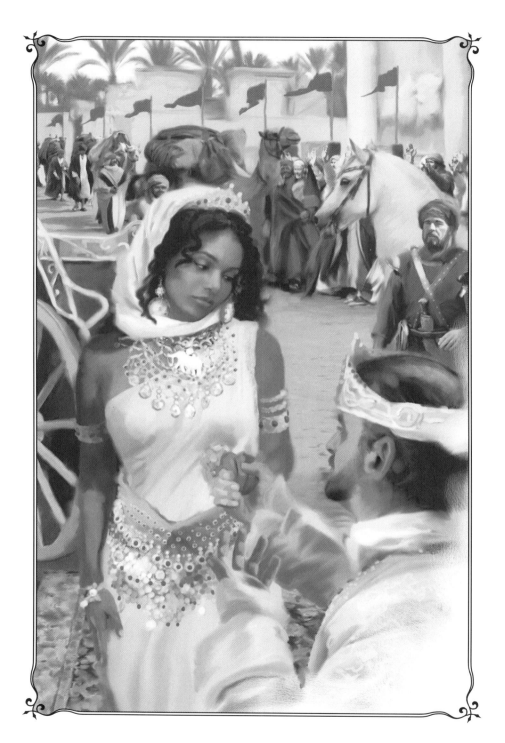

a wonderful, soothing experience.

Clean clothes seemed strange, but we wore them with delight as we walked into the next room, where the food seemed endless with fruit and wine and, of course, countless women waiting to serve us. We ate with wonder, savoring the taste of so many new foods from all over the world including food flavored with exotic spices from India.

Later that day the King invited us to walk with him in the palace, which seemed like a continuous dream. As we entered the court, string instruments with harps were playing soft music while sweet voices filled the air with songs of love. As Solomon led us to his throne room, we marveled at the beauty that surrounded us.

His throne was carved from ivory and inlaid with pure gold, with six steps and a footstool attached. Six lions were lined up against each of the six steps and one against each side of the armrest, all carved out of ivory.

From the throne room we went into another elegant setting, where we were to dine with the King. Queen Balkis, Kaleb, Jona, Ayaar, and I were seated at the King's table. Plates of fine porcelain were placed before us, and even the drinking vessels were made of gold, not silver. The floors were polished marble, and the marble walls were inlaid with gold leaf. I had no idea that such things existed.

After we finished eating, Solomon brought one of his wives to meet us, who he introduced as Makshara. She was a woman of striking beauty and slender stature, much like Sheba. Although her features were not as refined, as I gazed into her face, I couldn't help but think how much she resembled the Queen. As I glanced towards Sheba, I saw that her face had become very sullen as her eyes dropped to the floor. At that moment I was sure that Makshara was the Queen's twin sister, who had stayed in Egypt when Sheba left for the Hadhramaut.

Makshara did not recognize her sister, for Sheba had looked very common when she last saw her in Egypt 20 years earlier. I could see that Sheba was getting very upset as the evening progressed until finally she asked if the King would excuse her so that she could lie down because she wasn't feeling well.

King Solomon had invited Makshara to sit by him at the table. After the introductions and the musicians began to play again, he stood and walked over to me and asked if I thought he should send the priest to attend the Queen. I assured him that it was just exhaustion from the journey and the excitement of finally being in his court.

Makshara sat motionless at the table, like a piece of furniture. I could see that she was not a happy woman. Solomon was very vocal about his concern for Balkis. Changing the subject, he asked if this was my first journey to Israel. I answered, "Yes, Your Majesty." , The King stood up from the table and beckoned me to follow him. I could tell that he wanted to talk some more as we walked out onto the balcony to enjoy the fresh, night air filled with the fragrance of the flowers from the gardens below.

"Tell me, Commander, how long have you been with the Queen?"

"About six months."

"Is this her caravan or yours?"

"Half of the camels are mine."

"Have you been carrying frankincense and other spices to other ports?"

"Yes, Your Majesty."

"Have you traveled many trails?"

"Most of my travels have been out of the eastern Hadhramaut across the Empty Quarter to Gerrha and out of Fort Sumhuram to Marib and Najran. My father harvested myrrh and frankincense resins and brought them from the mountains to old Qana with a small caravan.

Solomon seemed genuinely interested as he continued with his questions. "Have you ever been to Nineveh?"

"No, Sir, I have not."

"How much frankincense, myrrh, and spices do you carry in a year?"

"Perhaps 1,000 tons and the demand is growing every year."

"Is there that much frankincense in the Hadhramaut?"

"Yes, there is. However, if we keep harvesting as much as we are now, in another 200 years I believe the trees will start to die."

"So do you think it could be a good business with my fleet of ships?"

"King Solomon, the Emperor of China has discovered frankincense, and the Emperors from the Indus Valley of India are demanding more every season. Egyptians are using it for mummification ceremonies and for many rituals in their temples. The Pharaoh and his royalty are using it for their beautification and personal pleasure. The price of frankincense is continuing to increase, and one day it will become a rare gift."

"Captain Shutran, do you see yourself bringing caravans to Jerusalem in the future?"

"No, but I do have a feeling that I will return for another reason."

"And what might that be?"

"I am not sure but I will tell you that I want to learn more about the One God and this Messiah about whom the prophets have foretold. Perhaps we can talk about that at another time."

"Captain, I have one more question. Does the Queen own the frankincense land?"

"Yes," I answered. "She has a very strong hold on it, and we all pay taxes in order to pass through her kingdom."

"So, if my army conquered that land or I took her in marriage, then I would own the land of incense, the richest land in all the world." Solomon was silent for a moment as though expecting me to respond. But I remained quiet, hoping he would change the subject. I could see that he was thinking about something and looking for the right words, "Captain, would you accept a commission in my army?"

"Your Majesty, I would have to think about that. I have a family and my caravan business."

"That is not a problem. Move your family to Jerusalem and I will give you one of my finest houses. Bring your caravan and I will put it to good use. In fact, I have merchandise that I need brought here from Nineveh. A caravan is coming across the Silk Road bringing porcelain, brass, silk, paintings, spices, and cotton. Would you take your caravan and bring those goods to me? I will reward you handsomely."

"King Solomon, you are a gracious man, and your offer is tempting. I could send my caravan, but I could not go at this time. Do you see the young man who was sitting on my left?"

"Yes."

"He is my oldest son, Kaleb. I promised him and his mother, sister, and younger brother that this would be my last long caravan that would take me so far away from home for months at a time. My little daughter is not doing well, and we do not know why. I must return home."

"Captain, I could have one of my ships take you home and save you four months if you would return and go to Nineveh for me. Please accept my offer and I will have my ship take you home."

"I could give Ibram charge as commander over my caravan and let him make the journey. I will take Jona and Kaleb with me."

"Captain Shutran, I can see that you are weary and need to rest. Let us meet for breakfast to have further conversation."

"Yes, thank you, King Solomon. We will talk in the morning. Good night." The King bid me good night and was then escorted to his chambers.

Kaleb and Jona were waiting for me in the courtyard with great curiosity. I told them about the King's offer and that we would talk first thing tomorrow to make our plans. We said good night and retired to our quarters. I was feeling like someone had blown out the flame on a candle as the exhaustion of the end of the journey came upon us. Our heads were filled with all the events of the day as we sunk into feather beds, something we had never felt before. It was like sleeping on a mountain of sheep fleece. Kaleb was asleep before he was fully stretched out.

I stood beside his bed and thought of the many experiences we had had together on the trail and felt such tremendous gratitude for this time together. Not only was he my son, but he had become a great companion and friend. Not one time did I have to wake him up or remind him of his responsibilities, nor was I ever disappointed because he had not done his job, and he was quick to complete all the assignments he was given.

He had helped Jona and Enos so much with anything they needed, and I was very impressed with how he befriended Enos and helped him to believe in himself. Kaleb even befriended Alimud, who was rejected and hated by everyone. He calmed down Queen Balkis and showed her respect and friendship, even when she didn't deserve it. He took such good care of Sultan and always had him ready for me. He held the captives together, and fought beside me in battle and saved my life.

Not once did he ever complain on the journey, even when he would get so tired that occasionally his chin would drop to his chest when he closed his eyes while in the saddle. He had brought so much joy and happiness to me on this caravan. Mirah would be just as proud of him as I am. My heart was so full that my eyes felt like rain was falling from them.

I kissed him on the forehead and whispered, "I love you, my son." Wiping the tears away, I went to bed and instantly my head was filled with thoughts of Mirah and the children. I thanked God for blessing my family and for such a great day. I had barely sent them kisses when I felt like I was floating into the clouds and was gone for the night.

As the sun heralded a new day, I awoke, wondering where I was. When I looked around and saw the beauty of my surroundings, I remembered I was in the King's palace. As I put my feet on the carpet, I remembered all that had transpired since we were invited into Solomon's court. I dressed and decided to go out for a walk before I met with Jona. I looked at Kaleb sleeping and chuckled, wondering if he was making up for all the early mornings on the trail. His job was to make the accounting of all the gifts, so I trusted he would wake up in time.

I checked on Sultan and was pleased to see that he was well taken care of with the other animals. Then I walked over to look at the majestic beauty of the temple Solomon was building, which was why he wanted the goods from Nineveh.

The temple was exquisite and almost took my breath away. The pillars had beautiful, bronze capstones on top. The network of lattice covered with a wreath of chain work and bronze pomegranates dazzled the eye. The Molten Sea of brass that rested on the backs of 12 bronze oxen next to the altar of gold was magnificent in both size and beauty. There were many tables, lampposts, and bowls with ladles made of gold. Even the door hinges were of gold. Surely, there was nothing as splendid. After I left, I wondered if the gift of white smoke would fill the air of this temple when it was finished. I pondered the riches that were being used to build this temple, only to find myself longing for my home in Al-Balid.

I sent Jona to have breakfast with Solomon to discuss the things we had talked about last night. I accepted Solomon's offer to have one of his ships take us home. We would leave in eight days after the giving of gifts and trading was completed. Ibram, Micah, Enos, Mohamed, and Alimud would take the caravan to Nineveh in about ten days, after all of the repairs were made and the camels were rested.

I asked Enos if he would like to return home with us. A look of sadness came over him as he stared into the distance and said, "I miss my mother and father a lot, but I am not ready."

"Enos, the caravan needs a good captain."

"Captain!" he yelled excitedly. "What do you mean?"

Jona spoke up, "You know, captain, like me."

"Enos, you have served well and I am proud to give you that position—a position of responsibility—one that I know you will take very seriously. I will tell your father and mother when I see them."

"I am honored, Commander; thank you."

"Now, men, Queen Balkis would like everyone to be in attendance when her servants present her gifts to Solomon."

"Have you talked with the Queen this morning?" Jona asked.

"No, I haven't but earlier I saw Solomon pacing like a stalking puma in the palace courtyard, expecting her at any moment."

"Shutran, has she said anything yet about him?"

"No, she hasn't but I'm sure this day will be very interesting. I'm going over to her quarters and wait for her to come out, because she wants me to go with her when she meets with the King. Sheba doesn't feel comfortable meeting him alone and wants me to go with her."

I walked over to meet her, and when she was ready, Solomon's servants escorted us to his private chambers. I bowed slightly to the King as they greeted each other. He hoped she was feeling rested after sleeping in such beautiful surroundings after her long journey. Solomon left us for a short time while we were served a lavish breakfast. Sheba and I talked about his magnificent palace and the reception that she had been given.

When the King returned, he invited her to go with him into the garden room, where they visited and enjoyed the view of the lake and where the birds were singing in the warmth of the morning sun. I stood a short distance behind her and quietly watched as she tried to determine how she was going to interact with the King. She seemed anxious but let Solomon think she was still recovering from the long journey.

Feeling a bit uncertain, Sheba started to make conversation with him. "King Solomon, you have not asked me why I have come to your court."

"That's true, my Queen, so why did you come?"

"I feared what I might feel about the magnificence of your wealth, your wives, your passions, and your wisdom. I had heard about your many servants and their apparel, your abundant tables of food, your lavish palace, and your powerful military. I have found that everything I have heard is true and beyond anything I expected. What I have seen far exceeds your fame, your wisdom, and your wealth. I thought your subjects would be ruled by an oppressive and controlling King, but I find that they are happy and delight in hearing the wisdom you speak. Your words are kind and carry great eloquence and charm. Your greatness is beyond anything that I have heard spoken of you."

"Queen Balkis, surely you didn't make a six-month journey with all of your gifts just to tell me that."

"No, my King, I want to trade my gifts for your wisdom, and walk beside you and learn great things from you—things of wisdom, knowledge, and the wonders of our world. But first, may I present my gifts?"

"Please, my Queen, as you wish." Solomon clapped his hands and servants appeared from every direction. He announced, "The Queen of Saba wishes to present her gifts. Let us make way to receive them." Solomon extended his hand to her, and she cautiously placed her arm on his as he led her into the great hall.

The musicians began playing their strings and harps as the parade commenced. Both the servants of Solomon and Balkis carried in the sacks of tons and tons of magnificent gifts from many kingdoms abroad as well as from the great land of the Hadhramaut of the Queen of Sheba.

Kaleb had found his way there and, as the scribe, was very busy making an accounting of everything that was laid before Solomon. The first and greatest gifts were the 20 tons of frankincense, 15 tons of myrrh, and 5 tons of balsam. Next came another 10 tons, which included the spices of cassia, cinnamon, pepper, jasmine, and rosewater. There were also 3 tons of spice teas from India.

Next, the servants laid precious metals and gem stones at his feet: 50 tons of gold, 1 ton of pearls, 1 ton of diamonds, 1 ton of sapphires, 1 ton of rubies, and ½ ton of turquoise. The 5 tons of ivory from Africa were most beautiful, as were the 5 tons of silk fabrics, 5 tons of cotton, 8 tons of goat and camel skins, 6 tons of flax and camel wool carpets, 5 tons of beautifully embroidered tapestries, and 2 tons of rolled paintings. Lastly came the 5 tons of brass wares, 10 tons of dates, and 10 tons of salt.

Her black Arabian stallion, Cassia, was brought into the courtyard for Solomon to see. The saddle was exquisite with the harness and bridle of inlaid gold and diamonds. Arabians are very smart horses, which was evident by the way Cassia held his head high as he pranced before the King as though he knew he was on display. As the stallion was led away, by the glance that Sheba gave me, I could see that she was not too happy about losing her prized stallion, but it was all part of her plan that had now been set in motion.

The mountainous amount that the Queen had carried to Jerusalem totaled 168½ tons. It took 250 men all day to carry all of the gifts into Solomon's court. By that afternoon Solomon had become very quiet as he watched the merchandise being laid before him. Solomon, with a tone of amazement, asked, "All of this for my knowledge and wisdom, or is it for my kingdom?"

"My King, it is my desire to please you. It is for you to decide the answer to your question."

"Queen Balkis, what game do you wish to play?"

"The game of riddles."

"I accept your challenge; please continue."

Sheba was certain that Solomon was no match for her clever riddles. She asked, "King Solomon, what is the most powerful part of the body?"

"The tongue," he answered. "Death and life are in the power of the tongue."

She smiled, "Very good. Here is another one. What is a vessel with a form that has ten openings? When one opening is open, nine are closed; when nine are open, one is closed. What is it?" she asked, knowing this would stop Solomon.

He paused for a moment and then answered, "The vessel is the womb. The form is a baby. The ten openings are the openings in the body. When the baby is in the womb, the navel is open and the other nine openings are closed. When the child is birthed, the navel is closed and the other nine openings are open." Sheba was extremely impressed. Except for Shutran, Solomon was the first to answer her riddles.

As she thought about his response, she decided to ask him one more. "What is the most unpleasant thing in the world, and what is the most rewarding? What is for sure and what is unsure?"

Solomon thought for a moment and then said, "The most unpleasant thing before God is a saint becoming a sinner. The most rewarding to God is the sinner repenting. Death is a sure thing, and our place in the world to come is the most unsure."

The intellect of Solomon was so impressive to her that his physical looks became unimportant. She was captivated by his intelligence. Sheba became Solomon's shadow and questioned him about everything, and he slyly probed her about the Kingdom of Saba. As the days passed, he subtly asked about the strength of her military, how many troops she had, and where her military outposts were positioned. However, Balkis was very guarded and clever with her answers.

At the end of the day, she would always seek me out and ask me what I thought. I cautioned her to be careful and reminded her how other kings and emperors desired her kingdom. On the fifth night while we were walking past the temple, I turned to her and asked, "Why are you here? You are as intelligent as Solomon, and you have riches that exceed his wealth. You are learning to let the woman inside you be a woman who can be more powerful than Solomon. If you rule from your heart and let your head bring balance, you will become a great and beloved ruler. Solomon doesn't have anything that you need."

With deep sadness in her eyes, she said, "Shutran, he has one thing."

"And what is that?"

"He is married to my sister without her consent. She hates him and hates her life. Our father arranged it, thinking this would bring peace with the Israelites, but Solomon has become proud and arrogant. He boasts about his 700 wives and 300 concubines and hasn't fathered a child with hardly any of them. He measures his power by the number of his women, horses, military, and possessions. My sister is not a possession to be owned or displayed like a tapestry on the wall."

I could feel her pain coming up as the anger in her voice intensified. "Have you spoken with her since you arrived?"

"No, I have not seen her since that first dinner. The other women have told me that he moved her to Megiddo, one of his chariot cities."

"Sheba, what do you want?"

"I want to free my sister and all of the other women he holds captive!"

"Just a minute. I do not see anyone forced to be here."

"Of course not, Shutran. Do you think he will let you or me talk to anyone here who is unhappy? Shutran, he is changing. He thinks that he is a god and is invincible. I came wanting to learn more about him and his God and find him worshiping idols with his foreign wives."

She grabbed my wrist, turned to face me, and reached out and grabbed my left hand. "Shutran, I feel betrayed again. You are my only true friend. You have taught me so much about life, honesty, and how to treat people," she said, looking up into my eyes with a longing to be loved. The pain that I felt for her with the intoxicating fragrance of jasmine and sweet myrrh stirred my blood.

"Shutran, I have never asked this of anyone, but would you hold me?" Without waiting, she hugged me like she did the night we crossed the slide together. I slowly put my arms around her, feeling pain in my heart for one of the most beautiful women in the world, who had never known what it is like for a man to love her, or shower her with beautiful gifts. She had never conceived the seed of the man who loves her, experienced the joy of life growing within her, or had a family to love.

My mind had wandered away thinking how painful it must be when the sound of her voice called me back to the moment, "Shutran, Shutran."

"Yes?"

"I started on this journey hating you, hoping to fall in love with who I thought would be the man of my dreams when I reached my destination. Now I am falling in love with you and hating the man of my dreams."

"Queen Balkis, you honor me with your words, but I can only love you as a sister or a daughter. A man can have no greater love than the love he has for his wife and the children she bore him. My Queen, as the person you have become, you will always have a place in my heart and will always be my friend. One day, the man you deserve will come.

"I need to tell you that in three days Jona, Kaleb, and I will leave for Aila and take a ship to return home to Al-Balid. My little Armin has been sick, and I need to go to her. Ibram and Mohamed will take my caravan to Nineveh for Solomon. They will leave two days after our departure. The caravan will take 8 to 12 weeks, depending on the arrival of the westbound caravan coming across the Silk Road. When they return, they have my orders to take you back home, if you are ready."

"Shutran, will you be coming back?"

"If all is well at home, yes."

The morning of our departure was a sad parting, and goodbyes were very difficult, knowing it could be a long time before we would meet again. In her finest gown Queen Balkis came into the courtyard to see us off. With tear-filled eyes, she gave Kaleb a big hug and kissed him and whispered, "Take care of your father and come back to take me home."

Hugging Jona, she smiled, "Big man, take care of Shutran; we all need him."

"Well, my Queen, trying to take care of Shutran is like trying to put a rope on an ibex. He always ends up taking care of us, but I'll do my best, God willing."

Sheba put her arms around my neck and held me close as if she were about to lose her best friend. She looked deep into my eyes and whispered, "Shutran, I do love you and it's all right. Now go to Mirah and your children. Mirah has to be the luckiest woman alive."

"No, my Queen, once you meet her, you will realize that I am the luckiest man in the world."

"Shutran, come back! Now go with God and be safe."

Looking down into her beautiful, dark eyes, I asked, "Sheba, which God?"

"Our God," she said as she squeezed my hand. "You made me believe, Shutran. You showed me the light. That is the gift you have left with me."

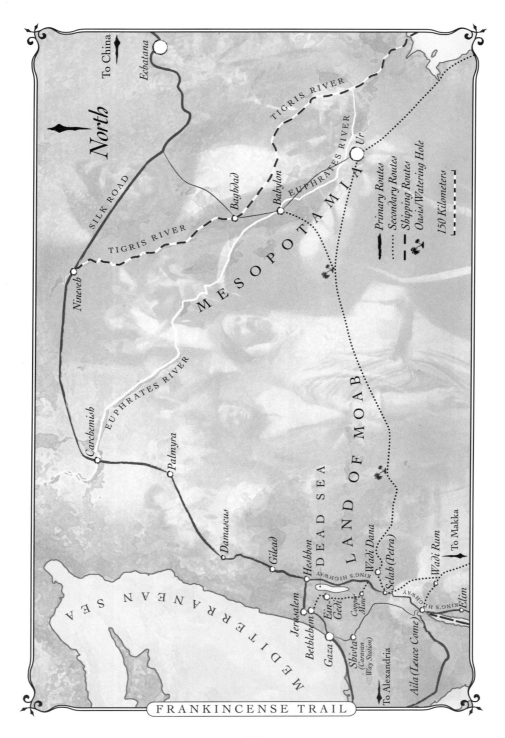

To China

Echatana

North

SILK ROAD

TIGRIS RIVER

TIGRIS RIVER

EUPHRATES RIVER

Ur

Nineveh

Bagdad

Babylon

EUPHRATES RIVER

M E S O P O T A M I A

Primary Routes
Secondary Routes
Shipping Routes
Oasis/Watering Hole

150 Kilometers

Carchemish

Palmyra

Damascus

Gilead

Heshbon

DEAD SEA

L A N D   O F   M O A B

Wadi Dana

Selah (Petra)

KING'S HIGHWAY

Wadi Rum

To Makka

M E D I T E R R A N E A N   S E A

Jerusalem

Bethlehem

Gaza

Ein Gedi

Copper Mine

Shivta
(Caravan
Way Station)

To Alexandria

Aila (Leuce Come)

KING'S HIGHWAY

Elim

FRANKINCENSE TRAIL

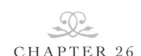

CHAPTER 26

Tamrin's Last Fight

expressed my thanks and deep gratitude to King Solomon, and then swinging into the saddle, I bid him farewell. Just as I gave Sultan my knee to ride, I heard a familiar voice say, "Captain Shutran, not so fast." I felt the hair on the back of my neck stand up, and my blood ran cold as I recognized Tamrin's voice. Turning Sultan around, I saw Tamrin boldly approaching as he rode across the square with two rough-looking Edomites, who had probably come with him from the village where he had been taken to heal.

"Shutran, have you forgotten our agreement about when we reached Jerusalem?"

I felt a coldness come over me. Things had been so good during the last few weeks. I asked myself, "Why did I let this man live?"

Queen Balkis spoke up immediately. "Tamrin, you are stripped of your command and dismissed from my military. Now, leave!"

"Well, well, my Queen, if I am stripped of my command and I am not *owned* by you, you have no control over me, and I can do as I please."

General Hiram, head of Solomon's military, walked over to Tamrin. "Sir, I do not know you, but it is a great offence to the King for someone to ride into his city uninvited and insult one of his guests."

"I beg your forgiveness. Let me introduce myself."

Queen Balkis quickly interrupted, "This is Tamrin of Saba, who was the captain of my caravan. He was directly under the command of Captain Shutran and intentionally disobeyed the Commander's orders, causing the death of one of my men. Captain Shutran should have killed him then but chose to let him live. I discharged him from his command, and Captain Ayaar has taken his place."

Tamrin cut her off, "This battle is between Shutran and me, and I make this challenge publically today. Shutran, I challenge you to fight to the death by the sword."

"Tamrin, I have put my sword to your throat, saved you from the thrust of Sleeman's sword, beaten you with my fists, and have let you live. I think it is time to let it go. You violated direct orders and have created your own outcome. However, I am willing to forget it, and you can ride on."

"No!" he yelled. "Just look at my face! Look, Shutran. I have to live with this every day."

"Well, it should be a reminder to never again do what you did. Tamrin, you can change your destiny now, but it's up to you."

"You are right and I am going to do that, right here!"

"No, Tamrin. You are on the grounds of the King. If you want to fight, then it must be taken outside the city."

General Hiram spoke up, "Captain Shutran, I can take him and have him put in prison so that you can ride."

"Yes, I know, but then I'll be looking over my shoulder every day. No! It has to end here, now! General Hiram, we must have King Solomon's permission to have the fight outside the city."

King Solomon had just come out to the courtyard and was listening. As we turned to acknowledge him, he called out, "Captain Shutran, you have my permission to fight here in the courtyard, if you desire. My servants would welcome the entertainment. I have no fear for you. There can only be one outcome for a man who chooses to fight out of revenge and hate when he could walk away. He came into my city uninvited, threatening my guest and violating the code of conduct. If you don't kill him, my officers will."

Tamrin, sitting arrogantly on his horse, yelled, "It is worth dying to kill you!"

Kaleb gave his horse a kick and rode up beside me. "Papa, if you get hurt, it will delay us getting home. Let the King put him in prison until we come back."

"Thank you for your concern, Son, but this is something that I have to finish. We will still ride this day." I turned my head and looked at Tamrin, who was impatiently waiting, and said in a loud voice so that everyone could hear, "The challenge is yours; how do you want it?"

"Any way you want it, Shutran."

"Then let it be sword to sword, Tamrin!"

"Shutran, I am going to carve you slowly into little pieces so that everyone can see who the real master is."

I looked over to the King, who was watching intensely, so I turned towards him and asked if I might have his permission to make a request.

Solomon motioned to me and said, "Commander, please, make your request to the court."

"Your Majesty, if Tamrin kills me, please let him go free. He will have earned that right."

"As you wish, Captain. Let it be written."

Turning back to Tamrin, I could see the color drain from his face, which I was counting on, since I knew that would unsettle him. It was hard to recognize him with his broken and scarred face, but his countenance and condescending tone of voice were the same. I called out, "General Hiram, clear the courtyard. This will be a battle from horseback."

"Yes, Captain."

He waved to the trumpeters to sound the call, which pierced the air, as both spectators and servants ran up on the steps and to the courtyard walls to make room. I rode up to Kaleb, who had now moved back. I winked at Jona and said, "Have no fear, my son," nodded my head to Queen Balkis, and rode back to Tamrin. "I have chosen to fight sword to sword on horseback. Are you man enough for that?"

I watched his ears turn purple and his bottom lip start to quiver. Hesitating only for a second, he yelled, "Prepare to die!"

I moved away and yelled back, "Draw your sword, Tamrin." I dropped the reins and clenching Sultan with my knees gave the signal with my right heel that was all too familiar to him. He lunged his right shoulder into Tamrin's unfamiliar horse, pushing him sideways and knocking Tamrin off balance.

As Tamrin drew his sword, Sultan stayed tight with the other horse. Then as I nudged him with my left heel, he turned inside to the right, putting Tamrin on my left. Gripping my sword handle, I drove my left fist into the same cheek that I had broken before, which was probably still healing. He yelled with pain and kicked his horse to get away, but Sultan stayed with him. As Tamrin came around swinging, I ducked down, watching for my opening.

His second backhand pivot was quick, and he opened up my right arm. When Tamrin saw the blood, the gleam came back into his eyes. I thought, "This is good. Now it will be a good fight to the death." Sultan charged again but Tamrin's horse moved fast to avoid contact. However, Sultan stayed against him as we clashed swords.

Tamrin's horse kept moving away from the fight, so now Tamrin was distracted while trying to keep his horse in close. As I blocked a high overhead swing, Sultan bolted forward, spinning to the left on his heels. I came down with a backhand swing just above the saddle and followed all the way through across Tamrin's stomach. He gasped and went forward in the saddle, grabbing his insides as the blood gushed out over his hands and ran down the saddle.

The horse slowly walked in the direction of the palace steps where King Solomon was seated. Tamrin became limp, leaned from his saddle, and fell face down in the dirt. He coughed and gurgled as the blood drained from his body, and with a last gasp for air, lay dead at Solomon's feet.

When I sheathed my sword, the trumpets sounded and the people cheered. Solomon rose from his chair, put his hand up to stop the noise, and said, "Because a man has died in battle is no reason to cheer."

I rode over to the King and bowed, thanking him for allowing the battle and for stopping the cheering. "Captain Shutran, this was obviously not your first battle."

"No, my King, and probably not my last."

"Captain, consider my offer. The world needs men who fight for the right reason."

"Thank you, Your Majesty; I will consider your offer." I bowed once more as I took my leave, rode over to Kaleb and Jona, and said, "Let's go home!"

"Papa, your arm?"

"It's just a scratch. We can tend to it on the trail."

Queen Balkis cried out, "Shutran, your arm."

"My Queen, thank you; it is nothing," and we turned and rode out, heading for the port city on the Aqaba coast.

As we came up over the ridge above Jerusalem, everyone, including Sheba, was standing in the courtyard waving. We waved back, feeling the excitement of returning home and the sadness of leaving the caravan. It felt very strange to be leaving our friends and comrades after spending eight months with them on the trail.

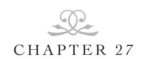

CHAPTER 27

Armin's Sky Father

told Kaleb it would be an easier and faster route for the horses if we traveled south through Jabal al-Fourdis southeast to the Salt Sea and then directly south to Aila. If we rode hard, we could reach the great water in five days. The winds were blowing out of the northwest, which was perfect for our journey home. Solomon sent a runner a week ago to have them prepare a ship so that we would be able to sail as soon as we arrived.

We rode out of Jerusalem at high noon and five days later rode into the old port city of Aila. I shuddered as I saw two of the burned ships resting half submerged on a reef near the port. The third ship must have sunk to the bottom. It was like a terrible dream that I didn't want to remember. King Solomon's runner had made arrangements to keep our horses there until we returned or Ibram picked them up with the caravan on his return to Marib with the Queen.

We stopped at the market long enough to buy some fruit and provisions only to discover that Solomon already had the ship well stocked with more than what we needed. We were under sail soon after our arrival.

This was our first time traveling by ship, and going out to sea was a bit unsettling for the three of us. The unknown with the caravan was an exciting challenge, but the unknown of the great water made us feel insecure, since we didn't know what to expect. The farther we moved away from the shore, the more uneasy we became.

Jona's face was pale as he said, "I don't know why I let you talk me into doing something strange like this. Listen, can't you hear my camel calling me?"

"Well, Jona, just think, you could be in the desert of Gilead with sand blowing in your face and bored out of your mind."

"Sure, Shutran, with you? Your life never slows down long enough for anyone to get bored or even take a bath."

"Oh, Jona, if you stayed home, you wouldn't know what to do with yourself, and besides, you would drive Salmah crazy."

"Maybe so, but I would like to try it just once."

The captain and his crew of ten men just laughed at us. "You'll get your 'sea legs' about the time we arrive," Captain Eilam told us. "If you want to see what it is really like to be bored, just sit here and watch the water for a few days. You'd better enjoy it because once we reach the breakwater coming out of the big sea into the ocean, we could hit a storm that would get rid of your boredom very fast."

"Thanks a lot," Jona quipped with his greenish, half-sick grin.

The captain continued, "With the Nabaioth triangular tracking sails, this ship can maneuver where the ships with the big square lug sails can't. The Egyptian and Roman square sails can only sail when the wind blows in the right direction, making it almost impossible to get into the Aila port."

The constant breeze blowing off the coastal mountains to the southwest provided steady sailing to the south. During the first four days at sea, the constant rocking and slapping waves dumping water into the ship brought us to our knees, spewing our breakfast, lunch, and dinner into the turquoise blue water. Jona looked pale and was as weak as a newborn camel.

"Shutran, I don't ever remember seeing each meal three times in the same day!"

"Jona, what do you mean three times a day?" Kaleb asked.

"First, when it's cooked, then when you eat it, and then when it comes back up."

By the second week we were adjusting and able to keep some food in our stomachs; and sure enough, just as the captain said, when we entered the ocean with a northwesterly breeze and high seas, we felt as though we were going in every direction all at the same time. All 14 of us were on the oars, fighting the storm with all we had.

We were very sticky from the waves of saltwater that crashed down on us for almost two days, but there was no way to wash it off. We needed just a gentle rain, but then the storm died out, the clouds broke, and the sun came out and dried the salt to our skin. Fighting the storm had been so exhausting that every man laid down on the deck and slept for one entire day, except for the captain and his first mate, who reset the sails, and two other men who traded off and on to man the rudder.

The ship clipped along at a remarkable pace, and on the 19th day at sea, the first mate yelled, "The cliffs of Zophar!" which meant only a half day more to Al-Balid.

We felt such excitement as we watched the shoreline. "Shutran, it is hard to believe that after traveling eight months to get to Jerusalem, it has taken us only four weeks to return."

"Yes, Jona, it's most amazing."

Captain Eilam explained, "It is not always like this. There are only two times a year when the winds are right. Most of the time the wind blows in the opposite direction, or there is no wind at all. It can take up to two months to navigate the red sea alone. With the new Nabaioth sails, we do much better, and on this trip we didn't encounter any pirates, as we often do."

When we sailed into port the next afternoon, several children were playing in the water. When they saw us, they started yelling and jumping up and down as they waved with excitement, but I know we were more excited as we waved back. Jona turned to the captain and asked, "What are your plans?"

"King Solomon has requested that we bring back more luban. We'll stay one week and then return. So, Jona, if you went back to Jerusalem, would you want to go back with the ship or on a horse?"

"If you had asked me three weeks ago, I would have said by horse, but now I think I would go back by ship."

We bid the captain and his crew farewell and anxiously left the ship. As we started up the beach to our house, I could hardly contain my feelings. My heart was pounding so loud that I couldn't hear anything else, and I was sure Kaleb and Jona were feeling the same thing. We embraced and parted as Jona went to his house.

"Shutran, see you tomorrow."

"Yes, Jona."

As we entered the village, I couldn't help but wonder, "What if I'm too late?" But I had to push that thought from my mind. It seemed unusually quiet as we walked through the village. When we reached our house, I knocked on the door, since I didn't want to startle anyone. There was no response so I opened the old, wooden door, and we went inside. Kaleb, looking around, said, "Mama isn't here and I can't find Armin and Joshua."

I could feel my heart throbbing in my temples as I fought my worst fear. I walked into the cooking area and could see that there had been a morning fire. Then I went into Joshua and Armin's room and could see that both beds had been slept in the night before, which helped me calm down. Kaleb asked, "Where could they be?"

"Let's go out and check the animals." I knew that we would have new ones, and when we went inside the stable, I was happy to see the young camels that were almost a year old and the two new colts from Sultan that looked just like him. It is so good to be home!

"Let's go to Jona's house and see if they are there." We rushed out the door and came around the corner only to meet Jona hurrying to our house. "Jona, they're not here."

"Let's go over to Ahsein's. He'll be home. He never goes anywhere," Jona anxiously suggested.

Sure enough, Ahsein was sitting in front of his house. As we approached, he jumped up, not believing his eyes. We weren't expected home for another eight to ten months. He was speechless and almost in shock as he reached out and grabbed me. He wanted to know how we got home.

"On a ship," I said. "Ahsein, do you know where Mirah, Salmah, and the children are? Have you seen them?"

"Yes, Shutran, calm down. Today is market day and all the ladies are there, including Mirah, Salmah, Samira, and the children." Ahsein began to sob, "I am so glad you are home. Shutran, little Armin has been sick almost the entire time you have been gone. It has been very difficult for Mirah. Come, I'll help you find them. Jona, you look a little sunburned," he said with a questioning look.

"Shutran thought I should go to sea like my namesake, the prophet, only he didn't put me in the belly of the ship. He left me out on the deck to bake." We all laughed.

Then Ahsein's expression changed as he asked, "How is Enos? I know his mother and father really miss him. I have heard that his mother often cries herself to sleep at night."

"I'll go to see his family in a few days. Maybe you could let them know that I am home."

As soon as we entered the marketplace, I could see Mirah beside Salmah buying some melons. Armin was standing next to Mirah, hanging onto her side, while Joshua was bartering with one of the merchants. Kaleb wanted to run to them, but I just wanted a moment to watch while choking back my tears of joy.

Jona's two children were playing near Salmah as she made her purchases. His son, Ezim, was the same age as Joshua. His daughter, Ahleeynh, was a year younger. Our children had grown up together and were great friends. Jona was so happy to see them but was in a state of amazement as he saw Salmah holding a baby. A son, he wondered? Was she with child when he left? "Shutran, do you see the baby?"

"Yes, Jona, I do. It looks like Salmah has a very special gift for you."

His eyes began to water as he anxiously moved towards her. "Shutran, how could we have the two most beautiful women in the world?"

"Good question; and to think, we're just a couple of old caravaners."

Mirah moved to pick up some more produce, but Armin just stood there and then laid down on some old wool sacks piled up next to her. It was easy to see something was wrong, which sent me into deep thought.

"Shutran, what's the matter?" Jona's voice snapped me back to the present.

I just looked at him and said, "Let's go surprise them."

As we came close, I said, "Excuse me, ladies. When will dinner be ready?" Joshua and Armin screamed and Mirah became faint and started to fall. I caught her just in time so that she fell against me, and we both went down.

I was on the ground holding Mirah as Joshua and Armin hugged and kissed me until I thought I couldn't breathe. Little Armin had lost a lot of weight. Her skin was a grey, ashen color, which told me she was not doing well. I fought back the pain of seeing her this way.

A bit bewildered, Mirah put her hands on her cheeks, and as she came to her senses, asked, "What happened? Salmah, I thought I heard Shutran's voice." She blinked her eyes as she cleared her head, realizing that she was on the ground and someone was holding her.

She turned her head and as she looked into my face, I said, "Mirah, I'm home."

She gasped and cried at the same time, throwing her arms around me. Both Armin and Joshua had their arms around my neck as Kaleb tried to put one arm around his mother while trying to hold onto his little brother and sister. Mirah reached out and put one arm around Kaleb so that we were all entwined and crying with great joy to be together again.

I could hear Salmah crying as she proudly presented Jona with his surprise gift, while the other children laughed with glee at their father's reaction.

Ahsein and Samira were asking questions as fast as they could without giving me time to answer. All I could say between tears was, "Let's go home." As we came to our feet, Jona, Kaleb, and I were smothered with the excitement of many family members and friends when they learned what all the commotion was about.

When we finally reached our house, Mirah was able to ask a few questions. They all wanted to know how we got home, did we go to Jerusalem, and what happened? I grabbed Mirah and sat her on my lap and said, "Listen to Kaleb tell his stories to the children."

Mirah heard the word ship. "What did he mean—ship?"

"King Solomon had one of his ships bring us home."

"So you did make it to Jerusalem?"

"Yes, we did," I said as Armin came over and crawled up into my arms, displacing her mother.

"Papa, thank you for coming home. God told me you would come. Papa, hold me. Just hold me, Papa, and never go away again."

"I promise you, my little princess, I will never leave you again."

Mirah looked at me in disbelief, "How can you say that?"

"Very easily, Mirah, very easily."

We sat on the pillows laughing and crying as Kaleb told stories until we all fell asleep. A few hours later I awoke with a very hot sensation only to discover that Armin, who was lying on my arm, was burning up with fever. I quickly awakened Mirah. "Armin is on fire."

"Yes, Shutran, this has been happening ever since you left. It comes and goes."

I placed Armin in Mirah's arms while I went to get some fresh water from the well. When I returned, Mirah started bathing Armin's little body in the cool water. I started a fire and then gathered some vernonia plants to make a tea with luban. This was a blood cleanser and was supposed to help calm the fever. She drank it slowly while Mirah bathed her with an extract of the fagonia plant. Her fever soon broke and she returned to sleep. "Mirah," I asked, "How often does this happen?"

"Maybe twice a week. I have talked to everyone in the village, and no one has any answers. The priest says she is possessed by an evil deity. It goes away for a few days and then seems to get worse when she gets excited. Shutran, this is different. She knows something. She said that when you came home, she was going to go live with her Father in the sky. She said she had something special to do, and when she's with her Sky Father, she won't be sick any more.

"Shutran, I am so frightened. I don't want to lose her."

"I don't either, Mirah. I have missed so much of her life already. Come, let's try to sleep while we can."

Armin didn't have another fever for several days, and Mirah was hopeful that she was over whatever it was. But something told me differently. Every day we went down to play in the sand and water, which seemed to be good for her. She loved the smell of the sea.

Jona had lined up a shipment of luban to go back to Solomon. The last evening before sailing, the ship's captain came to our home to share the evening meal. I wanted him to meet my family and then take a message for me back to King Solomon and Queen Balkis that Armin was very sick and that I wouldn't be returning.

Jona announced that he felt he should return to Jerusalem to bring the caravan home. "Shutran, I just feel I should go. I just get cranky worrying about the caravan, and Salmah will wish I had gone anyway." We walked outside to talk. "Shutran, what is it?"

"I don't know. Armin seems better since I have been home. We have been giving her the tea of vernonia and luban and bathing her in fagonia and myrrh, which have seemed to help, but I feel this is just the calm before the storm, and the next time could be much worse. I promised her that I wouldn't leave her again. Armin told Mirah that when I came home, she was going to go live with her Papa in the sky where she wouldn't be sick any more. She said that she had something special to do."

"Shutran, you feel so strongly about your God. Can't He help you?"

"Jona, He has already helped me. I have prayed so much for Armin, and even Kaleb and I have prayed together for her. I believe that God did answer our prayers and let her live until we came home. I do not have all the answers. I just know there is a plan, and God is in charge. If we trust in Him, whatever the outcome, there will be something we will learn that will be for our good. But right now I need to be here for Armin and give strength to Mirah and the boys. We all love Armin so much."

The next morning Jona was carrying baby Jashman as we walked with him, Salmah, and the other two children down to the shore to bid him farewell. "Shutran, thank you for bringing Jona home for this short time. He feels such a responsibility and knows that if he is there, you won't have to worry and will be able to give all your attention to Armin."

"Salmah, that is true. Thank you. He has always been there when I needed him whenever it was possible."

Jona put his little son into Salmah's arms, knelt down in the sand, put his arms around Ezim and Ahleeynh, and held them tightly. The children were crying and hanging onto him as they kissed and hugged each other. "I will be home soon, I promise. Take good care of Mama and help her with the baby." He stood and kissed Salmah and the baby once more and with a big sigh, resolutely turned towards me.

Jona and I embraced and then looking squarely at him with great trust and admiration, I spoke as the Commander, "Jona, take my cross belt. I know you will wear it with the dignity of the Commander and the responsibility it carries. You are the kind of friend that not many people have."

Jona lowered his eyes for a moment in deep thought, then lifted his head with the air of someone who was about to take control and boldly said, "Yes, Commander."

I put my hand on his shoulder and with much gratitude calmly said, "God be with you, Jona."

"And with you, Shutran." He then turned and crossed over into the ship. We all waved as the wind took to the sails and pulled the ship into the deep water and soon over the western horizon out of sight.

Three weeks later Armin still seemed to be improving, and then without reason the fever came back, and this time it was much worse, lasting all night and into the next day. We kept giving her pomegranate juice and the luban tea. That afternoon when the fever didn't break, I steeped the roots and leaves of the lycium shawii plant for her to drink. It was known to be a good blood cleanser as well, so I hoped it would help.

She drank a little at a time as I held her in my arms. As she looked up at me, I could tell that she was seeing something far away. She stared for the longest time and then gave a sigh that would bring her back to me. I asked her what she was seeing. "Oh, Papa, my new home is so beautiful."

"Armin, we want you to stay with us; Joshua and Kaleb would miss playing with you. You and Joshua helped Mama so much while we were gone. What would we all do without you?"

"I know, Papa, but in my new home I won't be sick, and I can see you every day. You won't be able to see me, but, Papa, I will be there."

If a camel had kicked me in the chest or a jambiyya had been buried in my heart, I could not have felt more pain as I did with the words my little Armin spoke. They were etched in my mind forever. I held her through the night, and by noon the next day, the fever broke. She was acting a little better but still seemed weaker. I had pleaded with God through the entire night to please heal her and let her stay with us.

I remembered my plea months earlier when I asked God to not take her home until Kaleb and I returned. I wanted to cry out loud or hit something but could find no relief for my pain. My plea to God was constantly in my heart, begging Him not to take her. Mirah put her arms around me and said, "Shutran, I pleaded with God to let us have her until you returned home, and He has granted that request."

I walked outside to the stable and sat down. I put my head in my hands and cried for what seemed like hours until I couldn't cry anymore. "Oh, Father, please just a little more time."

Then the words came in my head, "Yes, my son, a little more time, but I have a special mission for her. She will be in your hearts forever, and you will come to understand her purpose."

I hurried back to the house to get my family. "Come, let's go to the mountains and spend a few days. We gathered our blankets, packed some food, and rode the camels into the Zophar Mountains, which were coming alive with beautiful flowers and green grass. Khorf, the time of the great rains, had just finished and left the air fresh and pure. We picked flowers and put some luban resin that we had brought with us to burn in the fire as we cooked our meals.

We laid under the stars as Kaleb told stories about his experiences on the caravan and when he was captured by the pirates and then rescued. Armin cried and laughed with us. "Oh, Kaleb, I love your stories. Please, tell more." She seemed peaceful as she lay on my lap staring up into the star-studded sky with such wonder as they twinkled brightly.

Mirah lay beside me holding Armin's pale little hand as Kaleb continued to tell stories late into the night until Joshua and Armin both fell asleep. There we were together in God's living room, holding each other and wishing the night would never end. For three days we enjoyed our time talking, taking short walks, and gathering pomegranates and wild berries, and then we journeyed back home.

The next day Armin wanted to go down to the beach again. She loved to walk through the warm sand and feel the water run through her toes. The gentle waves were so calming as they washed sea shells up on the shore. We built palaces in the sand and drew pictures of the cave houses in Selah. For the next three weeks, we were rarely apart.

Salmah and the children visited us frequently. Baby Jashman brought laughter into our home with his discovery of new things and his playful nature. Armin loved the baby and was so motherly when she held him. I often wondered if she would ever have her own. Our families had become very close over the years and spent much time together. I could see the longing for Jona in Salmah's face, and I knew how much the children missed their father. I was always happy when they came, knowing that it helped them to be with us, especially since I was home.

When the children went outside to play, they made lots of noise while having fun, but Armin would lag behind and not join in very much. That night as Armin was lying on my lap, we listened to Kaleb telling Joshua again about his sword fight. Armin really wasn't listening as she looked into my eyes and said, "Papa. . . ."

"Yes, my little princess."

"My Sky Father says it is time for me to come home."

"Oh, Armin, I love you so much." I kissed her little cheek, trying to hold back my tears. "Thank you for coming to our home and being our little girl."

"Oh, Papa, I love you," and turning to Mirah, she quietly uttered, "I love you, Mama." Then she smiled at the boys and faintly whispered, "and Joshua and Kaleb, too." The air seemed still and the feeling was different. The boys were quietly watching as they came closer to Armin. She looked up at each one of us and touching our faces said, "I will always be with you."

Kaleb, so tenderhearted, felt the tears well up in his eyes as he realized what was happening. He cried, "Papa, do something. Please, Papa; God always hears you."

Joshua knelt beside Armin and held her limp little hand, crying, "I love you and I will miss you. Please come back and see me." Mirah put one arm around Joshua while holding onto Armin, who was still sitting on my lap.

Kaleb pulled on my hand, "Papa, please do something. Don't let Armin go. We love her. We need her. Oh, Papa, please."

Mirah put her arms around Kaleb and pulled him close to her, while Joshua gently caressed Armin's cheeks repeating, "Armin, I love you."

Kaleb continued to cry as Armin tried to comfort him. "Kaleb, I love you and will always be in your heart, and you can touch me when you touch your heart."

I looked into Mirah's eyes with a knowing and said, "Sing a song for us." The sweet sound of her voice filled the loneliness that we were beginning to feel in our hearts as Kaleb and Joshua softly cried themselves to sleep.

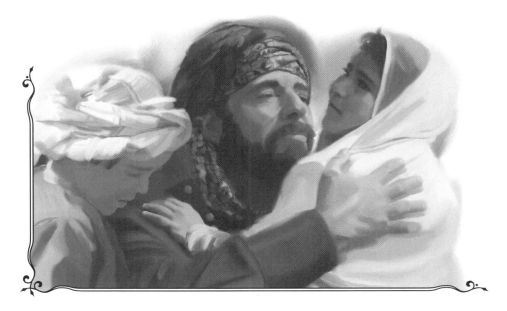

Armin looked into our eyes and again whispered, "I love you, Papa. I love you, Mama." With tears rolling down our cheeks, we could feel God's presence as Armin closed her eyes for the last time and left this world and returned to her Sky Father.

Mirah and I never moved. We just sat there not wanting to let go of our children. When daylight came, I took Armin's body to prepare it for her final journey. We loaded the wagon and drove to Armin's favorite place. Kaleb and Joshua never made a sound except for an occasional sob. It was unusually quiet during the two days that we were in the mountains as we all pondered our loss. I carved a special tomb deep into the limestone ridge under a giant luban tree that would be her guardian.

I made a beautiful box out of red sandalwood for her body and placed it inside the stone tomb. Then we all helped place a huge stone over it and sealed it with mortar, which was the most difficult task for all of us because it was so final. We sang Armin's favorite song, prayed for the angels to protect her resting place, and thanked God for sharing her with us for the short time that she lived, for the love she taught us, and for the trust she had in her Sky Father.

We stayed that night in the mountains close to Armin's resting place and journeyed home in the morning. Kaleb didn't speak for two days, just sorting out his feelings. We went down to the water to walk in the sand, wanting to pretend that Armin was still with us. We watched the waves and listened to the sound of the water, which only seemed to make it more painful. Kaleb started to cry and asked, "Papa, why?" And before I responded, he asked again, "Why?" By then Joshua was crying, too, but couldn't speak.

I remembered God's words to me when I was in the stable asking for a little more time. I put my arms around the shoulders of my boys and tried to console them. Speaking to Kaleb, I said, "Remember when we prayed and asked God to let Armin live until we came home? God did that."

"But, Papa, I thought that when you got home, you could heal her."

"I know, I hoped so, too. But listen, there are things about God's plan that I do not understand. I am learning, just like you, but what I can tell you is to never question God and never stop loving and trusting Him. God spoke to me before Armin left us and told me that she had something special to do. I can still hear His words in my head when he said that there would be a time when we would understand why. I know it is not the answer you want, but it is the only one I have. We must trust and know that Armin is watching over us right now and that she would not want us to be sad."

Mirah was very contemplative and hardly talked for a week. One night, as we were getting into bed, she asked, "Shutran, can you help me to understand something? I heard what you told the boys, but tell me."

"Mirah, I am just a tired, old caravaner without any book learning. All I can tell you is that I believe there is a higher law that has something to do with the choices we make before coming here. We don't know what choices Armin made before she came to us, but I believe that Armin had a greater purpose than what we know. I also believe that if we stay true, we will come to know."

The next day I had a strong desire to go to the mountains, so after breakfast, I saddled up and rode back to Armin's tomb. I sat down and took a deep breath of the fresh, mountain air. As the tears ran down my cheeks, I kept thinking about what God said to me. His words were comforting and gave me hope, yet I felt a terrible loss in my heart. I had to be strong for Kaleb, Joshua, and Mirah, but now it was my time to cry and come to an understanding of my feelings.

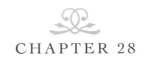
Finding Peace—
Life Goes On

I tied Yusal to a nearby frankincense tree and walked over to Armin's tomb. Being close to her resting place triggered that haunting pain all over again, which pierced my heart. "Why? Why did Armin get sick?" When she came into this world, she seemed different, special perhaps, as if she knew something we didn't.

She was so fragile, like a little doll. The boys were always so careful when they played with her. She would bruise and cut easily, not at all like the boys, who never noticed a scratch. She wasn't interested in physical things, even when the boys tried to include her.

I started to notice when she was about a year-and-a-half old that when Mirah and I talked about Abraham's One God, Armin would climb up in my lap and just listen and stare into my eyes as though she were looking through me. She always had such a peace about her, regardless of what was happening, like she had a connection to another world.

She would sit with me for hours and listen to me retell the stories that I had heard sitting around the campfire with other caravaners. She always seemed to be so fascinated to hear about the One God, the Creator of all things.

There were those who scoffed and laughed at such "nonsense." I remember an old Ishmaelite, who one night around the campfire, outside of Gerrha, was telling the story about the beginning of our world and how God created the earth with the great waters and then placed man, woman, animals, and birds on the land and fish in the sea in just six days. I was hearing these things for the first time, yet I had such a feeling of awe and truth about what he said.

At the same time a Sabataean from Marib, with disgust in his voice, said that anyone who believed such things had been in the desert sun too long. I remember how I felt the heat of a fire burst within me as I looked him in the eye and said, "So you think your sun gods and idols of rock could make the waters and the dark of night? Any man who believes in idols is the one who has been blinded by the sun."

While I told the story, Armin stared at me in silence as if in deep thought, which seemed so unusual for a child her age. When I finished, she would clap her little hands and with excitement say, "Yes, Papa, yes." Her response gave me chills. She seemed so much older, as if she had come to teach us something from another world.

Mirah said to me one night after putting Armin to bed when she was about two years old, "Shutran, Armin is different. She is such an unusual child and doesn't seem to connect with this world like our boys. Sometimes her eyes seem to go blank, and she looks like she is in a distant place. Is she too perfect for this world?"

"Yes," I thought, "Armin is too perfect."

I continued to ask God for understanding as I sat on the gentle, sloping hilltop, leaning against a big tree that shaded me from the hot sun and overlooked the valley below. It was so peaceful as I watched the birds glide through the air. I thought I could feel Armin's presence, like the "calm after the storm," reminding me how tired I was. It had been over nine months since I had really been able to sleep. My eyes became heavy and I found myself drifting in and out of the present moment until exhaustion took me into a long-awaited sleep. I sank deeper and deeper into a most vivid dream.

I saw my caravan going east out of Jerusalem through the land of Gilead. Kaleb and Enos rode ahead to check on the oasis where we were going to camp for the night. Kaleb's horse was farther ahead and ran into a pit of quicksand and couldn't get out. Kaleb fought to free his horse, but with no success. Enos was close but not close enough to reach Kaleb in time to save him. I could see Enos crying as he rode back to bring me the terrible news.

The dream was so vivid that tears actually started to run down my face while I was sleeping. The pain was becoming too real, when suddenly everything changed and I was on the ship with Jona returning to Jerusalem. A raging windstorm came up when we were in the Gulf of Aqaba. The waves came crashing so hard over the sides that the ship finally turned over. Jona was knocked unconscious when a piece of the broken mast hit him and knocked him into the sea. When I saw him sink, I let go of the plank I was hanging onto and went under the water to retrieve him. Using all the force I had, I pulled him up on top of a plank that had been caught in the back current of the ship. He had a sizable cut on the side of his head that was bleeding heavily.

I knew I had to get him on land to stop the bleeding. I fought the current and wind-driven waves with all the strength I had while trying to get to shore. I took off my gutrah and tied Jona to the plank to keep the waves from washing him off. After what seemed like hours, fighting against the roaring winds and pounding waves, I didn't know if I could hold on much longer. My arms just didn't have any more strength to keep towing the plank, when a huge tidal wave came over us, hurtling a piece of the ship's rudder that hit me on the back of the head, breaking my neck, while pushing the plank with Jona onto the shore.

I felt myself sinking deeper and deeper into blackness, as I fought to come awake. I broke out into a cold sweat as I yelled in my sleep, "No, it can't end this way," which snapped me into consciousness. My whole body was tingling as I shook my head, trying to get rid of the dream. Then I heard a voice again inside my head say, "My son, we are all interconnected and have different roles to play. Armin chose to come to your family, knowing she would be giving up her time with you in order to change your destiny and that of Kaleb's."

Just then I heard a horse coming and turned to see Mirah approaching. She climbed off her horse and embraced me with her gentle love and caring. I looked into her dark eyes that were red and swollen from crying and wondered how I could help ease her pain. I put my arm around her while we walked for a moment, and then I told her about this most amazing dream I had had. She listened quietly and then asked, "Shutran, what can it all mean? Are you all right?"

"Yes, Mirah, I am. But what about you, Kaleb, and Joshua?"

"They seem to be doing all right. They are home feeding the animals. I told them I was just going to bring you some food and water and a couple of blankets for the short time you would be here so that you could stay a couple of days to think and find some peace."

Then Mirah asked, "What do you mean, change your destiny?"

"If Armin had not been sick, Kaleb and I would have been on the caravan going to Nineveh. Had she become well, I would have been on the ship with Jona returning to Jerusalem."

Mirah thought for a moment and then said, "I don't know how to understand that, but surely it is something to think about. How do you feel?"

"I don't know, Mirah, but it makes me feel better to think that Armin had a purpose other than just coming to earth to be sick and die."

"Shutran, she brought us a gift, the gift of bringing the family together."

"Mirah, if there wasn't a purpose, then why wasn't she totally healed rather than just having her life extended until Kaleb and I returned home? What were the chances of her living for ten more months while I returned with the caravan? What was the chance that Solomon would have had a ship in the Aqaba bay and was willing to take us home at no cost? Mirah, look at all the miracles. I don't have the answers, but I know God is working in our lives. I carry a prayer in my heart and hope to find understanding.

"This may not be the right interpretation of my dream, but it gives me a place to go for some understanding. It helps me to let go of my pain, and besides, we have to go on with life for Kaleb and Joshua."

"Yes, you're right."

"It may not be the truth, but right now this is the only understanding I have. So it is my truth, and tomorrow, perhaps with more information, it could all change."

"Yes, Shutran. It does give me more to think about. I had better get back to the boys before dark," Mirah said as I helped her get on her horse.

"Don't worry, Mirah; I'll be home in a day or so."

"I know," she answered as an understanding smile came over her face. "You need this time."

I watched Mirah ride until she was out of sight in the canyon below. Walking over to Yusal, I took my saddle and bridle off so he could graze. Then I sat back down on my blankets to reminisce about the past nine months and think about the future.

"What is my purpose? And Kaleb's purpose? Did I have a dream about something that really happened? What about Jona; is he safe? Did someone else ride into the quicksand?" There were so many questions without answers. "What is the real gift, life or death?" I felt pain knowing my little girl was gone. Mirah was doubtful about my interpretation and was still looking for an answer. "What do I teach my boys? Where do I go from here? How do I get to know about this Messiah? There are no books and even if there were, I couldn't read them anyway."

My head was churning with a million questions. I felt a bit weak. I blinked my eyes at what looked like heat waves coming off the ground

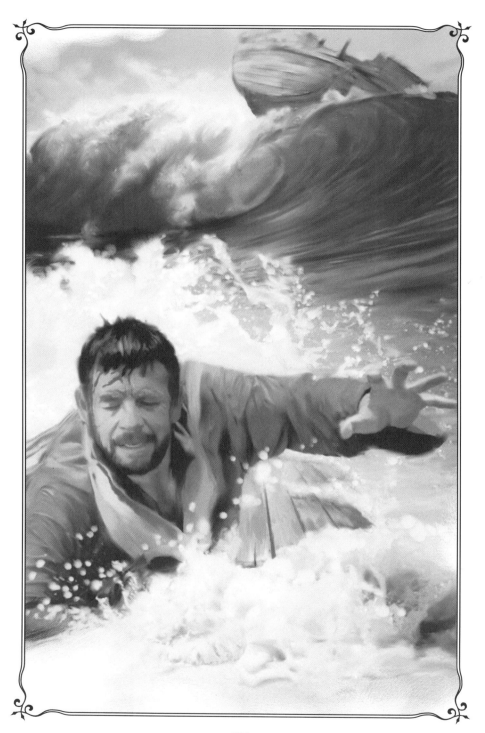

by Armin's little tomb. But it couldn't be. It wasn't hot enough. Closing my eyes and lying back on the blankets, I just wanted to be close to God and learn more.

"What was Armin's gift?" I wondered as I slowly sank into a deep, deep sleep like none I had ever had. I felt a different joy as Armin appeared in front of me. She was so pretty with her rosy cheeks and vibrant smile. My eyes filled with tears as I listened to her laugh and watched her play, doing all the things she had not been able to do before leaving her earthly life. Her eyes met mine as she came running towards me. "Papa, Papa, I told you I would never leave you!"

I stretched out my arms and beckoned her to me, "Yes, that is what you said." Just as I thought she would be in my arms, she vanished from my sight.

Instantly, my dream opened up again to the caravan, which had stopped moving. The men were standing close to the campfire as Micah ran towards them. "What's wrong?" Ibram asked.

"Oh, Captain, his horse!"

"Whose horse?"

"Jaaba's," Micah yelled, pushing through the men.

"Jaaba's horse ran into quicksand when he was riding ahead to check the campsite for tonight."

Just then Jaaba's face transformed into Jona's as the scene shifted again. He was standing on the shore, covered in blood. Only Jona, the ship's captain, and two others were washed ashore. I heard Jona say, "Captain, I felt someone pull me up as I was sinking down into the water and tie me onto the plank that was washed ashore."

The dream faded again into darkness. I began to toss and turn as the picture of my home in the village came into view. Mirah was talking with the boys about Armin and what she might be doing. I suddenly felt anxious to ride home so that I could tell them what I had seen in my dream. By then I was wide awake. I quickly gathered the blankets and saddled my horse.

I paused for a moment as I sat on Yusal and took a deep breath as if to take in the peacefulness of the mountain. I looked over at Armin's tomb with a longing for my precious gift that had been lost. But, no, she wasn't lost. She was with me. She would always be with me. I was grateful for this short time that I had spent with God opening my mind to greater understanding. But now it was time to go. My family needed me. As I rode off the mountain, I felt Armin close to me and rejoiced that she was happy and knew she would never be far away.

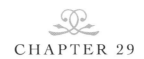

CHAPTER 29

Jona Brings the Caravan Home

It had been almost seven months since Armin's death. I spent a lot of time with Mirah and the boys, working in the garden. The boys and I made new pack saddles and took care of the animals. I was so happy with the quality of baby foals and baby calves from the camels that were being born.

Kaleb, Joshua, and I made a few caravan trips with 20 to 30 camels to Wubar and back, which we could do in three weeks. Once a week we would go to Fort Sumhuram to bring merchandise for the village, which meant an overnight stay at the fort. I enjoyed these trips because the boys loved the caravan, and they were able to be with me where I could teach them so much about caravanning. Sometimes the boys would talk Mirah into going with us to Fort Sumhuram.

She pretended that she wasn't interested in seeing the new porcelain dishes, teapots, spices, tapestry, paintings, copperware, and all the things in the market. She did like hearing about the ships that came in from India or China carrying sandalwood oil and the wood carvings from Java that were so beautiful. The only time she didn't like to go was when slave trading ships came in from East Africa with ivory and diamonds.

Time had passed quickly while I kept busy, and that was good. I was glad to be home to work with the ships bringing in their goods. According to Kaleb's records, the demand kept increasing for more frankincense, myrrh, copper, rose water, and other textiles. With all the orders, we needed to move more merchandise. We established regular trade schedules with Wubar, Wadi Hanoon, and Fort Sumhuram, which made our deliveries more efficient.

While we were in Wubar, I met with Muflek, who owned the caravan that ran from Wadi Andhur to Wubar. He was tired from a lifetime of caravanning and wanted to sell his business. His sons had all gone to sea, which had disappointed him greatly. Muflek had several offers from others but wouldn't sell to any of the men who wanted to buy. He said they told him they could push the caravan and make five trips a month rather than just the three he made.

While we were talking in the inn at Wubar that night, he said, "Shutran, some of my camels have been making this trek for 20 years and have another 10 years left in them, but if they get pushed really hard, they will die in 2 or 3 years. I can't let that happen to my camels. They are my most trusted friends." Looking into my eyes, almost pleading, he continued, "Shutran, please buy my caravan. I know my camels will be treated well, and I will enjoy seeing them from time to time."

"Muflek, let me talk it over with my sons. What will you do if you sell?"

He answered slowly, "My wife wants to move to Al-Balid, where she will be closer to our grandchildren."

"That's understandable. I'll let you know in the morning."

When Joshua and Kaleb came from taking care of the animals, we met at our tent. Kaleb asked, "Father, why did Muflek come to see you?"

"He wants us to buy his caravan with all his contracts, camels, and gear."

Kaleb said, "That would increase our business, but who would run it?"

"I was thinking of one of our men like Musilum, who has a lot of experience."

"Father, what about Enos? I really think he would be a good choice."

"Why?" I asked.

"Father, you saved his life twice, you treated him like a son—like one of us—you gave him value when he wanted to end his life, and most of all, you can trust him. Enos would do as you say and wouldn't betray you. You don't know what Musilum would do once he tasted the money. Besides, Enos is my friend and we can work together. Musilum would not want to listen to me, and besides, it would also make Enos' mother happy."

"Son, it's a very good idea. Let's sleep on it."

The next morning while eating breakfast, Muflek and I made an agreement. He would make four more trips with Enos, or whoever would take over, and teach him about his caravan and the personalities of his 105 camels and 8 horses. Enos was already a seasoned caravaner, so it would be easy for him.

On our return to Al-Balid, we traveled east with Muflek to meet the guard who was the gatekeeper and the scribe who did the accounting at the Wadi Andhur Treasury House and the apothecary. Everything was in place, and as we learned how the demand for different merchandise had increased, it became very clear that we would need to add another 25 camels to the caravan.

Muflek was very happy when we made the agreement so that he could head back to Wadi Andhur, knowing he had to make only another four trips, and then in about six weeks he could be home with his family.

When we returned home, the village had come alive with excitement as the news spread from house to house that the caravan would be arriving in two more days. All the people including the children were out cleaning the streets, hanging banners and ribbons, and setting up the marketplace. There was singing and dancing as the festivities were being planned and the fire pits were made ready for a great feast.

It had been a total of 17 months since the caravan had left, and now they were almost home. A strange feeling came over me as I thought about it. Yes, it was my caravan, but I was not with them. I would just be waiting with the villagers to welcome them. I would not be the Commander bringing them home.

The returning of a caravan had always been one of the most exciting times of my life. It was such an exhilarating feeling to see all the villagers waving in the distance. I rejoiced to see my family, how the children had grown, and the changes that had taken place in their young lives. Listening to all of them talk at the same time with such excitement was intoxicating.

But this time Jona would bring them into the village. I could feel myself starting to choke up as I thought about the sacrifice my great friend had made for me and the rest of the caravan. Yes, it was my caravan, they were my men, and we would have a great reunion. But I knew what a great moment this would be for Jona.

It seemed like the biggest event of the year for the village. Everyone was there: our families, neighbors, and friends. Mirah's father was excited to see new goods that would be going into the Treasury House. He had never been outside of Al-Balid. He had always wanted to travel but was very afraid to leave home and didn't like to ride, except when it was absolutely necessary.

I was always amazed at those who told me how much they wanted to travel with a caravan and see the world, but because they had so

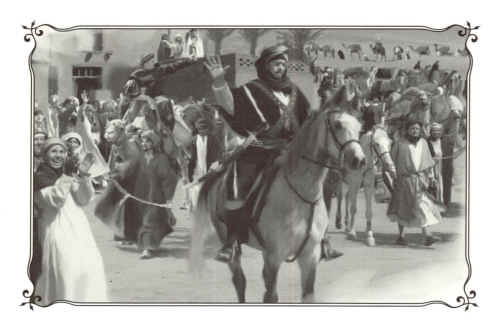

much fear, they never had that opportunity. There was so much in life to experience, and yet too many chose to live in fear and regret and often tried to live the adventure through someone else's experience.

In anticipation of the arrival of the caravan, many families that had been waiting since daylight were lining the sides of the road leading to the village square.

Kaleb, Joshua, and I rode out of Al-Balid before daylight to meet the caravan. When we spotted them in the distance, Kaleb became very animated in his excitement to see everyone again.

When Jona spotted us, he started to ride faster as we rode at a gallop towards him. It was such a wonderful feeling to see my most trusted friend and to know he was safe and almost home. We jumped off our horses and embraced. Jona looked at me and then turned to hug Joshua and Kaleb. He stumbled over his words as he tried to speak.

"Shutran, you can't imagine how happy I am to see you. He unbuckled the commander's cross belt to hand back to me.

I shook my head, "No, Jona. You are the Commander of this caravan. You brought it this far and now you will take it home. Everyone is waiting." Jona embraced me again with such a feeling of gratitude and respect.

"Let's go home," I said, slapping Jona on the shoulder as we turned to mount up. I laughed, "I didn't know I would be so happy to see such an old, dirty caravaner as you."

"Me? Who's the old caravaner here? Shutran, you look great. The rest has been good for you."

Kaleb laughed, "What rest? Father has had us pushing caravans to Wubar, Fort Sumhuram, and Wadi Andhur ever since you left."

"What have you been going up there for?"

Kaleb looked sideways while Joshua blurted out, "Father bought another caravan."

Jona, shaking his head, said, "Let me guess. Muflek's caravan!"

"Yes, that's the one," Kaleb answered. "Why would you think Father would rest?"

"Oh, that hit on the head must have altered my thinking."

A chill ran through my body. "What hit on the head?" He slid his gutrah back a little so that I could see the scar. When I looked at it, I felt a little dizzy as a queasy feeling passed over me. I started to ask more questions when Ibram, Ahmad, Mohamed, Micah, and Enos came riding up.

My heart started to swell with such joy that I could hardly keep it inside. As I got off my horse, they got down at the same time, and we all embraced together. "I am so proud of all of you. You have done a great job. Welcome home!" It seemed like we were all trying to hold back our tears.

I turned to embrace Enos and said, "I am so glad you came home."

"I am, too, Captain. I feel I am ready to face whatever Ahsein wants to do to me."

Joshua said excitedly, "Oh, Enos, Father has a big job for you." Enos had a puzzled look on his face.

I just grinned at him and looked down at Joshua and said, "Just wait; we will talk about that later."

More of the men came walking up to greet us, as well as our scouts, Ali, Musilum, and Hussin. "It is so good to see you."

"Captain, we are so sorry to hear about Armin."

"Yes, it has been difficult, but we are doing well, thank you."

Just then Alimud rode up. I shot a glance at Jona, who nodded his head and winked in approval. Alimud swung out of the saddle, walked over to where I was standing, and offered his hand to greet me. As I took it, he said, "Captain, thank you for giving me back my life."

"I thought you were going to stay in Damascus."

"I thought so, too, but things have changed for me. I felt I needed to come home and do the right thing, as you said, and heal the past."

"Alimud, your decision is good. Surely God smiles upon you. You have made me proud."

I looked up at everyone with excitement in their faces. "Well, men, the entire village is anxiously waiting. Let's ride. This is a great day!"

As we entered the village, it was hard to determine what was loudest, the crying or the shouting for joy from excitement as family members greeted their loved ones coming home. There were enough tears to quench a camel's thirst for a week.

The parents of Enos were standing together with Ahsein and Samira. Enos came down out of the saddle and embraced his mother and father, who were both teary-eyed. "Enos," his father said, "welcome home, Son. I have missed you so much. You have made your father so proud. Please forgive me for not standing by you and helping you through that terrible time."

His mother was holding him tight and crying, "Oh, Enos, I am so happy that you have come home." While other family members came to greet him and rejoice in his safe return, Enos felt nervous as he glanced over to Ahsein, wondering what was coming.

Ahsein now had his chance and stepped over to Enos before he could say anything. Wrapping his arms around Enos, with tears running off his face, he cried, "Enos, can you ever forgive me for the horrible things I said and the anger I displayed towards you? Enos, I was so wrong. I have caused you and your family so much hurt and anguish that I deeply regret." Enos bowed his head in gratitude as Ahsein embraced him.

Salmah was crying with joy as little Jashman went running to his papa. As Jona scooped his little son into his arms, Jashman squealed with delight when Jona tossed him into the air. When Ahleeynh and Ezim reached him with Salmah, they were all hanging on so tightly that Jona looked like he was practically being choked with their hugs. Jona's deep laugh told me how happy he was to be home.

The fires were burning and the smell of roasting goat and camel meat filled the air. The lentils and beans were cooking in the kettles with apples and pineapple. It made everyone feel hungry and anxious to start eating.

Incense burners were sending billowing clouds of the white smoke of frankincense into the air. I thought about how my life had evolved into such a demanding business because of that aroma. I thought of all those camels and the heavy bags of resin that we carried for Sheba to give to Solomon. So much work and so much of my life had been given to this gift from God.

It was beautiful to watch the smoky trails waft throughout the village, bringing such peace and contentment. Yes, it was peaceful and we were content, but it wasn't just because of the frankincense. We were happy because we were home, and we were together.

It was getting dark before all of the villagers finished their greetings. The music was playing and families were now eating and enjoying being with each other. Seth's family also came, although they were still suffering from their terrible loss. I had been with them several times while I was at home, wanting to give them any comfort I could. I shared my feelings with them about Armin, which did seem to give them more peace.

While everyone had gathered to eat, Alimud had asked the priest if he would call them to attention. At the sound of his voice, they quickly became silent, turning their heads to hear what he was going to say. The priest held his arm out to the young man walking towards him and said, "This young man has something that he would like to say to all of you," and stepped down as Alimud walked up the steps near the well.

He turned to look into their inquisitive faces and was obviously deep in thought. It was easy to see that he was having difficulty trying to find the right words. He took a deep breath and began, "I have a great need to speak to all of you here in Al-Balid. Some of you don't know me, but those of you who do, know me as Alimud. I am responsible for and caused the death of some of your family members, and I want to express my deep pain for what I have brought to your families.

"I used to be one of Commander Shutran's captains. But in my arrogance, I betrayed him in Gerrha and started my own caravan almost three years ago. I was full of pride and thought I could do a better job than the Commander. He always made it look so easy.

"My caravan was attacked in the desert by raiders, who killed almost all of my men. I wanted to die in their place. I wanted to die and couldn't, nor could I find any escape for my tortured soul. I didn't come back to Al- Balid because of the shame I felt and the embarrassment to my family. I didn't think I could ever look into the faces of the families who lost a loved one because of me. I begged the Captain to let me work for my journey to Damascus, where I thought I would try to build a life where no one knew of my past.

"The Captain gave me another chance, even though most of the men silently resented his decision. When I arrived in Damascus on our return from Nineveh, I knew that I couldn't run any more. I knew I had to come back and ask you all for forgiveness. I owe the village a great debt and wish to pay it however I can. If you wish to take my life, I am ready."

His voice broke and everyone could hear that it was hard for him to talk. With tears in his eyes, he was almost at a whisper, and there was not a sound to be heard except for the crackling in the fire pit. "My heart is heavy and without your forgiveness, there is no reason for me to live."

He regained a little more control, and looking directly at me, he continued, "First, I want to thank Captain Shutran for giving me a chance to own my mistakes and the opportunity to go forward and try again on the caravan, to give up my arrogance, and most of all, for what he taught me about Abraham's God. He has given me much hope.

"Second," with a big sigh, he turned to Jona, "I want to thank Captain Jona for trusting me on our return journey and showing me how to lead, how to be a man. He gave me a lot of courage to return. My family is here and I want to be with them and feel their love; but most of all, I am here to pay the price for my mistakes."

Ahsein walked up and put his hand on Alimud's shoulder as he stepped down and turned to face those listening. "I know Alimud's experience has affected so many of you, but I would also like to speak to you about my heartache. Many of you blame Alimud for the death of one of your family members, a father or a brother. Please, just think about how you feel while I speak.

"I blamed Enos for the death of our son, Nahor, who most of you knew from the time he was a small boy. My hatred for Enos was eating me alive and nearly destroyed our two families. I wanted him dead like my son. I wanted his family to hurt as I hurt. Yet, Enos has become a fine, young man, as fine as any who have walked in our village.

"Many of you, including my own wife and children, have been so patient and loving with me. Shutran, my longtime friend, and his family have trusted me and taught me about the One God, and as I came to know Him, it changed me inside. Now I feel only love for Enos and ask his forgiveness for my anger and the terrible things that I said to him. My heart was cold and hard.

"My family is together again and we are happy, as you all have seen. God has blessed us as I have reached out, wanting to help those in need. If you need help, if your heart is hurting, come and let us talk. Let me share your pain. Please, let me help. That is the least that I can do. We all make choices and we all make mistakes. God knows us and will use us to help each other and will take our pain, if we will just let Him."

After Ahsein finished and everyone returned to the festivities, the air was again filled with music and laughter. I watched two men walk over to Alimud whose sons had died on that fateful caravan two and a half years ago. As they stood in front of him, I wasn't sure what they would do. They could have run their jambiyyas through him, but instead I saw them extend their hands and reach out to him. I could see the rigidness in Alimud's shoulders relax as he conversed with them. They even began to smile as they talked.

Jona and I had been sitting on a couple of big rocks a short distance from where everyone was eating. We had so much to talk about. I wanted to hear about the caravan and the journey Ibram made to Nineveh and what happened with Sheba and Solomon and her return home. It surprised us when the priest brought everyone to silence in the middle of the celebration. But as I listened to Alimud and Ahsein express themselves with such humility to the villagers, my soul was filled with gratitude, and I silently thanked God, knowing that I had made the right decisions. If I had chosen to reject them both, the outcome would have been very different.

I nudged Jona with my elbow. "What happened to Alimud that made such a difference?"

"The caravan was crossing the Euphrates River at Carchemish without knowing that a flash flood from upstream was dumping into the big river. The men didn't see it coming, and it caught the last five camels crossing. The water hit with such force that it started to push the camels with two of our men downriver. The camels were fighting the current as the men hung on, trying to grab branches that were hanging over from trees in the water not too far from the shore.

"Without hesitating, Alimud jumped into the water and swam out into the swirling current, risking his life. He was able to get a hold of one of the ropes trailing in the water and wrapped and wedged it around a tree growing up out of the water near the riverbank, securing it long enough for the other men to grab hold and finish bringing the camels and the men across.

"Ibram had been impressed with the way Alimud had helped on the caravan, offering assistance whenever necessary. He was quick to respond and made good decisions. It was obvious that he could be a good leader. When this happened at the river, which could have cost the lives of several camels and men, Ibram was so impressed with the way Alimud took charge of what could have been a disaster that he made him a captain to be responsible over his own group. He has come home a changed man."

"It's amazing to see how much good comes when one can let go of hatred. Now, tell me about the scar."

"Remember when Captain Eilam warned us about the big storms they often encountered on the big sea? Well, this storm was one of the worst. It slammed the ship so hard that it turned it over. I was hit in the head and was sinking in the water when I felt a hand grab me, pull me up, and then tie me to a plank. Shutran, I know this sounds impossible, but I was sure it was you. I could hear your voice telling me to hang on for Salmah and the children."

My eyes dropped down as I stared in amazement at the ground, searching for understanding. His words pierced the depth of my soul. The pain of so many unanswered questions flashed through my mind. Was this a possible answer? My heart was pounding and I felt my throat tighten. I couldn't talk and I didn't want Jona to hear me struggle to try to get the words out with my "broken" voice.

"Shutran," Jona continued with a strange tone of questioning, "there was something else that happened that was very sobering. It was when the caravan was crossing Gilead going to Damascus. Jaaba had galloped ahead to look for a campsite for the night when his horse rode into a quicksand pit. Jaaba, being older, knew to throw himself from the saddle, and the others got there in time to help him, but he lost his horse."

I could hardly breathe as his words shook my sense of reality. I was mystified by the memory of my dreams and just kept staring at the dirt and stirring it with my toe. Jona felt something unusual in my silence and sensed that I couldn't speak for whatever reason, and so he just kept talking.

"Shutran, a chill went up my spine knowing who would have run into that quicksand if you and Kaleb had been there. Not having experience, Kaleb would not have thrown himself off his horse. He would have tried to get his horse out, and we would have lost them both." Jona paused for a moment to reflect and then said, "As strange as it sounds, somehow, I feel Armin had something to do with all of it."

I was so overwhelmed by the realization that had just come to me that I had to stand and turn away. Jona quickly came to his feet, put his hand on my shoulder, and came around, looking me in the face. Anxiously wanting an answer, he said with an astonished tone, "Shutran, you know, don't you?"

With tears streaming down my cheeks, I looked deep into his eyes, "Yes, Jona, but I thought it was a dream."

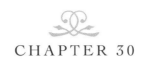

CHAPTER 30

Twenty Years Later

The sun had not crested over the horizon when I went out to the stable to check on the animals. I walked among my horses and camels, feeling great satisfaction with the quality of new stock being born. I couldn't help but reflect on how fast the time had gone by. It had already been 24 years since Armin had passed into the next life.

The year was 967 when Jona, Kaleb, and I came home on Solomon's ship. Time seemed to rush by with increasing speed after Jona went back to Jerusalem to bring the caravan home and return Queen Balkis and her caravan to Marib. So many things had happened, so many changes, and the boys had grown up so fast that it seemed like we had passed through all these years in a short moment of time.

King Solomon had passed away two years ago, and all of Israel was in an upheaval. Rehoboam, Solomon's son, had been crowned King of Israel, but because he would not lighten the people's burdens, ten tribes pulled away, leaving him as the King of Judah, which included only Judah and some of Benjamin. The people of Judah hoped that he would walk in his father's footsteps, but to their disappointment, he never carried his father's greatness. His leadership skills were questionable and the people turned against him.

Jeroboam, who was once favored by Solomon but then had displeased him, had fled to Egypt. After Solomon died, Jeroboam came back and was made the King of Israel. The ten tribes, led by Jeroboam, raised up rebel forces in the north to fight against Rehoboam, bringing great turmoil to the Israelites and ending the peace of 40 years.

Solomon had wanted to find out about the Queen's military strengths, with the intent to conquer the Hadhramaut and take over the incense trade. But Solomon had lost himself in his own passion and was so smitten with desire for the Queen that he didn't realize that he was giving her strategic military information that would eventually bring down his own kingdom.

The Queen had very cleverly discovered Solomon's military weaknesses, and out of her desire to get revenge for her sister, she later gave her half-brother, Shishak, who was now the Pharaoh of Egypt, her priceless information that enabled him to march his army into Judah through the unguarded passes and conquer Rehoboam's kingdom without the loss of a single man.

After the Queen returned to Marib, Solomon fabricated the lie that she carried his child, from which many untruths were spun. He wanted to show the world his superiority and how irresistible he was to all the women. It was said by many that Solomon was cursed by God and became impotent, because he turned away from God and started worshiping idols and false gods. It was astounding to think that everything his father, David, had worked for—building one of the most powerful kingdoms in the world—was now beginning to fall and would soon be lost.

The caravaners spread many stories that probably grew every time they were told, but it was rumored that King Solomon, until his death, was still in love with the one woman he was never able to conquer.

Queen Balkis, the Queen of Sheba, remained true to her agreement with her father, which was that she would never marry. It was said by Captain Ayaar, "There was only one man in her life for whom she would have given up her kingdom, and that was Captain Shutran; but Captain Shutran's wife, though not a queen of the richest kingdom in the world, commanded greater power than the Queen herself."

I never saw the Queen again. Kaleb, however, made several caravan treks with Jona to Marib and had supper with the Queen in her palace. She would always say to Kaleb, "Ask your father to come with the next caravan."

Queen Balkis ruled her kingdom with honesty and integrity, treated her people well, and died the beloved Queen of the land of Saba. Her sister, Makshara, returned to her homeland of Egypt but never came out of her deep sorrow.

I reflected on how things had changed over the 50 years that I had been leading caravans and had fought in battles, the things that I had seen and experienced. "If only I could write about them," I thought. "Oh, well, no one would believe my stories anyway," I chuckled to myself.

Mirah called for me to come and eat. When I entered the house and saw her getting the food ready, my pulse raised with a little excitement as I watched this beautiful woman with whom I had shared a bed for 40 years prepare our evening meal. I called to her, "I'm here."

I thought about Jona's comment years ago before he married Salmah. "Shutran, as beautiful as Mirah is, how can you stand to leave home?" I smiled to myself. After all these years of being together, she still stirs my blood, even though Father Time is showing signs around her eyes. Yet after three children, she still has a young-looking, slim body.

I asked one day, "Why do you always look so good?"

She looked up and smiled, "You deserve to have the same woman you married. Why would I change if I love you?"

I thought about the statement that Queen Balkis made, "Mirah has to be the luckiest woman alive."

But as we sat down to eat, I said to myself, "If Sheba had known Mirah, she would have understood why I am the luckiest man in the whole world."

I looked admiringly into Mirah's face and said, "After breakfast, let's walk down to the water. I think two of our ships came in last night from the east."

"Yes, Kaleb and Joshua stopped by earlier and said they were going down to oversee the unloading. You know Kaleb; he has to keep perfect records. I know you are anxious to see the ships, so you go on ahead and I'll come down as soon as I finish here."

When I arrived, Kaleb was making an inventory as he directed the merchants with the goods coming off the ships. Joshua came walking up, calling to Kaleb, "We need eight more camels. More merchandise is being unloaded than we expected."

Kaleb asked, "Joshua, do we have more camels? We just sent 200 to Shabwah for Ibram, and 350 went to Mohamed in Aila. Oh, yes, and last week 321 camels went to Micah in Damascus, and 45 camels went to Enos in Wadi Andhur."

Joshua laughed, "I bought 600 camels at the market last week when Father and I went to Masqat. We have what we need."

Kaleb was managing the shipping along with the K & J Caravan business, and Joshua was managing the camels, horses, and pack station equipment and leading caravans, just like I had. Kaleb waved me over while he and Joshua were discussing news about one of the ships. When we finished talking, I turned around to look for Mirah and saw her standing beside Kaleb's wife, Alorhyee, who was holding their firstborn, a beautiful baby girl, healthy and full of life, who they named Armin. Mirah was so happy being a grandmother and now having two "daughters."

Jona enjoyed his time at home and often helped Salmah with her new herbal business. Their young son, Jashman, who was born while Jona was with me in Jerusalem, had grown into a fine, young man and worked with Jona in the business. Jashman's wife, Taneeyha, had blessed their family with twin boys, Fishtahr and Asher, who were a great joy to Jona. He spent a lot of time playing with his grandsons and telling them stories of his days on the caravans.

Two ships had come in from Java with sandalwood and spices, and one ship had come from the Socotra Island with myrrh. Kaleb was busy getting all the merchandise logged in so that he could have it dispatched within four days.

The myrrh was going by ship to Aila. Then Mohamed would take it with a caravan over the Sinai Peninsula to Egypt. The caravans were busier than ever, so Joshua would often go to check on our pack stations, the camels, and the equipment. He always returned with great news. "Father, you trained the men well."

After spending some time with Kaleb and Joshua, I decided to go to the stable to catch Bahkit, one of Sultan's offspring, and ride out to our farm in the mountains, where I was building Mirah a new home of limestone and marble.

The white limestone was quarried at Aila and brought on one of our ships to Al-Balid along with copper from Wadi Dana, silver from Solomon's mine, and salt from the Salt Sea. The cedar wood came from Lebanon and was brought by caravan over the mountains through Damascus to Aila and loaded on one of our southbound ships.

The marble and granite, the finest in all of southern Arabia, came from Sharjia, one of the oldest cities on the peninsula. There were fine porcelain dishes, silk window hangings, tapestries that came from China, and beautiful woodwork that was carved from sandalwood.

I wanted a beautiful home for Mirah, the children, and the grandchildren when they came to be with us. I wanted it to be a home that we all loved and enjoyed. After all the hard times and our humble beginning, Mirah deserved the best.

How little I realized at that time that my businesses would create interest among so many other people in our little village, which had now grown into a thriving, industrious city. As the news traveled to Masqat, people from all over Arabia came to the office to ask Kaleb and Joshua questions about the marble, limestone, cedar wood, and woodwork made from sandalwood that was now being transported on our returning ships.

One day when we were all together talking, Mirah commented, "Can't you ever stop creating other businesses?"

Jona laughed, "Mirah, when he does stop, you'll have to send Joshua to come and get me so that we can dig a hole and plant him in it."

I just chuckled, "Have you all forgotten? Some of our ancestors lived to be 400 to 500 years old, so I figure I have another good 10 to 12 businesses in me." We all laughed.

Salmah spoke up, "Why don't you two just go fishing?"

I looked at Jona and replied, "I never thought of that."

"What, Shutran, a fishing business?"

"Come on, Jona; let's go check it out. We could sell our fish in Selah or Jerusalem."

Mirah shook her head laughing as she walked back into the house with Salmah. "His ideas never stop."

"I'm sorry, Mirah, I shouldn't have said anything."

"No, don't even give it a thought; besides, you know it wouldn't change anything anyway. Just don't suggest that he start selling your ointments or the incense that he's extracting. I can just hear him, 'Buy your liquid gold now before it's all gone.' What would happen if he got the idea to start shipping liquid incense around the world?"

Yes, life was good. Jona and I enjoyed our time at home; but every three or four months, we would feel the desert calling us, so we'd go with Kaleb, Joshua, and Jona's son Jashman on a caravan trip up to Wubar and back. The caravans had been such a major part of our lives. Caravanning was in our blood. Besides, we had a great time being with our sons and telling stories around the campfire.

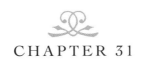

CHAPTER 31

The One Gift

I have been in Ein Gedi for the last 12 years and have had a rewarding experience with the development of the extraction chamber for distilling the resins of frankincense and myrrh. The oils are so rich in their ability to heal physical ailments and bring peace to the soul. I feel such a spiritual presence when I distill them. Now I also have the balsam oil and a new world of healing to discover. The resin is not as abundant as frankincense and myrrh, which makes its value beyond anything that I know. This golden oil is truly a gift.

In my growing-up years, I traveled with my father as he led his caravans from the Hadhramaut Mountains across the wilderness of the Empty Quarter. I developed such a great love and respect for the mountains and the desert like my ancestors before me.

There are times when I long to be with the caravans, but I do not miss the long days of endlessly blowing sand, unrelenting heat, and the packing and unpacking of the camels every morning and night. It was a constant fight for survival to deliver the frankincense and myrrh to the next destination and to know that a life wasn't worth a kilo of resin.

Ein Gedi had become a welcome change, working in the distillery and learning the extraction process of the resin. The constant breathing of the aromas was so uplifting and made the challenges of the days easier to overcome. Over the years many caravaners have brought me resin to distill. There was such a fascination for the oils from which exotic creams, lotions, and perfumes were made and highly sought after, which meant that I needed to distill more resin.

When the caravaners arrived, I was excited to see what resin they brought for me to distill. They always allowed me to keep a little of the oil for myself, which was my treasure. We had many trees that grew on the terraced side hills across from the Treasury House, so we had a nice harvest of balsam and frankincense resins, which I was able to distill and sell.

I walked outside to feel the coolness of the fresh, night air and to see if any more changes were in the western sky. For the past six months, the stars had been unusually bright, and I had noticed a triple star configuration that appeared to be moving. It gave me a feeling of great anticipation—a feeling of excitement—like something was about to happen. Perhaps it was just the anticipation of the arrival of the caravans that were due any day. They would be bringing resins for me to distill, for which I was most grateful.

I noticed how quiet the night was as my gaze wandered across the ravine to the terraced balsam groves that extended down to the old village below. I marveled at how many of the beautiful balsam trees were still growing that my ancestors had brought here from the western Hadhramaut over 900 years ago. I was amazed that the trees survived after their bark had been so overcut in years past because of the great demand for their precious resin. Kings, queens, and rulers of many kingdoms sought to possess it.

Caesar Augustus of Rome was the largest purchaser of the frankincense and myrrh resins. He also wanted more balsam than was harvested because he loved the exotic smell. He bought all that I would sell to him, but I always kept some for my family. We had discovered that the oil soothed the pain in our arms and backs after working in the fields all day, and we never wanted to be without it.

We loved the smell of incense burning in our home, and my wife liked to mix the oils of balsam, myrrh, and frankincense together and make an ointment with rose and coconut oil to put on her skin, which was so soft and youthful looking. The aroma filled me with such peace and tranquility.

I loved watching the golden liquid of the balsam oil come to the top of the water when the resin was boiled. It was easy to pour off and separate from the water. The scent was so soothing as it permeated the air and made me feel like I was the master of my own destiny. The aroma brought a feeling of peace and strength, similar to when I cooked frankincense, a tradition that had been passed down from my ancestors for more than 1,000 years.

I wanted to experiment with the golden oil in the apothecary and make ointments and medicines. Those of us who grew up in the Land of Frankincense where the resins were part of our lives knew they had special powers, and we used them in many different ways.

My grandfather told us stories about how the ancient people believed that the smoke of frankincense became the white wings that forged a link between them and God and carried their prayers to heaven. My father taught us that the smoke would help clear our minds and that we might even see things beyond this world.

Stories were told about how the resins could heal different maladies and how royalty even bathed in the resin water to maintain youth and beauty. I watched my mother boil myrrh resin and make ointments with the oily liquid to put on infections and boils. She loved to put it on her skin, and she always used it for the lotus birth. Sometimes she boiled the resins together and made ointments with coconut, flax seed, and olive oils mixed with beeswax, coconut, and goat fat. I was very drawn to the ointments and wanted to make my own mixtures.

Those early years shaped my destiny and brought me from my homeland with my father's caravan to the Treasury House in Ein Gedi to learn about balsam and how to extract the liquid from all the resins. I knew the oils were special, especially with the spiritual feeling that was as empowering as the miraculous healings I saw. It was amazing how the demand for frankincense had grown throughout the world.

I thought about the prophets of old as they spoke of a new King soon to be born—a Messiah. The words of Micah resounded in my head, ". . . among the thousands of Judah, yet out of thee shall he come forth unto me that is to be ruler in Israel. . . ."

The Prophet Isaiah said this newborn King would be like none before, for he would bear our griefs and carry our sorrows. He would be wounded for our transgressions, and we would be healed.

Grandfather said the prophets foretold that this time was coming and that we would recognize it by the signs in the heavens. I wondered, "Is this how the wise men will know when to come? Surely they will stop here to rest before their final journey. I know many will want to take gifts, just as I do." My thoughts went to the distillation that was just finishing, and the feeling came over me to give my precious liquid gold—the balsam oil—as my gift to the newborn King.

But what would be the gifts of the wise men? And who would bring them? Would they come from the great commanders of the caravans that I knew would be arriving soon? Would they bring the resins of frankincense and myrrh for me to distill? What heavenly gifts these would be. Yes, how fitting for the new Messiah!

These holy oils would be very special gifts that no one else had. Although the balsam resin was known to the world, no one had the liquid gold that came from it. What a rare and treasured gift. Is this my purpose for being here, to bring such beauty to the world—such a joyous discovery for God's children? How is it that I am so blessed?

My father taught us about the One God, and each time he returned with the caravan, he brought more stories of the prophets and the legends that were passed down from Abraham, Moses, Isaiah, Micah, and others about a great event that was to take place in my lifetime. It was also foretold that three men, one from the east, one from the south, and one from the west, would each bring gifts for the new King, who was not yet born. But who would they be?

How many people really knew of the old prophecies and the event to come? The caravaners carried the words of the prophets to distant places as they traveled far and wide, and wondrous stories were told around the campfires. There were many, like my people, who anxiously waited for the prophesied time to come, and yet others laughed and scoffed at those who believed.

Surely it would be caravaners who would bear the gifts. But would their gifts be the precious oils of frankincense and myrrh that I would distill for them? From what distant lands would they come? Would they carry my precious gift to our newborn King? The questions just kept turning over and over in my mind. In my heart I *knew* that I would play a part in this sacred event.

I walked back inside to check on the distillation of the balsam that, after ten hours, was almost finished. Because the resin had become so scarce, I did not want to lose a single drop. I treasured the golden balsam and knew it would be used for something very special.

When I went outside to refuel the firebox, I noticed some movement along the shoreline. The moon, reflecting off the water, illuminated the caravan that would soon be here. It thought to myself, "How interesting—a full moon to light the way of the caravan." I hurriedly sent the cooks off to put on more tea and prepare some leavened bread, as the caravaners would have traveled all night and would be hungry.

We didn't have to wait long for them to arrive. Most of the caravan had probably stopped in Heshbon, as only the commander and his guards came to the palace. He looked very tired as he got down from his camel as he must have journeyed through the night with his three loaded camels. In a very quiet voice, but one of strength and conviction, he said, "I am Caspar. Is this the Palace Treasury House of Ein Gedi?"

"Yes, it is, Commander. Welcome, I have been expecting you! Come inside and sit down and eat a little. I have prepared a place for you to rest. My servants will attend to your camels and packs."

"Thank you. I will tell my guards to give your servants the packs that I have brought. They are filled with the finest silk, polished cotton, jasmine oil, and small gifts of porcelain. I would be most grateful if your servants could wrap and prepare them for the last part of our journey. They are my gifts for the new King, for the stars in the heavens now tell us that He will soon be born."

"Yes, of course. It is my honor that I might serve you."

After giving his instructions, he followed me into the room where the food was ready. As he sat down, I asked him, "From where have you come and how long have you been traveling?"

"I have traveled for eight months and come from the Indus Valley near Kashmir, ruled by King Gondophares."

"Did your king send you?"

"No."

"Then how is it that you come here?" I inquired.

"For many years as I traveled with my caravan across the Silk Road to Nineveh and Damascus, I heard the stories that were told around the campfires and talked about in the marketplaces of a great event that would come to pass in our time.

"When I returned to my country, I told my people and our king what I had learned. They laughed at me and said I had been in the desert sun too long, but I believed it to be true. The storytellers always told us to watch for the signs in the heavens. As a caravan commander, I constantly watched the sky. It was normal to follow the stars as the guiding light to our destination. That was how we lived.

"Eight months ago I began watching three stars that seemed to be moving together. Every night there was more change than the night before. After 21 days they were in perfect alignment with what appeared to me to be an illumination that was growing brighter. I knew this was one of the signs of which they had spoken. For this reason I have come. I know that I am to help fulfill a prophecy told long ago. According to the legend, two others will come with gifts. I am certain they also will have seen the same stars."

A look of wonder must have been obvious on my face as Caspar paused for a moment and then asked, "And what is your name, Sir?"

"My name is Shutran Ali Abdulla Ismelacor. I am the overseer of the Palace of Ein Gedi, the great Treasury House, where we extract the holy oils of balsam, frankincense, and myrrh. I have waited long for this time to come, as the prophets have foretold."

Caspar again spoke, "This is most interesting. Stories are still told around the campfires about a great caravan commander whose name was also Shutran Abdulla Ismelacor. It is said that he was very wise and led with powerful discernment. He was fearless and journeyed many times across the Empty Quarter. It was his caravan that carried 50 tons of incense, plus many other beautiful gifts of great value, for the Queen of Sheba to present to King Solomon in Jerusalem. It has been said that Shutran's descendants still own caravans today."

"Yes, that is true," I answered. "Shutran, the great caravan commander, is my ancestor. The caravan business has been run by our family for over a thousand years." My grandfather was a commander and my father still leads the caravans today.

"But what about you? You don't seem to be leading a caravan."

"That is also true. I grew up in the Hadhramaut and crossed the desert many times with my father. As a family, we would go to the hills to gather the resins. We would burn frankincense resin at home to fill the air with the sacred smoke. My mother often boiled myrrh resin in water and soaked up the liquid that came to the surface with a cloth. Then she put it on her skin, which is perhaps why her skin always looked so beautiful to me. We also discovered that the oils cool the sting and ease the pain of scorpion, snake, and spider bites.

"I felt something very different with the resins and wanted to know more about the oily liquid that was within each crystal. So when I was old enough, I came here to work in the Treasury House to learn how to extract the oil from the resin. It is here that I built the extraction chamber. I have been here for many years and am now the overseer. My father named me after my 12th great-grandfather, Shutran Abdulla Ismelacor. I carry his legacy and his love for the resins.

"God has blessed me to live at this time and to be in this place that I might help prepare the gifts that you will carry. But now I must take leave to attend to my duties. Eat and rest. I will return soon."

The sun was still climbing in the sky when the second caravan arrived. The lead camel stopped and knelt down so that the weary traveler could step away. He said to me, "I am Melchior and have traveled for three months from the Hadhramaut, the land where God created man, ruled by King Yada'il Darih II. The gift that I bring comes from Eden, which is part of the prophecy to be fulfilled."

"And what is this gift?"

"I have brought the sweet myrrh of Eden that represents sacrifice and suffering. I would be most grateful if you could distill it for me so that my gift may be made ready for the mother of our new King."

"Ah, yes, the sweet myrrh of birthing," I said as I pondered for a moment. "Your arrival is important that the new mother may use the myrrh in the tradition of the Queen's lotus birth.

"Come, you have traveled far. I have prepared food and drink and a place for you to rest. My servants will attend to your camels and carry the resin inside. We must hurry to begin the distillation."

"Thank you, I am most grateful." After the camels were unloaded, Melchior turned to his second-in-command and said, "Take the caravan to the old copper mine to get supplies, secure the new load, and wait for me there. I will join you in a few days when my journey here is completed."

"Yes, Commander," he said, and then he turned to start down the wadi. A moment later he looked back over his shoulder and with a tone of wonder and respect said, "I know little of your One God, but I feel something different here that I cannot explain. Perhaps it is the beautiful smell that is carried on the breeze." He appeared to take in a deep breath and called out, "Commander, we await your return."

Melchior watched for a moment and then turned to me and said with a voice of great urgency, "When I saw the signs in the heavens, I knew it was time to start my journey. The stars have guided me here that I might be ready when the time is right." I nodded in agreement and led him inside the Treasury House, where Caspar was sitting. They greeted each other as I invited Melchior to sit down and eat.

"It is good to rest for a moment. Thank you for your kindness."

"I am blessed to be of service." When I was certain that his needs had been met, I bowed my head slightly in respect to Caspar and Melchior and said, "I must take leave now to see to the distillation. I shall wrap and prepare all the gifts for their final journey. Rest in peace; I shall return soon."

My servants had already put the myrrh in the bubbling, hot water, as it would take a few hours before the oily liquid would start to separate from the resin. I wanted to be finished with the myrrh so that we could be ready to distill the frankincense that I was certain the third caravan would be carrying. I knew we would have to distill during most of the night in order to extract the precious oil and have it ready by morning. That meant I had to make sure that the water continued to boil so that the myrrh extraction would be finished in time.

The afternoon passed as the sun faded into the shadows, and still no sign of the third caravan. But I could feel that it would come soon, so I sent my servant to gather more wood to put on the fire. My servant had just gone out when he came running back, calling to me, "Master Shutran, the caravan is in the wadi."

I felt a burst of excitement as I went out to greet the riders who were approaching. The one who appeared to be the commander inquired in a rather loud voice, "Is this the Palace Treasury House of Ein Gedi?"

"Yes," I answered.

"Good, the time is right. I bring with me the finest hojari in the entire world from out of the Zophar Mountains—frankincense, the symbol of divinity. May I trust that the oil will be distilled for the morrow? I desire to carry my gift of the holy oil to our newborn Messiah."

"Yes, it will be ready. Commander, may I ask your name?"

"I am called Balthazar and have been traveling for three months. I am from the Land of Frankincense, ruled by King Aretas, the IV, and I have come to fulfill the ancient prophecy."

I hesitated for just a moment, looking up in awe at this powerful presence. He was large in stature and had a look of determination in his face. I wondered how this great commander came to fulfill his destiny. I motioned towards the Treasury House and said, "My servants will take care of your camels and take the packs of resin to the distillery chamber. Please come inside. Food, drink, and a place to rest have been prepared for you."

I introduced Balthazar to Caspar and Melchior, who were still eating. They greeted each other as though they were kindred spirits with an anticipation of knowing that they had all come for the same purpose.

I knew little about Balthazar, but he had a wise and engaging presence, and I found myself wanting to know more about him. He seemed to know what I was thinking and answered my unspoken question. "My family comes from Al-Balid. I descend many generations from Joshua, the second son of the great caravan commander, Shutran Abdulla Ismelacor."

With great surprise I responded, "We are of the same blood. My father is Yakrid, who is generations descended from Kaleb, the first son of Shutran. We are kin. How long have you been leading caravans? What news do you bring from our homeland?"

Balthazar just smiled. He was much older and seasoned by his travels. "I have led my caravan out of the great Zophar Mountains, which you may know from your youth, and have crossed through the Empty Quarter to Yathrib to bring the frankincense from our country. I was taught the words of the prophets as a young boy traveling with my father. In every city I heard talk about the new King who was to be born.

"My father said that the new King would be born in my time and that I would celebrate His birth and bring Him gifts. For many years I didn't understand, but I believed in the one God and in the prophecies, and as I grew, that *knowing* grew within me, and I began to watch for the signs. When I saw the new stars, I was filled with a *knowing* that the time had come and began my journey, which has brought me here. I felt the truth of what I had heard and wanted to know more."

With great admiration, I responded, "I am filled with joy to share with one of my blood this glorious event in our time, and I am honored to prepare the gifts that will be taken to the new King."

Melchior stood up and said, "Is this not a wondrous sign that we have come from different lands for the same purpose and have arrived just three days apart? Please, tell me, how is it that you come here?"

Caspar again told of his experience and how many of the people in his country believe that the old prophets were talking about the birth of a new prophet, not a Messiah. They ridiculed and scoffed at him when he tried to tell the stories he had heard, saying that the heat of the desert and endless swirling sand had made his mind spin.

He told us that he had seen three unusual stars in the sky that appeared to be moving together. "I remembered the stories passed down by my ancestors that new stars appearing in the heavens would be the first sign. Every night for 21 days, I watched them move slowly until they came together. I knew it was time to start preparing another caravan trek to Damascus, and here I am."

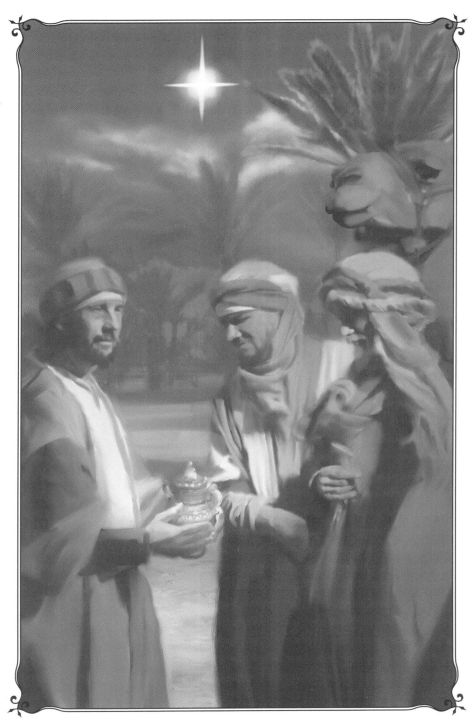

"This is most interesting," Melchoir said, "because I, too, saw three stars moving and coming together, only it was just four months ago. I knew it was the beginning of the fulfillment of legends that had been passed down for generations to my father and now to me."

I turned from Melchior and looked at Balthazar. A slow smile of *knowing* broke out on his lips as he began to speak. "Surely, the Spirit of the Almighty has brought us here. I also watched the three stars as they moved and knew that the prophecy of old would soon come to pass. My grandfather always said, 'Follow the stars. Every night you must watch and look for the signs that will one day appear in the heavens.' Now we are here together to await the third sign."

A tingling shiver raced up and down my spine as the men told of their experiences. I wondered how many other people would recognize the signs and bring gifts. The people had been waiting a very long time for the Messiah, who would free them from the cruel aggression of Herod's army. I remembered the words of the ancient prophet Balaam, who said, ". . . there shall come a Star out of Jacob, and a Scepter shall rise out of Israel, and shall smite the corners of Moab, and destroy all the children of Sheth."

Was this the hope of Israel? Certainly, there would be many who would come with their gifts, expecting that this would be the beginning of their deliverance. But only these noble Magi would be able to take the gifts that had been given to me to prepare.

We all felt the same truth—a truth believed by many of our great ancestors hundreds of years ago. Now this same truth that has shaped each of our lives has brought us here this day to begin new friendships that will bridge the eternities.

I felt very humble as I reflected on the immense sacrifice of our great ancestors—the caravaners. Had it not been for their strength and relentless determination, we probably would not be sitting here now. They had fought many battles and given so much to make this world a better place. What they believed and taught, as uneducated caravan commanders, had helped to prepare us for one of the greatest events that would affect the lives of millions of people.

That realization pierced the very depth of my soul as the question came into my mind, "Shutran, what have you done that will change the world and make it a better place?" I pondered my own question as I looked at Caspar, Melchior, and Balthazar. Then I knew: We have shared in the preparation of God's powerful healing oils—His holy oils—that have been extracted from the precious resins that the commanders had carried from afar. No others can bring such gifts to the newborn King. Our hearts are bonded forever in His love and in His gift to us.

I looked down, not wanting these great commanders to see my tears. But quickly regaining control, I lifted my head and saw that they were also wiping their eyes. "Shutran," Balthazar said, "it seems we all have inherited this same, deep, profound respect for our ancestors."

The spirit of kinship was strong as we stood and embraced with a knowing of the heritage we shared and the knowledge of prophecy about to be fulfilled. I spoke softly, "You must rest; we will talk again. The hour is late and I must finish my work. The time is nigh."

As I completed the distillation and collected the beautiful frankincense oil, my head servant, Samah, having great concern for me, said, "Master Shutran, Sir, you have not slept for three nights. Let me finish so that you may rest."

Raising my eyebrows, I looked at him and said, "Samah, and neither shall I sleep this night. Come! Let us make ready." I took the hojari frankincense oil into the apothecary, where our finest bottles were kept. All the gifts had been gathered to be prepared for the journey.

The frankincense and myrrh resins that had not been distilled were placed in one alabaster box, neatly wrapped with beautifully colored silk ribbons. The oils that had just been extracted from the frankincense and myrrh resins were poured into beautiful containers, which were placed in a second alabaster box and wrapped similar to the first one.

Then I took another alabaster box that was lined with an exquisite, white, silk cloth into which I placed my beautiful bronze vessel—my precious gift—filled with the sacred liquid gold of balsam. Next, I wrapped the box with white and gold ribbons and placed it in a special pouch that I would give to Balthazar to carry for me.

The other gifts for the mother and father of the new King were wrapped in special cloths and placed in the packs to go on the camels. The gifts were all so majestic.

As I walked outside, the smell from the Salt Sea, mixed with the aroma of frankincense, lingered in the air. There was a calmness beyond description, and I marveled at God's creations as I watched the stars shimmering in the immensity of the sky. They seemed so close that I felt I could reach up and touch them.

The night had such a feeling of serenity, a peace as if being in the presence of God that enveloped my whole being. It was transforming and I never wanted it to go away. An overwhelming feeling of love swelled within me; I just knew my heart would burst. I thought to myself, "Surely, this is like being with God." I took another deep breath and then turned to go back inside, when an extraordinary shimmering brightness caught my eye.

My eyes searched where the three stars had been, but now they had become one — a single blinking star! Yes, this was the beginning of the third sign, a brilliance that would soon grow and fill the sky.

I felt the tears of joy begin to run down my cheeks. My feet felt as though they weren't touching the ground as I turned to run back to awaken my guests. While hurrying down the hill where I had been standing, I called to my servants to bring the commanders' camels.

When I entered the Treasury House, I found that my guests were already dressed. Their robes were made with the colors of royalty, and their heads were wrapped like the majesty of kings. They were ready and carried a magnificence like the gifts they were to bear.

We went outside the Treasury House and found the camels waiting. My servants carried out the packs in which I had placed the gifts and carefully loaded them. Everyone from the palace was there to see what was happening. My wife came out to see if she could help in any way. I smiled at her with that *knowing* as I held our precious gift in my hand. She watched with joy as I walked toward the commanders, who were now ready for their final journey.

With a questioning look toward Balthazar, I raised my hand that was holding my special pouch. He nodded and motioned to me to put my gift in the pack with the other gifts. I felt my heart go with it as I stood back to bid my new friends farewell. We all felt a reverent excitement as the camels lifted their travelers into the air.

Balthazar looked down and saw the longing in my face. To my surprise, he reached back and put his hand on the pack and asked, "Shutran, would you like to carry your gift to our new King?" My longing turned into amazement as I nodded my head, trying to find words to respond. "Come. Join us for the final stretch of our journey."

I humbly said, "It is a great honor, but I am not ready. I thought I was only to help you prepare for your final journey to carry your gifts to the Christ Child."

Balthazar turned to Caspar and Melchior, who also seemed to be thinking the same thing as they nodded to each other. Then Balthazar turned back and with a deep voice that touched my very soul said, "Shutran, we will wait for you."

When I saw they were all in agreement, I felt my heart begin to beat faster. I quickly called to Samah, "Please prepare my donkey and bring her to me. I have a journey to make." My wife hurried with me to the Treasury House to help me gather a few things and went out with me to meet Samah, who was waiting for me with my donkey. As he handed me my staff, an overpowering feeling of being a part of something great caused a tingling sensation all over my body with the expectation of that which was to come.

We could hear what seemed like faint singing in the air. I embraced my wife, reassuring her that I would return soon with all the news. As I turned and looked into the village below, I could never remember so much excitement, as the villagers gathered their gifts for the journey. Yes, they, too, had seen the star that was shining brightly in the sky and were coming from all around to follow the caravan.

An indescribable feeling of expectation was in the air of what the newborn King would bring to the people. As the singing increased, my throat swelled as I choked back the tears of a thousand years.

I looked up at these three wise men, the Magi, who sat so proudly on their camels, ready for their greatest journey. As Balthazar's eyes met mine, tears were rolling down his cheeks. The heart of this tough, hard-as-granite commander, whose blood I shared, seemed to melt into tears that he could not hold back as the sound of the music on the breeze penetrated his very being. He had such a look of *knowing*, and an essence of light seemed to illuminate around the three of them as they were filled with the Spirit.

Balthazar nodded in acknowledgment that it was time to go. My heart was so full, knowing that my dream was about to be fulfilled—to carry my gift to our new King.

I wanted to shout for joy, but the lump in my throat would not let anything come out. I nodded back to Balthazar and could barely whisper, "Yes! Yes, Commander. It is time to ride. Let us follow the star to the One Gift!"

About the Author,
D. Gary Young, N.D.

oming from a very humble beginning in the mountains of the Frank Church wilderness of northern Idaho, D. Gary Young rose from the depths of depression and hopelessness after a logging accident left him paralyzed and confined to a wheelchair for life, according to all medical prognoses. His sheer will to walk again or die drove him on a quest to find a natural way to heal his body. His journey of 13 years in learning to walk again, from crutches, to a walker, to now being able to ride his horse, is nothing short of a modern miracle.

His insatiable desire "to know and see for himself" has led him to the far corners of the world in search of truth and knowledge. He has studied in various universities in the world with renowned doctors and scientists, attending courses in specialized medicine, science, and technology, working in hospitals and laboratories, and earning his doctorate degree in naturopathy and master's degree in nutrition. Since 2005 he has been a Deputy Member of the National Assembly of the International Parliament for Safety and Peace, headquartered in Palermo, Italy. In April of 2008 he was appointed Professor in the Field of Natural Health Sciences by Metropolitana Universidad in Guayaquil, Ecuador.

He was pioneering essential oil usage and making discoveries in the world of health and beauty that would someday bring hope to millions, while others considered them to be a fad or have little or no value. As the founder and president of Young Living Essential Oils, the largest privately owned essential oil company in the world, he is respected as one of the leading authorities on essential oils in modern times.

Secrets of the unknown that were hidden in the ruins and the ancient caravan trails led him on a journey into the "forbidden territories" of Yemen and the mountains and deserts of Oman, Saudi Arabia, Socotra Island, Egypt, Jordon, and Israel. With the help of God, he has been able to conquer the impossible as his path of discovery has taken him back through the pages of history.

Gary was in awe when he realized that his early years in the wilderness of the mountains, tracking wild animals, packing horses and mules, and following the stars when there were no signs to point the way would bring him into an ancient world, as though he were coming home.

He feared nothing and welcomed the challenge of the unknown. His desire to bring to life the mysterious world of the incense trade and the caravans that carried the precious cargo evolved into the writing of this book.

Shutran, the greatest commander of his time, epitomizes the same determination and dedication to his mission as does the writer of this novel in modern times. Their similarity of personalities, their grit, their way of dealing with human emotion, their immense vision and insight into the future, and their love of God are inspiring.

The wit, intrigue, action, sorrow, romance, and love experienced through the pages of this most unique novel challenge our imagination as we travel through the ages of time as an ancient world reveals its gifts.

Mary Young
June 1, 2010

Glossary of Terms

Abaya: an enveloping outer garment worn by women in some Islamic traditions; also called a burka.

Achillea: *Achillea biebersteinii*, an herb used in folk medicine for diarrhea and abdominal pain.

Al-Balid, Oman: once a thriving city of commerce on the Arabian seacoast with great wealth because of its trade industry of frankincense, myrrh, and Arabian horses. Known anciently as Zofar, its ruins are on the outskirts of Salalah.

Al-Hasik Mountains: a mountain range near the fishing village of Hasik, Oman.

Aila: known as the "White City" and anciently called Leuce Come, a Nabataean trading city on the Red Sea built of white limestone.

Al-Mawsaqah Mountains: a primary myrrh-growing region 100 miles south of Marib, Yemen.

Al-Ula, Saudi Arabia: a stop on the way to Selah (Petra); also called Dedan.

Bayhan, Yemen: a caravan way station and the gateway to the myrrh kingdom.

Bedouin: desert-dwelling Arab tribes, which are mostly nomadic.

Black Fattail scorpion: one of the most dangerous scorpion species in the world that has a sting from which several people die annually.

Bolster: fits over the axle assembly and supports a wagon bed. Two-wheeled wagons have one bolster; four-wheeled wagons have two bolsters.

Boswellia carteri(i): the botanical name for one of the species of frankincense grown in Yemen and Somalia.

Boswellia elongata: a species of frankincense found only on Socotra Island off the coast of Yemen.

Boswellia frereana: this frankincense species is not found in Oman, only in Somalia; in the 16th century it was called elemi.

Boswellia papyrifera: a frankincense species native to Ethiopia.

Boswellia sacra: the only frankincense species that grows in Oman. As the Latin name of this frankincense species implies, sacred frankincense could be linked to the frankincense taken to the newborn Messiah.

Boswellia socotrana: a species of frankincense found only on Socotra Island off the coast of Yemen.

Burka: an enveloping outer garment worn by women in some Islamic traditions; also called an abaya. A head scarf (hijab) is also worn, which in some Muslim countries covers all but the eyes.

Camel spider: a fictionalized predator in this novel. Found throughout Southern Arabia, Iraq, and Iran, it grows to a size between 6 and 8 inches long. Its bite is painful and can be bloody but is not life threatening.

Dedan, Saudi Arabia: a stop on the caravan trail north; anciently called Al-Ula.

Denarii: coinage for monetary exchange used around 300 B.C.

Edomite Kingdom: existed from the 11th century B.C. in the area of the Dead Sea and Jordan.

Ein Gedi, Israel: at the time of the birth of Christ, the Ein Gedi Treasury House Palace was five stories high and was used for the distillation of balsam, frankincense, and possibly other aromatic plants. It had a complete apothecary where ointments and medicines were made and sold to traveling merchants on caravans. It was also known as the bank building because it stored the precious and highly valued resins and oils and perhaps other valuable commodities and merchandise.

Elim: a location in present-day Saudi Arabia believed to be an encampment for the Israelites when Moses brought them out of Egypt and was perhaps the beginning of the King's Highway.

Empty Quarter: also known in Arabia as the Rub al Khali, a vast desert that spreads over approximately 600,000 square kilometers (approximately 250,000 square miles) in parts of Oman, Yemen, Saudi Arabia, and the United Arab Emirates.

Fagonia plant: common to Arabia and used for healing wounds and infections.

Fort Yabrin, Saudi Arabia: today known as Fort Jabrin; one of the first forts on the caravan trail built in the Empty Quarter at a small oasis as a caravan stopover; a major crossroad for caravans traveling from Najran to Gerrha and from Fort Sumhuram to Gerrha.

Fort Sumhuram, Oman: a major port city of commerce for merchandise coming in and going out of the Hadhramaut, located at the Khor Rori inlet or bay and under the rule of the Queen of Sheba.

Galabeya: the robe Arab men wear; also called a thobe. In modern times, women also wear a galabeya, especially in Egypt.

Gerrha, Saudi Arabia: believed to be located along the Persian coastline somewhere near present-day Bahrain; a strategic crossroad for international trade of the lucrative resins and goods coming from India and elsewhere.

Gilead: a mountainous region east of the Jordan River that extended from present-day Petra to Amman, Jordan.

It is possible that balsam trees grew in Gilead and that the resin was traded by the Ishmaelites who lived there, who were also the first people recorded to carry incense to Egypt.

Gutrah (or ghutra): a scarf that wraps around the head to protect it from the intense heat and covers the face from the reflecting sun and blowing sand. When needed, it can be used for a variety of things such as a wrap or sling for injuries.

Habban: a main supply station on the Frankincense Trail northwest of the port of Qana, located in present-day Yemen.

Hadhramaut: known as the land of frankincense that ranged from western Yemen to central and eastern Oman, once ruled by the Queen of Sheba. It was the richest production area of frankincense and myrrh in the world.

Hijab: a large scarf worn about the head by Arab and Muslim women, sometimes covering all but the eyes.

Hojari: the clear, white frankincense crystals cut from the trees found in the Al-Hasik Mountains in Oman. At one time, anciently, when there was so little hojari, only royalty was allowed to possess it. However, with time and increased production, it became highly prized and sought after by many. Today it is regarded as the world's best quality of frankincense, containing the highest levels of boswellic acid. It is presently being distilled for the first time in hundreds of years in Oman by the author of this book.

Ibex: a relative to the goat and is found in the mountainous desert and areas of the Arabian Peninsula. It is widely known for its large horns and weighs 60–80 kilos.

Ishmaelites: one of 12 Arab tribes that are descendents of Ishmael; known in the Bible as the caravaners coming from Gilead and going to Egypt with "spicery, balsam and myrrh" and to whom Joseph was sold as a slave (Genesis 37:25, Darby Translation). Balsam is referred to as "balm" in many other translations.

Jambiyya: the traditional, curved dagger used by Arabs, especially in Saudi Arabia, Yemen, and Oman.

Jebel Al-Lawz Mountain: now believed

by many to be the true Mt. Sinai, located east of the Gulf of Aqaba in Saudi Arabia.

Jilbab: a long, loose-fitting garment worn by some Muslim women and girls (see galabeya).

Ka'aba: a focal point of worship in Mecca, Saudi Arabia; a cube-shaped building containing a black stone thought to be a meteorite for which, the legend states, Abraham built the original sanctuary.

King's Highway: an ancient trade route from Egypt through Saudi Arabia, Jordan, Israel, and Syria, ending at Resafa on the upper Euphrates. Many historians believe that this is the highway on which Moses led the Israelites. The Bible tells how the Edomites refused to allow the Israelites passage on this highway (Numbers 20:17-21).

Khor Rori, Oman: a major sea port for international trade of frankincense, myrrh, spices, and many other commodities, located about 40 kilometers east of Salalah, the site of Fort Sumhuram.

Land of Midian: homeland of the nomadic Midianites, believed to be in northwest Arabia on the east shore of the Gulf of Aqaba and the northern Red Sea; the land to which Moses returned with the Israelites.

Land of Punt: many believe it was in Africa or Ethiopia. In the Omani Museum of the Frankincense Land book *The History Hall*, the text states that Dhofar has had numerous names including "the country of Punt." Omani author and archaeologist Ali Ahmed Al-Shahri says there is an ancient word "pint" (peent) that he thinks is the Shahri name for Punt and that it was in Oman. However, the Land of Punt most likely was the area of the Hadhramaut, which is part of present-day Oman and Yemen.

Levonah: Hebrew equivalent of the Arabic word "luban," meaning frankincense.

Luban: the Arabic word for frankincense.

Lycium shawii: this plant was recommended to fight inflammation by the Roman historian, Pliny the Elder.

Mablaqah Pass: located in the Al-Mawsaqah Mountains in modern-day Yemen, through which the myrrh caravans crossed.

Makka, Saudi Arabia: Mecca, the holy city of Islam.

Marib, Yemen: a taxation point on the Frankincense Trail; a verdant oasis because of the dam built by Sabaeans; also believed to be where the Queen of Saba (Sheba) lived.

Masqat: Present-day Muscat, Oman.

Menthe: a version of the botanical name for peppermint, *Mentha piperita*.

Mesopotamia: now modern Iraq and part of Turkey.

Najran, Saudi Arabia: the last important stop on the frankincense route before heading to Gerrha or Egypt.

Nard bush: an aromatic bush found throughout Israel and Arabia, also called spikenard; a ground bush that is used for its calming properties and relaxation. Historically, it was used to anoint the feet of people who had been traveling for long distances before entering a house, as it was soothing and calming to the weary traveler. It was also used by caravaners for relaxing and for healing wounds.

Nabaioth: also spelled Nebajoth (Gen. 25:13). According to the Bible, he was the first-born son of Ishmael from whom the name Nabataeans is derived. The Nabataeans began the building of Petra and developed the lateen triangular sails.

Qana: anciently, an important seaport on the coast of Yemen for international trade of frankincense and myrrh, now called Bir Ali, but which has long been deserted.

Qat: a slightly narcotic plant, its leaves are chewed as a stimulant.

Queen Hatshepsut: the Egyptian queen who transported frankincense and myrrh trees from the land of Punt to Egypt, although the trees eventually died.

Qur'an: the holy book of Islam; also spelled Qu'ran, Quran, and Koran.

Reach: the wooden shaft that connects the two axle assemblies of a wagon.

Rub al Khali: known throughout the modern world as the Empty Quarter and is considered to be the most wicked and treacherous desert in the world. It spreads over parts of Oman, Yemen, Saudi Arabia, and the United Arab

Emirates, encompassing approximately 600,000 square kilometers (approximately 250,000 square miles).

Ruta: an aromatic plant that still grows in Yemen and can be found in the street markets today. It is sold as a remedy for fear, anxiety, and depression and for driving away "evil spirits."

Saba: a kingdom in Yemen; also the name of a famous queen (Sheba in the Bible).

Sabaeans: the people of Saba who lived in southern Arabia (now the country of Yemen), who became rich by trading in the very lucrative spice and aromatic industry.

Salalah, Oman: the largest port city in the Dhofar province, which controls the Land of Frankincense today.

Sana'a, Yemen: the capital city of modern Yemen, founded by Noah's son Seth.

Selah, Jordan: ancient name for Petra, meaning "red rock."

Shabwah, Yemen: once the capital of the Hadhramaut, a major city of commerce in ancient Yemen. It became very rich because of the trade of spices and the resins of frankincense and myrrh. It was a major taxation way station for the caravans.

Shekel: an ancient unit of currency coming from Mesopotamia around 3000 B.C. (about 11 grams or .35 troy ounces). It was common among western Semitic peoples, Moabites, and Edomites. Solomon paid 600 shekels for his chariot from Egypt.

Shishak (also known as Shishank): son of Siamun and was the Egyptian Pharaoh who marched on Judea following Solomon's death (2 Chronicles 12:9). In this novel he is fictionalized as the half-brother of Sheba.

Siamun: Pharaoh of Egypt who reigned from 986 to 967 B.C., fictionalized as having fathered Sheba and her twin sister, Makshara, who became one of Solomon's wives.

Socotra Island: an island 250 miles off the coast of Yemen, where seven unique species of frankincense and four unique species of myrrh grow that are found nowhere else.

Taiz (Ta'izz modern spelling): the early capital of Yemen, between Sana'a and Aden; primary region for growing myrrh and balsam.

Tathlith, Saudi Arabia: a caravan way station between Najran and Makkah (Mecca); crossroad to Gerrha.

Terebinth tree: also known as the pistachio nut tree that grows in the Middle East. Its leaves were used for healing anciently as well as today; also produces an aromatic resin.

Thobe: another name for Arabic men's clothing.

Timna, Yemen: a caravan way station and gateway to the land of the myrrh trees.

Tongue: connects a wagon to the animals such as mules and horses that pull it.

Ubar or Wubar: richest trading city in the Arabian world for over 3,000 years. According to the Qur'an, it grew to become a wicked and decadent city before it was destroyed by an earthquake.

Vernonia plant: also known as ironwood, is a medicinal plant native to Arabia and Africa, used for persistent fevers, headaches, and joint pain.

Wadi Andhur, Oman: a grand fortress much like Fort Sumhuram for caravans on the way to Ubar. It was on top of a mountain and had extraction chambers and apothecary rooms similar to Ein Gedi.

Way stations: between Marib and Gaza there were 65 way stations, where the caravans stopped, rested, and replenished their food and water supply, according to Pliny the Elder.

Yathrib, Saudi Arabia: a stop on the way to Selah (Petra), now called Medina, one of the holy cities of Islam. It was a major crossroad for caravans traveling north, south, east, and west.

Zamzam Well: just a few meters from the Ka'aba. Muslims believe that the well was sent by Allah to save Hagar and Ishmael when they were dying of thirst.

Zophar Mountains: today called Dhofar in the country of Oman.

Weights and Measures

Kilogram or kilo: 1 kilogram = 2.2 pounds
Kilometer: 1 kilometer = 0.62 statute miles
Meter: 1 meter = 3.28 feet